Challenging Concepts in Respiratory Medicine

Titles in the Challenging Concepts in series

Anaesthesia (Edited by Dr Phoebe Syme, Dr Robert Jackson and Professor Tim Cook)

Cardiovascular Medicine (Edited by Dr Aung Myat, Dr Shouvik Haldar and Professor Simon Redwood)

Emergency Medicine (Edited by Dr Sam Thenabadu, Dr Fleur Cantle and Dr Chris Lacy)

Infectious Diseases and Clinical Microbiology (Edited by Dr Amber Arnold and Professor George Griffin)

Interventional Radiology (Edited by Dr Miltiadis Krokidis, Dr Irfan Ahmed and Dr Tarun Sabharwal)

Neurology (Edited by Dr Krishna Chinthapalli, Dr Nadia Magdalinou and Professor Nicholas Wood)

Neurosurgery (Edited by Robin Bhatia and Ian Sabin)

Obstetrics and Gynaecology (Edited by Natasha Hezelgrave, Dr Danielle Abbott and Professor Andrew Shennan)

Oncology (Edited by Dr Madhumita Bhattacharyya, Dr Sarah Payne and Professor Iain McNeish)

Oral and Maxillofacial Surgery (Edited by Dr Matthew Idle and Group Captain Andrew Monaghan)

Respiratory Medicine (Edited by Dr Lucy Schomberg, Dr Elizabeth Sage and Dr Nicholas Hart)

Forthcoming titles

Challenging Concepts in Cardiovascular Medicine, Volume II (Edited by Aung Myat and Shouvik Haldar)

Challenging Concepts in Paediatric Cardiology (Edited by Salim Jivanji and Michael Rigby)

Challenging Concepts in Critical Care (Edited by Reston Smith, Justine Barnett, Timothy Cook and Jerry Nolan)

Challenging Concepts in Respiratory Medicine

Cases with Expert Commentary

Supervisory editor

Dr Nicholas Hart

Clinical and Academic Director, Lane Fox Respiratory Service, St Thomas' Hospital, Guy's and St Thomas' NHS Foundation Trust; Reader in Respiratory & Critical Care Medicine, Department of Asthma, Allergy and Lung Biology, King's College London, London, UK

Co-editors

Dr Lucy Schomberg

Respiratory Consultant, Frimley Park Hospital, Frimley Health NHS Foundation Trust, Frimley, UK

Dr Elizabeth Sage

NIHR Academic Clinical Lecturer and North West Thames Respiratory Registrar, University College London, London, UK

Series editors

Dr Aung Myat BSc (Hons) MBBS MRCP

BHF Clinical Research Training Fellow, King's College London British Heart Foundation Centre of Research Excellence, Cardiovascular Division, St Thomas' Hospital, London, UK

Dr Shouvik Haldar MBBS MRCP

Electrophysiology Research Fellow and Cardiology SpR, Heart Rhythm Centre, NIHR Cardiovascular Biomedical Research Unit, Royal Brompton and Harefield NHS Foundation Trust, Imperial College London, UK

Professor Simon Redwood MD FRCP

Professor of Interventional Cardiology and Honorary Consultant Cardiologist, King's College London British Heart Foundation Centre of Research Excellence, Cardiovascular Division and Guy's and St Thomas' NHS Foundation Trust, St Thomas' Hospital, London, UK

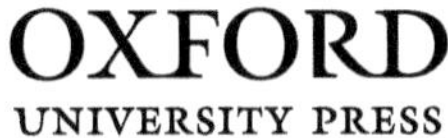

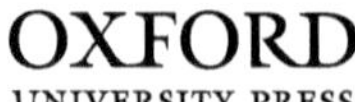

Great Clarendon Street, Oxford, OX2 6DP,
United Kingdom

Oxford University Press is a department of the University of Oxford. It furthers the University's objective of excellence in research, scholarship, and education by publishing worldwide. Oxford is a registered trade mark of Oxford University Press in the UK and in certain other countries

© Oxford University Press 2017

The moral rights of the authors have been asserted

Impression: 3

All rights reserved. No part of this publication may be reproduced, stored in a retrieval system, or transmitted, in any form or by any means, without the prior permission in writing of Oxford University Press, or as expressly permitted by law, by licence or under terms agreed with the appropriate reprographics rights organization. Enquiries concerning reproduction outside the scope of the above should be sent to the Rights Department, Oxford University Press, at the address above

You must not circulate this work in any other form
and you must impose this same condition on any acquirer

Published in the United States of America by Oxford University Press
198 Madison Avenue, New York, NY 10016, United States of America

British Library Cataloguing in Publication Data
Data available

Library of Congress Control Number: 2016944783

ISBN 978–0–19–965774–2

Printed in Great Britain by
Ashford Colour Press Ltd, Gosport, Hampshire

Oxford University Press makes no representation, express or implied, that the drug dosages in this book are correct. Readers must therefore always check the product information and clinical procedures with the most up-to-date published product information and data sheets provided by the manufacturers and the most recent codes of conduct and safety regulations. The authors and the publishers do not accept responsibility or legal liability for any errors in the text or for the misuse or misapplication of material in this work. Except where otherwise stated, drug dosages and recommendations are for the non-pregnant adult who is not breast-feeding

Links to third party websites are provided by Oxford in good faith and for information only. Oxford disclaims any responsibility for the materials contained in any third party website referenced in this work.

CONTENTS

EXPERTS

Ronan Breen
Consultant in Respiratory Medicine
Guy's and St Thomas' NHS Foundation Trust
London, UK

Jeremy Brown
Professor in Respiratory Infection,
Honorary Consultant in Respiratory Medicine
University College London
London, UK

Martin Carby
Consultant in Respiratory and Transplant Medicine
Royal Brompton and Harefield NHS Foundation Trust
London, UK

Christopher Corrigan
Professor of Asthma, Allergy and Respiratory Science
King's College London, UK
Consultant in Allergy and Respiratory Medicine
Guy's and St Thomas' NHS Foundation Trust
London, UK

Paul Cullinan
Professor in Occupational and Environmental Respiratory Disease
National Heart and Lung Institute,
Honorary Consultant Respiratory Physician
Royal Brompton and Harefield NHS Foundation Trust
London, UK

Craig Davidson
Oxygen Lead for NHS England,
Specialist in Intensive Care and Respiratory Medicine,
Former Director of the Lane Fox Respiratory Unit
Guy's and St Thomas'
NHS Foundation Trust
London, UK

Seamus Donnelly
Professor of Medicine
Trinity College Dublin, University of Dublin
Dublin, Republic of Ireland

Mark J Griffiths
Honorary Reader in Critical Care Medicine
National Heart and Lung Institute,
Imperial College London
London, UK
Honorary Reader in Critical Care Medicine and Consultant Physician
National Heart and Lung Institute and Royal Brompton Hospital
London, UK

John Hurst
Reader in Respiratory Medicine
University College London
Honorary Respiratory Consultant
Royal Free London NHS Foundation Trust
London, UK

Nick Maskell
Professor of Respiratory Medicine
University of Bristol
Bristol, UK

Andrew Menzies-Gow
Consultant in Respiratory Medicine,
Director of the Lung Division
Royal Brompton and Harefield NHS Foundation Trust
London, UK

Robert F Miller
Professor of Clinical Infection and Honorary Consultant Physician
University College London Hospital
NHS Foundation Trust
London, UK
Honorary Professor
London School of Hygiene and Tropical Medicine
Honorary Consultant Physician
Central and North West London NHS Foundation Trust
London, UK

Onn Min Kon
Consultant Respiratory Physician and Chief of Service for TB
Imperial College Healthcare NHS Trust,
Adjunct Professor of Respiratory Medicine
National Heart Lung Institute
Imperial College London
London, UK

Neal Navani
Consultant in Respiratory Medicine
University College Hospital London
London, UK

Mike Polkey
Consultant Physician and Professor of Respiratory Medicine
Royal Brompton and Harefield NHS Foundation Trust
London, UK

Paul Reading
Consultant Neurologist
James Cook University Hospital, South Tees Hospital NHS Foundation Trust
Middlesbrough, UK

Joerg Steier
Consultant in Respiratory Medicine
Guy's and St Thomas' NHS Foundation Trust
London, UK

David Treacher
Specialist in Intensive Care and Respiratory Medicine
Guy's and St Thomas' NHS Foundation Trust
London, UK

Athol Wells
Professor of Respiratory Medicine
Royal Brompton and Harefield NHS Foundation Trust
London, UK

Adrian Williams
Professor of Sleep Medicine
Guy's and St Thomas' NHS Foundation Trust
London, UK

Matthew Wise
Consultant in Critical Care and Respiratory Medicine
University Hospital of Wales
Cardiff, UK

John Wort
Consultant in Pulmonary Hypertension and Intensive Care Medicine
Royal Brompton and Harefield NHS Foundation Trust
London, UK

CONTRIBUTORS

Saima Alam
Previous Specialist Registrar in Allergy
London Deanery, UK

Mark H Almond
Welcome Trust Clinical Research Fellow
Airways Disease and Infection Section,
National Heart and Lung Institute
Imperial College London
London, UK

Jessica Barrett
Infectious Diseases Specialist Registrar
University College Hospital
London, UK

Chloe Bloom
Specialist Respiratory Registrar
North West Thames
London, UK

Simon Brill
Specialist Registrar in Respiratory Medicine
North East Thames
London, UK

Jim Brown
Consultant in Respiratory Medicine
University College London
London, UK

Dami Collier
Infectious Diseases Specialist Registrar Division of Infection and Immunity
University College London
London, UK

David Dobarro
Consultant Cardiologist
La Paz University Hospital
Madrid, Spain

Johanna Feary
Respiratory Physician and Honorary Clinical Research Fellow
Royal Brompton and Harefield NHS Foundation Trust
London, UK

Justin Garner
Specialist Respiratory Registrar
Royal Brompton Hospital
London, UK

Amina Jaffer
Specialist Respiratory Registrar
Barnet Hospital
Royal Free London NHS Foundation Trust
London, UK

Swapna Mandal
Consultant in Respiratory Medicine
Royal Free London NHS Foundation Trust
London, UK

Rory McDermott
Specialist Respiratory Registrar
University College Hospital
London, UK

Anant Patel
Consultant Respiratory Physician
Royal Free London NHS Foundation Trust
London, UK

Marcus Pittman
Consultant in Respiratory Medicine
Basildon and Thurrock University Hospitals
NHS Foundation Trust
UK

Michelle Ramsay
Consultant Respiratory Physician
Guy's and St Thomas' NHS Foundation Trust
London, UK

Clare Ross
Consultant in Respiratory Medicine
Imperial College Healthcare NHS Trust
London, UK

Georgina Russell
Consultant in Respiratory Medicine
Imperial College Healthcare NHS Trust
London, UK

Lucy Schomberg
Respiratory Consultant
Frimley Park Hospital, Frimley Health NHS Foundation Trust
Frimley, UK

Anand Shah
Consultant in Respiratory Medicine
Royal Brompton and Harefield NHS Foundation Trust
London, UK

Janet Stowell
Wellcome Trust Clinical Training Fellow
Imperial College London
London, UK

Joanna Szram
Consultant Respiratory Physician and Honorary Senior Clinical Lecturer
Royal Brompton and Harefield NHS Foundation Trust
London, UK

Georgia Tunnicliffe
Respiratory Consultant
Frimley Park Hospital, Frimley Health NHS Foundation Trust
Frimley, UK

Sophie Vergnaud
Specialist Respiratory Registrar
North East Thames Deanery
London, UK

Dave Walder
Specialist Respiratory Registrar
Kent, Surrey and Sussex Deanery, UK

ABBREVIATIONS

A–a	alveolar to arterial
A&E	accident and emergency
AAFB	acid- and alcohol-fast bacilli
AASM	American Academy of Sleep Medicine
ABG	arterial blood gas
ABPA	allergic bronchopulmonary aspergillosis
ACE	angiotensin-converting enzyme
ACQ	asthma control questionnaire
ACR	acute cellular rejection
ACV	assist control ventilation
AECC	American-European Consensus Conference
AF	atrial fibrillation
AFB	acid-fast bacilli
AHI	apnoea–hypopnoea index
AHRF	acute hypercapnic respiratory failure
AICU	adult intensive care unit
AIDS	acquired immune deficiency syndrome
AIP	acute interstitial pneumonia
ALAT	Latin American Thoracic Association
ALI	acute lung injury
ALP	alkaline phosphatase
ALT	alanine aminotransferase
ANA	antinuclear antibody
ANCA	anti-neutrophil cytoplasmic antibody
AP	anteroposterior
APACHE	Acute Physiology and Chronic Health Evaluation
APRV	airway pressure release ventilation
APTT	activated partial thromboplastin time
AQLQ	Asthma Quality of Life Questionnaire
ARDS	acute respiratory distress syndrome
ARIA	*Allergic Rhinitis and its Impact on Asthma*
ART	antiretroviral treatment
AST	aspartate transaminase
ASV	adaptive servo-ventilation
ATS	American Thoracic Society
BAL	bronchoalveolar lavage
BCG	bacille Calmette–Guérin
bd	twice daily
BHIVA	British HIV Association
BIPAP	biphasic positive airways pressure ventilation
BLVR	bronchoscopic lung volume reduction
BMI	body mass index
BNP	brain natriuretic peptide
BOS	bronchiolitis obliterans syndrome
BTS	British Thoracic Society
CAP	community-acquired pneumonia
CAT	COPD assessment test
CBCT	cone beam computed tomography
CCP	cyclic citrullinated peptide
CCPA	chronic cavitatory pulmonary aspergillosis
CFA	cryptogenic fibrosing alveolitis
CFPA	chronic fibrosing pulmonary aspergillosis
CGI-S	Clinical Global Impression of change
CHART	continuous hyperfractionated accelerated radiotherapy
CI	confidence interval
cm	centimetre
cmH_2O	centimetre of water
CMV	cytomegalovirus
CNPA	chronic necrotizing pulmonary aspergillosis
CNS	central nervous system
CO	carbon monoxide
CO_2	carbon dioxide
COP	cryptogenic organizing pneumonia
COPD	chronic obstructive pulmonary disease
CPAP	continuous positive airway pressure
CPET	cardiopulmonary exercise testing
CRP	C-reactive protein
CRQ	chronic respiratory questionnaire
CSA	central sleep apnoea
CSF	cerebrospinal fluid
CSR	Cheyne–Stokes respiration
CT	computed tomography
CTD	connective tissue disease
CTEPH	chronic thromboembolic pulmonary hypertension

CTG	cardiotocography
CTPA	computed tomography pulmonary angiogram
CVVHDF	continuous veno-venous haemodiafiltration
CXR	chest X-ray
4DCT	four-dimensional computed tomography
DcSSc	diffuse cutaneous systemic sclerosis
DEXA	dual-energy X-ray absorptiometry
DIP	desquamative interstitial pneumonia
dL	decilitre
DLCO	diffusing capacity of the lungs for carbon monoxide
DNA	deoxyribonucleic acid
DPLD	diffuse parenchymal lung disorder
2,3-DPG	2,3-diphosphoglycerate
DRESS	drug reaction, eosinophilia, systemic symptoms
DVLA	Driver and Vehicle Licensing Agency
EBUS	endobronchial ultrasound
EBV	Ebstein–Barr virus
ECCOR	extracorporeal carbon dioxide removal
ECG	electrocardiogram
ECLS	extracorporeal life support
ECMO	extracorporeal membrane oxygenation
ED	emergency department
EEG	electroencephalography
eGFR	estimated glomerular filtration rate
EMG	electromyography
EMGdi	diaphragm electromyography
EN	erythema nodosum
ENT	ear, nose, and throat
EOG	electro-oculography
EPAP	expiratory positive airways pressure
ERA	endothelin receptor antagonist
ERS	European Respiratory Society
ERV	expiratory reserve volume
ESBL	extended-spectrum β-lactamase
ESICM	European Society of Intensive Care Medicine
ESR	erythrocyte sedimentation rate
ESS	Epworth sleepiness scale
ET-1	endothelin-1
ET_A	endothelin A
FDG	[18F]-fluorodeoxyglucose
FEV_1	forced expiratory volume in 1 second
FFP3	filtering face piece 3
FiO_2	fraction of inspired oxygen
fL	femtolitre
FRC	functional residual capacity
ft	foot
FVC	forced vital capacity
G6PD	glucose-6-phosphate dehydrogenase
g	gram
GABA	gamma aminobutyrate
GA^2LEN	Global Allergy and Asthma European Network
GCS	Glasgow Coma Scale
GFR	glomerular filtration rate
GGO	ground glass opacity
GGT	gamma-glutamyl transpeptidase
GMP	guanosine monophosphate
GORD	gastro-oesophageal reflux disease
GP	general practitioner
Gy	gray
HA	haemagglutinin
HCAP	health care-associated pneumonia
HCO_3	bicarbonate
HDU	high dependency unit
HFOV	high-frequency oscillatory ventilation
HIV	human immune deficiency virus
HLA	human leucocyte antigen
HMM	high-molecular mass
HPLC	high-performance liquid chromatography
HR	hazard ratio
HRCT	high-resolution computed tomography
HRQoL	health-related quality of life
HSCT	haematopoietic stem cell transplantation
HSP	hypersensitivity pneumonitis
Hz	hertz
ICP	intracranial pressure
ICS	inhaled corticosteroid
ICU	intensive care unit
IDSA	Infectious Diseases Society of America
IFITM3	interferon-induced transmembrane protein 3
IFN-γ	interferon gamma
IgE	immunoglobulin E
IgG	immunoglobulin G
IGRA	interferon-gamma release assay
IIP	idiopathic interstitial pneumonia
IL	interleukin
ILD	interstitial lung disease
INR	international normalized ratio

IPA	invasive pulmonary aspergillosis
IPAH	idiopathic pulmonary arterial hypertension
IPAP	inspiratory positive airways pressure
IPF	idiopathic pulmonary fibrosis
IQR	interquartile range
IRIS	immune restoration inflammatory syndrome
ISG	interferon-stimulated gene
ISHLT	International Society for Heart and Lung Transplantation
IU	international unit
IV	intravenous(ly)
JCVI	Joint Committee on Vaccination and Immunization
JRCALC	Joint Royal Colleges Ambulance Liaison Committee
JRS	Japanese Respiratory Society
JVP	jugular venous pressure
KCO	transfer coefficient for carbon monoxide per unit lung volume
kDa	kilodalton
kg	kilogram
kPa	kilopascal
L	litre
LABA	long-acting beta-agonist
LAMA	long-acting muscarinic antagonist
LDCT	low-dose computed tomography
LDH	lactate dehydrogenase
LEV	local 'exhaust' ventilation
LFT	liver function test
LIP	lymphoid interstitial pneumonia
LIS	Lung Injury Score
LMM	low-molecular mass
LRTI	lower respiratory tract infection
LSCS	lower segment Caesarean section
LTOT	long-term oxygen therapy
LVEDP	left ventricular end-diastolic pressure
LVEF	left ventricular ejection fraction
LVRS	lung volume reduction surgery
6MWD	6-minute walk distance
6MWT	6-minute walk test
m	metre
MAC	*Mycobacterium avium* complex
MAP	mean arterial pressure
MDR	multidrug-resistant
MDT	multidisciplinary team
mEq	milliequivalent
mg	milligram
MGIT	Mycobacterial Growth Indicator Tube
min	minute
mL	millilitre
mm	millimetre
mmHg	millimetre of mercury
mmol	millimole
mMRC	modified Medical Research Council
MODS	microscopic observation drug susceptibility
mPaw	mean airway pressure
MPE	malignant pleural effusion
MRC	Medical Research Council
MRI	magnetic resonance imaging
MRSA	meticillin-resistant *Staphylococcus aureus*
MSLT	multiple sleep latency testing
MSM	man who have sex with men
MTB	*Mycobacterium* tuberculosis
MWT	maintenance of wakefulness test
MxA	myxovirus resistance gene A
NA	neuraminidase
NAAT	nucleic acid amplification testing
NAC	N-acetylcysteine
NARES	non-allergic rhinitis with eosinophilia
NBL	non-bronchoscopic lung lavage
ng	nanogram
NHS	National Health Service
NICE	National Institute for Health and Care Excellence
NIV	non-invasive ventilation
NLST	National Lung Screening Trial
nm	nanometre
NNT	number needed to treat
NO	nitric oxide
NSBHR	non-specific bronchial hyper-responsiveness
NSIP	non-specific interstitial pneumonia
NTM	non-tuberculous mycobacteria
NT-proBNP	N-terminal prohormone of brain natriuretic peptide
NYHA	New York Heart Association
OA	occupational asthma
OAS	oral allergy syndrome
OB	obliterative bronchiolitis
od	once daily
ODI	oxygen desaturation index
OHS	obesity hypoventilation syndrome

OSA	obstructive sleep apnoea
OSAHS	obstructive sleep apnoea hypopnoea syndrome
$PaCO_2$	arterial carbon dioxide tension
PAH	pulmonary arterial hypertension
PAMP	pathogen-associated molecular pattern
PaO_2	arterial oxygen tension
PAP	pulmonary arterial pressure
PBMC	peripheral blood mononuclear cell
PCP	*Pneumocystis* pneumonia
PCR	polymerase chain reaction
PCWP	pulmonary capillary wedge pressure
PE	pulmonary embolism
PEEP	positive end-expiratory pressure
PEF	peak expiratory flow
PEFR	peak expiratory flow rate
PET	positron emission tomography
PFT	pulmonary function test
pg	picogram
PGD	primary graft dysfunction
PH	pulmonary hypertension
pmol	picomole
PO	orally
PPI	proton pump inhibitor
PRA	polymerase chain reaction restriction endonuclease assay
pre-hab	preoperative pulmonary rehabilitation
PRR	pathogen recognition receptor
PSG	polysomnography
PTLD	post-transplant lymphoproliferative disease
PVR	pulmonary vascular resistance
qds	four times daily
RADS	reactive airways dysfunction syndrome
RAST	radioallergosorbent test
RB-ILD	respiratory bronchiolitis-associated interstitial lung disease
RCP	Royal College of Physicians
RCT	randomized controlled trial
RDI	respiratory disturbance index
rDNA	ribosomal DNA
REM	rapid eye movement
RERA	respiratory effort-related arousal
RF	rheumatoid factor
RFA	radiofrequency ablation
RGM	rapidly growing mycobacteria
RHC	right heart catheterization
RIG-1	retinoic inducible gene 1
RPE	respiratory protective equipment
RSVP	right ventricular systolic pressure
rt-PCR	reverse transcriptase polymerase chain reaction
RV	residual volume
RVESP	right ventricular end-systolic pressure
s	second
SAFS	severe asthma with fungal sensitization
SBRT	stereotactic body radiotherapy
SBT	spontaneous breathing trial
SCBU	special care baby unit
SD	standard deviation
SGRQ	St George's Respiratory Questionnaire
SHO	senior house officer
SIGN	Scottish Intercollegiate Guidelines Network
SIMV	synchronized intermittent mandatory ventilation
SLE	systemic lupus erythematosus
SOREM	sleep-onset REM sleep
SPC	Standards of Practice Committee
SP-D	surfactant protein D
SPN	solitary pulmonary nodule
SPT	skin prick test
SSRI	serotonin-selective reuptake inhibitor
sTREM-1	soluble triggering receptor expressed on myeloid type 1
SUV	standardized uptake value
SUVmax	maximum standardized uptake value
TAPSE	tricuspid annular plane systolic excursion
TB	tuberculosis
TBBx	transbronchial biopsy
tds	three times daily
TGF	transforming growth factor
Th	T helper
Ti	inspiratory time
TLC	total lung capacity
TLCO	transfer factor of the lung for carbon monoxide
TLR	toll-like receptor
TMP-SMX	trimethoprim–sulfamethoxazole
TNF	tumour necrosis factor
TPC	tunnelled pleural catheter
TST	tuberculin skin test
TU	tuberculin unit
UIP	usual interstitial pneumonia

UK	United Kingdom
UPP	uvulopalatopharyngoplasty
US	United States
VA	venous–arterial
VAP	ventilator-associated pneumonia
VATS	video-assisted thoracoscopic surgery
VILI	ventilator-induced lung injury
V/Q	ventilation–perfusion
VV	venous–venous
WASOG	World Association for Sarcoidosis and Other Granulomatous Disorders
WCC	white cell count
WHO	World Health Organization
WU	Wood unit

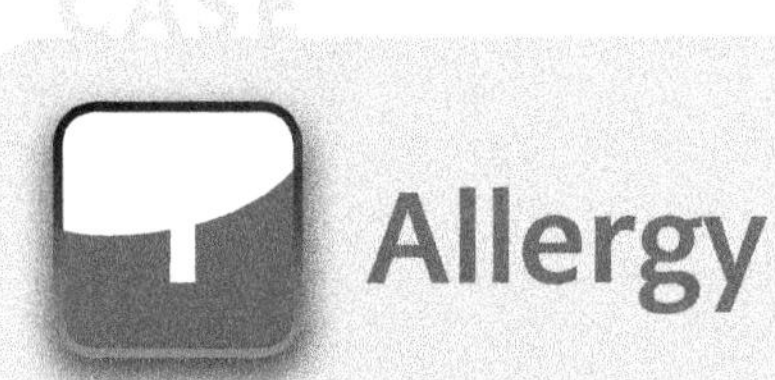

Allergy

Saima Alam

Expert commentary Christopher Corrigan

Case history

A 25-year-old female was referred by the ear, nose, and throat (ENT) team to the allergy clinic with a 2-year history of persistent nasal obstruction, rhinorrhoea, and sneezing. She had a seasonal (springtime) increase in her symptoms which were worse at home and more noticeable in the morning. She had a past medical history of eczema and asthma. She had also reported allergies to various fruits, nuts, and vegetables. She had a family history of atopy. Her father and paternal uncle had severe asthma, and her mother and sister had mild hay fever. She had been in contact with pets, in particular cats and dogs.

Examination showed mucosal swelling without any evidence of polyps. She had used topical nasal steroids and antihistamines for a few weeks only in the recent past. Her medications included two puffs twice a day of budesonide 200 micrograms and formoterol 6 micrograms combined in a dry powdered inhaler, and a salbutamol inhaler as required. She was a civil servant and had never smoked.

Learning point Allergic disease

Allergic disease affects 15–20% of the population in industrialized countries, as estimated in a report by the Royal College of Physicians (RCP) [1].

- It results from inappropriate production by the immune system of IgE antibody against particular protein antigens (termed 'allergens') presented to the mucosal surfaces of the skin, conjunctiva, and respiratory and gastrointestinal tracts, either as inhaled airborne particles or in foodstuffs.
- IgE binding to mast cells in tissues or basophils in the blood causes them to degranulate acutely, following further allergen exposure, releasing histamine and causing what is described as type I ('immediate') hypersensitivity. The propensity of some individuals to produce IgE inappropriately is termed 'atopy'.
- For as yet unexplained reasons, not all atopic subjects develop allergic diseases. Allergic diseases may have a profound effect on quality of life. Box 1.1 identifies the commonest IgE-mediated diseases referred to an allergy clinic.

Box 1.1 Common IgE-mediated conditions referred to a specialist allergy clinic

Common IgE-mediated diseases:

- Allergic rhinitis
- Immediate hypersensitivity to foods
- Immediate hypersensitivity to drugs
- Atopic asthma
- Atopic dermatitis

(Continued)

- Anaphylaxis to food and drugs
- Insect venom allergy
- Allergy to latex

Urticaria and angio-oedema

The symptoms of allergic rhinitis may be seasonal (caused by seasonally present allergens, typically pollens), and/or perennial (caused by allergens present all the time), and/or occupational (allergens encountered in the workplace). In 2001, the World Health Organization (WHO), in collaboration with other groups, drafted a document referred to as *'Allergic rhinitis and its impact on asthma'* (ARIA). This document proposed the use of the terms intermittent and persistent rhinitis and the grading of the severity of symptoms as mild or moderate/severe [2]. Whatever system is adopted, the aim is to take a careful history to define symptoms and their severity, and to link them with allergen exposure.

In clinic, the case study patient confirmed she had suffered from mild nasal and ocular symptoms since her late teenage years. She was symptomatic all year round, with noticeable worsening in spring (March to May), especially in the past 2 years. She also reported worsening of her asthma, diagnosed by her general practitioner (GP) a few years ago, during exercise and in springtime. Interestingly, her nasal symptoms improved when she was away from home. Direct questioning also revealed that she had been suffering from post-nasal discharge (drip) and a dry cough in the spring and had been prescribed a nasal topical steroid spray 3 years ago, which, with regular use, had improved symptoms considerably. Her sense of smell remained intact. Her parents-in-law owned a cat and two dogs, and she was exposed to these sources of allergen occasionally when she visited, although her symptoms did not worsen on exposure to the pets. She also reported having noticed severe itching of the inside of her mouth on eating apples, cherries, apricots, peaches, almonds, hazelnuts, and celery. She could eat apples in pies, tinned apricots, and peach and cherries in desserts. She had never had more severe or systemic symptoms when eating these foodstuffs.

Clinical tip History and examination

A **careful history** should focus on symptom timing:

- diurnal and seasonal variability;
- acute exacerbation on exposure to sources of allergen such as pets;
- symptoms in the working environment and when on holiday;
- duration and severity of nasal and ocular symptoms and their effects on quality of life;
- past medical history of associated atopic disorders such as eczema and asthma;
- family history of asthma, rhinitis, and eczema;
- focussed dietary history for food-related reaction;
- environmental history should include asking in detail about:
  - soft furnishings at home;
  - respiratory sensitizers at work;
  - animal dander.
- medications: clear record of 'what', 'when', and 'for how long' should be recorded accurately.

Clinical examination should look for 'classical' (not always seen!) signs of chronic allergic rhinoconjunctivitis:

- allergic crease (horizontal line across the nose caused by repetitive rubbing);
- Denny's lines (a double crease under the eyes for the same reason);

(Continued)

- the skin should be examined for eczema;
- nasal endoscopy is essential if rhinosinusitis or mechanical blockage of the nose, for example by polyps (often these patients have an impaired ability to smell and taste), is suspected, in which case an ENT referral is indicated.
- examination of the chest for wheeze;
- in children, height and weight measurements if they are using topical steroids [3].

Expert comment

Accurate allergy diagnosis relies almost invariably on the taking of an accurate history.

Symptoms result from histamine release in the short term, which may be local or systemic, depending on the severity of the reaction. Histamine when released locally into the conjunctivae causes running and itching; into the nose causes running, itching, and sneezing; into the bronchial tree causes wheeze and chest tightness (usually significant only in patients who also have asthma); and into the skin causes urticaria (nettle rash, hives) and angio-oedema (swelling). Nasal blockage in allergic rhinitis and increasing bronchial hyperreactivity in asthma are longer-term symptoms caused by ongoing T-cell activation and mucosal oedema and remodelling, and they are less amenable to histamine blockade; these symptoms require anti-inflammatory (typically topical corticosteroid) treatment.

Severe allergic reactions causing systemic histamine release may, in addition, cause hypotension (with dizziness, fainting, and collapse), laryngeal oedema (causing alteration, particularly croakiness of the voice and a sensation of blockage of the airways at the level of the voice box), generalized urticaria and angio-oedema, and occasionally bowel upset (diarrhoea). These are the only symptoms of allergic reactions. Typically, but with important exceptions, these reactions are immediate following exposure to the triggering allergen(s) and reproducible, at least in the short term, within patients. Their severity varies between patients for reasons which are still very poorly understood. In the longer term, symptoms may regress or disappear. Again the mechanisms of this regression are unknown but do not depend on reduction or cessation of allergen-specific IgE production.

ENT examination revealed hyperplastic lower turbinates bilaterally and hyperreactive nasal tissue. In the clinic, the patient had positive skin prick tests to Timothy grass, silver birch, hazel tree, house dust mite, cat and dog dander, apple, cherry, apricot, peach, almond, and hazelnut. A typical panel of common allergens used to investigate sensitization in patients with allergic rhinoconjunctivitis is seen in Box 1.2. She declined a nasal provocation test. Pulmonary function tests revealed moderate/severe reversible obstructive airways disease.

Box 1.2 List of common aero-allergens

- Grass pollen
- Silver birch pollen
- Plane pollen
- Alder tree pollen
- Hazel tree pollen
- House dust mite (*Dermatophagoides pteronyssinus*)
- Cat
- Dog
- *Aspergillus*
- *Cladosporium*
- *Alternaria*

Learning point Skin prick testing—simple and quick

Skin prick testing is the simplest and quickest method to demonstrate that an individual is producing IgE against one or more suspected allergens.

Skin prick tests are highly specific for individual allergens, and, when properly performed with intact allergens, they have a very high negative predictive value (in other words, patients with negative skin prick tests are not sensitized).

It is essential to remember, however, that positive skin prick tests (and blood tests) are poorly predictive of the likelihood and severity of clinical symptoms in those patients who make IgE antibodies. Many patients who make IgE against grass pollens, for example, never develop hay fever. Thus, skin prick tests are used to **confirm** sensitivity to allergens only when their involvement in the patient's symptoms is suspected from their history. They **cannot** be used to predict the presence and severity of allergic symptoms.

Glycerinated extracts of allergen solutions are placed on the skin, then lightly punctured under the skin with a lancet. This produces a wheal-and-flare reaction as a result of the interaction of IgE bound to mast cells in the skin with the allergen, causing histamine release (Figure 1.1).

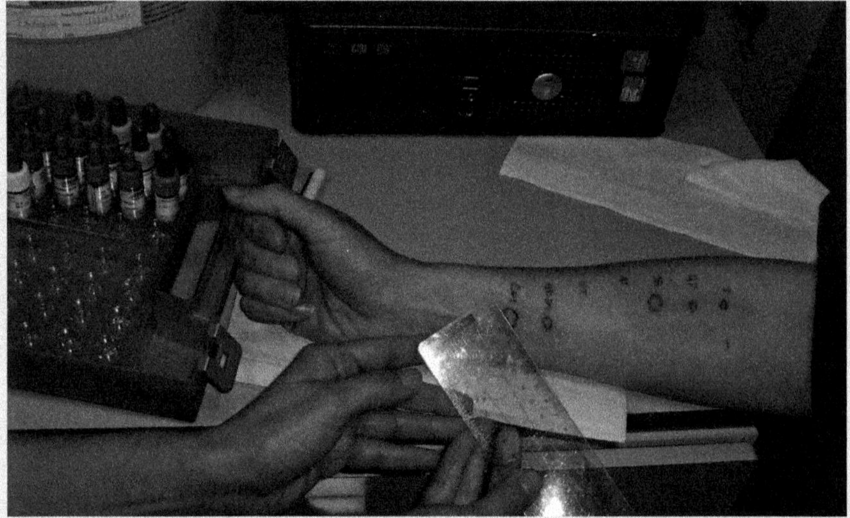

Figure 1.1 Positive skin prick tests to grass pollen, silver birch pollen, house dust mite, and cat dander.

Taking antihistamines and some antidepressants or using steroid creams on the skin may depress skin test reactions; this is usually monitored by including a concurrent positive histamine control test. Patients with widespread eczema and dermographism (which produces false positive reactions, monitored by including a concurrent negative allergen diluent control test) should have blood tests.

The reaction is read after 15 minutes, and a wheal diameter of 3 mm greater than a concurrent negative (diluent) control is considered positive [4, 5].

Learning point The more expensive tests

Laboratory tests: Allergen-specific IgE can be measured in the patient's serum, using a variety of commercial kits, based on incubation of the serum with a series of allergens immobilized on a solid phase, washing, and then adding a second layer of anti-IgE antibody coupled to an enzyme which changes the colour of a substrate. *In vitro* tests are less sensitive than skin prick tests, although their sensitivity has greatly increased over the years. They are also less reliable for some allergens, especially

(Continued)

some food allergens which are unstable *in vitro*. Although semi-quantitative, they are no more predictive of the presence and severity of allergic disease than skin prick tests (with the exception of certain food allergies in young children where high IgE against some foods is somewhat predictive of food allergic reactions).

Laboratory tests for allergen-specific IgE production are also much more expensive and do not produce an immediate result. Consequently, they should be used only in special circumstances or when skin prick testing is impossible or uninterpretable, as described in Learning point, p. 4. As with skin prick tests, laboratory tests are generally directed at unseparated allergenic proteins from a single source (such as grass or tree pollen or house dust mite extracts). Component resolved diagnosis is a novel technique whereby individual component allergens from a given source are microdotted onto an absorbent substrate, then incubated with the patient's serum. Binding of allergen-specific IgE is detected with a second layer of fluorochrome-conjugated antibody detected by a photomultiplier. This technique allows a complete component allergen profile and may prove useful in the future for delineating sensitization of patients to cross-reacting allergens from different sources.

The total serum IgE concentration is of no diagnostic value in allergy diagnosis. The blood eosinophil count is rarely elevated in allergic rhinitis but may be raised in associated atopic diseases such as eczema, asthma, drug allergy, and allergic bronchopulmonary aspergillosis (ABPA). There are various non-allergic causes of raised blood eosinophil count which should be borne in mind such as parasitic infestations, lymphoma, connective tissue disorders, and hyper IgE syndrome.

Other tests are available in situations where routine tests fail to identify allergic triggers of nasal symptoms. The preparation of nasal smears is a time-consuming procedure designed to delineate and approximately quantify the kinds of inflammatory cells infiltrating the nasal mucosa and can be used to diagnose diseases such as non-allergic rhinitis with eosinophilia (NARES). Allergen nasal challenge involves direct nasal provocation with increasing concentrations of a suspected allergen under controlled conditions and allows for objective measurement of the nasal response by various techniques such as rhinomanometry, acoustic rhinometry, and measurement of nasal nitric oxide and nasal inspiratory peak flow, as well as documentation of nasal symptom scores [6, 7]. These techniques are used in research settings or for difficult-to-treat patients in a specialist rhinology clinic [7, 8].

Three aspects of this lady's history are of particular interest. Firstly, perennial symptoms of rhinoconjunctivitis with deterioration in springtime suggest clinically significant polysensitization with multiple allergens. Common perennial allergens in the United Kingdom include house dust mites (*Dermatophagoides pteronyssinus* and *farinae*), moulds such as *Aspergillus*, *Cladosporium*, and *Alternaria*, and animal 'dander' (a mixture of hair, which is not allergenic, and shed epithelial cells and gut and urinary proteins).

House dust mites live in soft furnishings in the home, especially bedding. Perennial symptoms of rhinoconjunctivitis which are worst in the morning suggest significant house dust mite allergy. Moulds may be rife in the walls of chronically damp homes.

It is important to remember that chronic nasal inflammation with blockage is quite frequently not caused by allergy. Isolated congestion with blockage of the nose severe enough to cause loss of the senses of taste and smell, which often suggests the development of nasal polyps, especially in the absence of sneezing and itching, abundant clear rhinorrhoea, and ocular symptoms, is more suggestive of a non-allergic aetiology.

Secondly, the patient's increased shortness of breath in springtime strongly suggests seasonal exacerbation of atopic asthma. If she was not known to have asthma, this might suggest a diagnosis of concomitant seasonal ('pollen') asthma.

Learning point Seasonal allergens in the UK

- Tree (principally birch, alder, hazel, and plane) pollen produced in spring (February to April)
- Grass pollens produced in summer (June to August)

Expert comment

It is important to be wary of 'seasonal' or 'pollen' asthma; some patients have few, if any, asthma symptoms for most of the year but have severe symptoms during the tree and/or grass pollen seasons when their hay fever is also typically very bad. These patients should have peak flow monitoring to establish the diagnosis and the severity of the problem, then regular anti-inflammatory asthma therapy for the duration of the relevant seasons if they are not receiving it regularly anyway.

And thirdly, the patient's history of oral symptoms with fruits, vegetables, and nuts is suggestive of **oral allergy syndrome** (**OAS**).

Learning point Oral allergy syndrome

This condition is increasingly common and reflects cross-reactivity of certain allergens, particularly in tree pollens, such as silver birch (pollens are actually small fruits), with those in larger fruits (typically apples, pears, and any fruit which contains a pip or a stone) and sometimes certain vegetables and ree nuts. Some individuals may not have overt symptoms of hay fever but still experience oral symptoms with certain food ingredients [9]. Confirmation of sensitization to pollens and foodstuffs causing symptoms requires appropriate skin prick tests using either an allergen extract in the conventional way or performed as a prick–prick test directly with suspect fresh fruits. Component resolved diagnosis may also be used to identify cross-reactivity in more molecular detail which may, in the future, have implications for treatment, for example by directed immunotherapy [10].

In this case, a diagnosis of atopic asthma, perennial allergic rhinoconjunctivitis with seasonal exacerbation, and OAS was made.

Based on these symptoms and investigations, the patient was commenced on a regular non-sedating antihistamine (cetirizine 10 mg daily), as well as a topical nasal corticosteroid (fluticasone nasal drops twice daily (bd)). The dosage of her inhaled combined steroid and long-acting beta-agonist therapy was increased (two puffs daily of budesonide 400 micrograms and formoterol 12 micrograms combined in a dry powdered inhaler). She was strongly advised to take all of these medications regularly, shown how to use the devices properly, and warned to be aware of the possibility of the need for extra asthma treatment in springtime. She was advised to reduce exposure to animal dander (although she had no overt symptoms on exposure, the development of sensitization on continued exposure is likely in these patients) and was given information about house dust mite prevention/control measures. She was given information leaflets about allergen immunotherapy, since, if her responses to allergen avoidance and regularly and properly used pharmacotherapy were to prove unsatisfactory, she might then benefit from desensitization to house dust mite and tree and grass pollen allergens. She was finally advised to be wary of exposure to all fresh fruits causing oral symptoms and that eating cooked, tinned, or otherwise processed fruits is usually safe because these food allergens are easily degraded by heating. Follow-up was arranged in 4 months.

Expert comment

Oral allergy syndrome, caused by IgE production to components of fruits of the *Rosaceae* family (a large family containing, amongst others, common fruits which have pips or stones such as apples, pears, peaches, cherries, grapes, etc.), is usually seen in the UK and Scandinavia in the context of primary sensitization to tree and, less commonly, grass pollen allergens in patients with hay fever, although concomitant hay fever symptoms are not universal. Symptoms are a nuisance but rarely, if ever, life-threatening. In contrast, in southern Mediterranean, fresh fruit allergies tend to reflect primary sensitization and are typically much more severe. There is no cure, as yet, for oral allergy syndrome, although, with increasing understanding of the relevant components causing sensitization, it may be possible to design immunotherapy vaccines in the future. Patients should be advised to rub suspect fruits around their lips if they are not sure if they will react, or to lick the fruit cautiously. Fruit allergens, unlike some other food allergens such as nut allergens, are highly labile and typically denatured by any sort of cooking, canning, or heating process (most commercial fruit juices are safe, unless squeezed directly from the fruit into the glass, since they are pasteurized to prevent bacterial contamination before packaging).

At follow-up 4 months later, the case study patient reported some, but not complete, improvement in her nasal symptoms, but her asthma control remained poor. She had attended accident and emergency (A&E) on one occasion and had also been reviewed by her GP twice and prescribed a course of oral prednisolone for asthma control on each occasion. She could not identify any specific triggers, other than waking up with significant nasal congestion. She denied any nocturnal asthma symptoms. She was also using her rescue inhaler prior to starting exercise sessions at the gym. Spirometry revealed a forced expiratory volume in 1 second (FEV_1) of 55% predicted, significantly lower than that observed 4 months previously. She reported minimal improvement with the inhaled corticosteroid and long-acting beta-agonist device. Her inhaler technique was verified as good, and her compliance with therapy satisfactory.

The patient was advised to continue to take the antihistamine and topical nasal steroid. For better asthma control, she was switched to ciclesonide 80 micrograms and salmeterol 25 micrograms bd, both delivered with an Aerochamber Plus® spacer device. Instruction on the use of these new devices was provided. She was finally prescribed a leukotriene antagonist (montelukast 10 mg nightly) and advised to keep a peak flow and symptom diary.

The total serum IgE concentration was requested, in anticipation of a possible need for anti-IgE therapy if her asthma remained poorly controlled, necessitating frequent visits to the A&E department and/or hospital admissions. In view of her severe seasonal exacerbations of allergic rhinoconjunctivitis in spring and summer and her marked additional perennial symptoms, which her history suggests are attributable to house dust mite allergy, this lady would also benefit from desensitization immunotherapy for both tree and grass pollens, as well as house dust mite, if her symptoms remain inadequately controlled by regular, properly administered pharmacotherapy. This would have the additional advantage of reducing the severity of her seasonal exacerbations of asthma. Unfortunately, it is unwise to commence immunotherapy, a procedure in which purified allergen extracts are administered subcutaneously or sublingually, in patients with severe or unstable asthma, given the remote, but tangible, possibility of systemic anaphylaxis. If feasible, this would have to be commenced at a stage when her asthma is as well controlled and stable as possible and outside the pollen season.

This lady might also be considered for omalizumab (anti-IgE) therapy in the future, especially if her quality of life is impaired by frequent visits to the A&E department or hospital admissions. Omalizumab treatment is currently indicated, according to the National Institute for Health and Care Excellence (NICE) guidelines in England (different guidelines apply in Wales and Scotland), for severe atopic asthmatics who suffer from three such events or more in a typical year despite taking maximal anti-asthma therapy regularly and reliably, with all known disease-exacerbating factors (including allergen exposure and smoking) minimized or excluded. It is a humanized monoclonal antibody which binds to the constant region of the human IgE molecule, thereby preventing its binding to IgE receptors on a range of cells, including mast cells, basophils, B cells, and antigen-presenting cells. It therefore inhibits, after a lag period of some weeks, IgE-mediated reactions to allergens. Because the treatment is expensive, strict eligibility criteria have been set out by NICE [11]. The main benefit of omalizumab therapy is reduction of asthma exacerbations, although some patients are also able to reduce their therapy (a blessing if the patient is taking oral corticosteroid) while preserving their lung function.

Evidence base Innovate

INNOVATE was a randomized, double-blind, placebo-controlled trial of the efficacy of omalizumab in atopic patients with difficult-to-control asthma. A total of 438 patients in 14 countries participated. The primary outcome measure was improvement in clinically significant asthma exacerbations. Patients on omalizumab showed a significant improvement, compared to those on placebo treatment. Significant improvements were also recorded in secondary outcomes (less severe exacerbations and symptomatology) [12].

Learning point Omalizumab

Current licensing and NICE guidance restrict the use of omalizumab to patients >6 years of age, although this is presently under review.

Patients must have a definitive diagnosis of asthma with ongoing airways obstruction (peak expiratory flow (PEF)/FEV_1 <80% predicted) and a positive skin prick test to at least one perennial allergen if the total serum IgE concentration is <76 IU/L.

Dosing is calculated to neutralize all circulating serum IgE, which, in turn, depends on the patient's weight and total serum IgE concentration.

Some patients (those with high weight and/or high serum total IgE concentration) are excluded because they would require dosages outside the licensed range.

Exclusion criteria include pregnancy and breastfeeding and unwillingness to cooperate with regular disease monitoring.

Omalizumab is administered in specialist asthma/allergy centres, usually by a trained specialist nurse. Depending on the dosage, this may require up to four subcutaneous injections administered every 2 or 4 weeks. Patient response (lung function, symptoms, exacerbations, and hospital admissions) is monitored and reviewed at 16 and 26 weeks in the first instance. The treatment can be administered long-term if the response is good and well tolerated, or discontinued in the 20–30% of patients who, for as yet undefined reasons, fail to respond.

Expert comment

Omalizumab is an expensive treatment which currently only just meets NICE's threshold for cost-effectiveness, as assessed by their 'cost per quality of life years gained' technique. It is currently not available for children under the age of 6 years because it was licensed based on the results of INNOVATE (see Evidence base, p. 8), in which all the participants were aged 12 years or more. The future of omalizumab, including whether or not it will be made available to younger children, is currently under review.

Discussion

Therapeutic approaches to allergic rhinoconjunctivitis fall under the categories of allergen avoidance, pharmacotherapy, surgical intervention, and immunotherapy.

Allergen avoidance can be difficult but reduces symptoms of rhinoconjunctivitis, and there is some evidence that it also reduces the likelihood of asthmatic symptoms. Reducing humidity and the ambient temperature in bedrooms reduces house dust mite multiplication. Washing bed linen weekly at high temperatures (60°C) kills mites and is an additional means of reducing exposure [13, 14]. Close-woven barrier bedding over pillows, duvets, and mattresses can reduce exposure in bed. Keeping pets out of the home is easy, although many patients choose not to do so. There is little point in patients taking house dust mite avoidance measures in rooms also visited by domestic animals to which they are also clinically sensitized. Cat dander is light and tenacious, sticking to clothing, and therefore quickly becomes distributed throughout the house, typically requiring months to clear after the animal is removed [15].

Pollen allergen exposure can be reduced by simple measures such as avoiding obvious pollen sources, such as grasslands, and avoiding going out in the middle of the day when the pollen is high in the air, compared to early mornings and evenings when it falls. Bedroom and car windows should be kept closed. Changing clothes after washing hair and showering when coming in from work can reduce symptoms. Car ventilation systems should incorporate a pollen filter. For activities where pollen exposure is anticipated, such as mowing the lawn, nasal air filters are available which can be worn temporarily to keep pollen out of the nose; a generous smear of petroleum jelly around the borders of the nostrils has a similar effect.

Mould avoidance is difficult, but improving ventilation and reducing humidity and damp can reduce symptoms. Regular nasal washing with an isotonic saline solution is beneficial in sufferers from chronic rhinitis, and there are various devices available which facilitate this.

Evidence base ARIA

Pharmacotherapy for allergic rhinoconjunctivitis includes antihistamines, topical and oral steroids, cromoglicate, vasoconstrictors, and cholinergic and leukotriene antagonists. A number of double-blind, placebo-controlled clinical trials, as well as a meta-analysis, provide evidence to support the use of these therapeutic agents [16–23]. A landmark review document [24], published in *Allergy* in 2008, was produced in collaboration with the WHO, the Global Allergy and Asthma European Network (GA^2LEN), and the AllerGen NCE Incorporation (Canadian Research Council).

The ARIA (*Allergic Rhinitis and its Impact on Asthma*) document was intended for the specialist, the GP, and other health-care professionals:

- to update their knowledge of allergic rhinitis;
- to highlight the impact of allergic rhinitis on asthma;
- to provide an evidence base and regularly updated commentary on diagnostic methods;
- to provide an evidence base and regularly updated commentary on treatments;
- to propose a stepwise approach to management.

The present management guidelines are based on recommendations put forward in this document.

Antihistamines block histamine-induced symptoms of allergic rhinoconjunctivitis (sneeze, run, itch) but are less effective at preventing chronic nasal blockage which results from chronic inflammation of the nasal mucosa. First-generation histamine H1 receptor antagonists, such as chlorphenamine, are rapidly absorbed and act quickly, although briefly. They are very prone to causing sedation and should not be used when driving or carrying out any other activity which requires complete mental alertness. Some first-generation antihistamines, such as diphenhydramine, terfenadine, and astemizole, can block potassium channels in cardiac smooth muscle, prolonging the QT interval on the electrocardiogram (ECG), which is occasionally a prelude to cardiac dysrhythmia. For all these reasons, first-generation antihistamines are best avoided when treating allergic rhinoconjunctivitis.

Second-generation drugs (cetirizine/levocetirizine, loratadine/desloratadine, and fexofenadine) have much longer half-lives, are much less likely to cause sedation (although this is not unknown), and do not cause ECG abnormalities. Because of their long half-lives, they act more slowly and take several days to reach their full therapeutic concentration in the plasma. For this reason, they are much more effective when taken regularly (daily), and patients should always be advised to do this, unless they have very mild and intermittent symptoms. Topical antihistamine preparations (drops or sprays) may be useful for histamine-induced ocular and nasal symptoms not sufficiently controlled by regular oral drugs, usually as an adjunct to the latter [22].

While antihistamines blunt immediate symptoms of histamine release, topical nasal corticosteroids should be considered first-line therapeutic agents for patients with anything other than very mild symptoms of seasonal or perennial allergic rhinoconjunctivitis. These agents reduce nasal mucosal inflammation, and thus swelling and blockage, which antihistamines do not. In addition, when used prophylactically (that is, every day, commencing a few weeks before the onset of a pollen season through to the end of the season, or every day of the year in the case of perennial allergens), they drive out mast cells from the nasal mucosa, thus preventing histamine release in the first place. They have no immediate effects on symptoms, requiring several weeks to reduce nasal mucosal inflammation and mast cell numbers, which is why patients often believe they are not effective.

In addition to regular usage, correct technique when using nasal sprays or drops is imperative and should always be explained to the patient very carefully. Commonly used corticosteroid sprays or drops include beclometasone dipropionate, budesonide, fluticasone propionate and furoate, and mometasone furoate. There is minimal systemic absorption from the nose, and systemic side effects are rarely seen at routine dosages, although occasionally regular usage can render the mucosa friable and prone to minor bleeding which can be distressing. Sprays are of limited effectiveness when the nose is physically blocked, as, for example, by severe turbinate hypertrophy or nasal polyps. Drops are more likely to be successful in these cases.

Rarely, limited courses of oral corticosteroids may be justified to treat very severe symptoms, for example to alleviate severe nasal blockage prior to using drops or during periods where freedom from symptoms is highly desirable, for example during holidays or examinations [25–29].

Cromoglicate is poorly absorbed and is available as nasal or ocular drops. It inhibits mast cell histamine release and is generally used for relief of mild nasal or ocular histamine-induced symptoms, especially in children, as it is essentially devoid of unwanted effects. The major disadvantage of cromoglicate is its short duration of action; it should be administered ideally every 1–2 hours to be fully effective. Topical vasoconstrictors decongest the nose by constricting mucosal blood vessels. Their usage should be limited to temporary symptomatic relief for a severely congested nose at the beginning of conventional treatment and should be limited to a maximum of a few weeks, since long-term use can cause rebound structural nasal congestion which is difficult to reverse by any means. Oral vasoconstrictors have significant systemic unwanted effects in larger doses and are therefore rarely used [30–40].

The cholinergic antagonist ipratropium bromide, available as a nasal spray, is sometimes useful for managing excessive watery rhinorrhoea of whatever cause (often an isolated problem in the elderly). It can cause excessive nasal dryness [30–40]. Leukotriene antagonists, such as montelukast and zafirlukast, are now widely available in the UK. Although not specifically licensed for the treatment of allergic rhinoconjunctivitis, when used to treat concomitant allergic asthma, they provide additional and useful symptom relief because leukotrienes, also released from degranulated mast cells, contribute to symptoms. They are therefore particularly useful in patients such as this lady with marked allergen-induced asthma and concomitant allergic rhinoconjunctivitis, and add to the benefits of antihistamines for the latter [41].

Allergen immunotherapy is a means of desensitizing patients to the clinical effects of exposure to one or more specific allergens. It can be administered subcutaneously or sublingually. At present, in the UK, sublingual therapy is available for a limited range of allergens. Further details are provided in later text. Patient education particularly centered on allergen avoidance and the efficient and regular use of pharmacotherapy is essential for successful outcomes, as is true in any chronic disease. Clear explanation of the nature of the disorder and possible complications improves compliance with medical therapy. Providing leaflets and useful web addresses improves concordance further.

Surgical intervention is rarely necessary when medical management fails. Surgery is aimed at re-establishing the patency of physically blocked nasal airways (typically by enlarged turbinates or nasal polyps) and dealing with complications arising from this such as secondary chronic rhinosinusitis. The benefits may last from months to years.

Immunotherapy is a procedure in which a purified allergen extract is administered by subcutaneous injection or sublingually (tablets or drops held in the mouth before swallowing). Exposure of patients to an allergen in this way, rather than by inhalation, alters their immune response to the allergen. The end result is that clinical symptoms on allergen exposure are considerably reduced and occasionally abolished. In addition to reducing nasal symptoms, it is often particularly useful for troublesome conjunctivitis and associated seasonal exacerbation of asthma. It is most effective in patients whose severe symptoms are clearly related to exposure to one particular allergen, although desensitization with several allergens is also feasible. It can be used for any patient over the age of 5 years, although the elderly tolerate it less well and the outcome is usually less impressive [42].

The precise mechanism of action of immunotherapy is unclear but has been postulated to involve skewing of the cytokine profile of allergen-specific T cells from T helper (Th) 2 (including interleukin (IL)-4 and IL-5 which promote IgE synthesis and eosinophil and mast cell activation) to Th0 or Th1. There is also some evidence that the procedure generates allergen-specific regulatory T cells which produce cytokines, such as IL-10 and transforming growth factor (TGF)-beta, which inhibit the functions of mast cells and other granulocytes, as well as dampen down allergen-specific immune responses generally. As with any mechanism of 'vaccination', especially when the allergen extracts are injected subcutaneously along with adjuvants such as alum, there is a brisk allergen-specific IgG response which may also contribute to inhibition of the established allergen-specific immune response, for example by preventing the capture of allergen by antigen-presenting cells [42].

Immunotherapy is available for seasonal and perennial allergens. In the UK, it tends to be reserved for patients who retain debilitating symptoms, despite all attempts to avoid allergen exposure, where feasible, and an adequate trial of regular, efficiently administered pharmacotherapy. In cases of domestic animal allergy, avoidance of exposure (by removing the animal) is the preferred approach, but immunotherapy is sometimes offered to individuals in occupations, such as farming, laboratory animal husbandry, and veterinary practice, where avoidance is impossible. House dust mite desensitization is of proven effectiveness, especially in young individuals with severe rhinitis. It is worth noting again, however, that there are many other non-allergic causes of chronic nasal inflammation and rhinosinusitis and that these do not respond to immunotherapy. The patient must give a convincing history of symptoms upon allergen exposure (in a patient with house dust mite allergy, this is typically a history of marked acute nasal symptoms—sneeze, itch, run—and ocular symptoms—itch, run) first thing in the morning (exposure is generally highest in bed). As emphasized repeatedly, a positive skin prick test to house dust mite alone does not guarantee clinically significant house dust mite allergy.

Immunotherapy 'vaccines' are typically purified aqueous protein extracts of allergens (pollens, animal dander) collected in the field (although house dust mites can be grown in the laboratory). Since such extracts will contain variable quantities of individual allergens, they are uniformized for 'biological activity', usually by testing their ability to inhibit the binding of IgE in a reference serum to the specific allergen. This process is not directly comparable between manufacturers. For subcutaneously administered vaccines, extracted allergens are often combined with an adjuvant (alum or L-tyrosine) which delays absorption and also enhances a Th1 immune response, and may be modified by fixation with glutaraldehyde or a similar compound which chemically cross-links the allergenic proteins, altering their shape and therefore reducing their ability to bind to IgE, but retaining their T-cell epitopes [43–46]. This makes them safer (modern vaccines are extremely safe) and more effective.

Subcutaneous immunotherapy typically involves two phases: up-dosing, then maintenance. During up-dosing, typically administered weekly, the concentration of allergen is increased progressively over a period of 8–12 weeks to the maintenance dosage which is then repeated every 6–8 weeks for a total of 3 years. Pollen immunotherapy can also be administered pre-seasonally which involves weekly up-dosing for a period of 4–7 weeks prior to the relevant pollen season each year for 3 consecutive years. For most patients, unwanted effects are limited to local itching and swelling at the injection site and occasional transient urticaria or exacerbation of symptoms of rhinitis (for pollen-allergic patients) on the evenings of the injections. Subcutaneous immunotherapy is inconvenient because it involves multiple visits to a hospital clinic, essential because of the small, but finite, risk of systemic reactions which requires that the treatment be administered by trained specialists in allergy centres which have access to resuscitation facilities. On the other hand, current evidence suggests that subcutaneous immunotherapy is more effective than sublingual, although this situation may change as vaccines improve and further evidence accumulates. The principal contraindication is concurrent, poorly controlled, or unstable asthma, since these patients are at significant risk of life-threatening bronchospasm in the unlikely event of systemic anaphylaxis. Asthma should first be controlled or, if seasonal, treatment should be initiated outside the relevant season. It is also advisable to make sure that patients are not taking drugs which inhibit the actions of adrenaline, such as beta-blockers, since again adrenaline is required to manage systemic reactions [44–46].

Sublingual immunotherapy is available for an increasing range of seasonal and perennial allergens [47]. Typical regimens may or may not include a short up-dosing period (typically 2–4 weeks), in which increasing concentrations of the allergen are taken daily by the patient in drop or tablet form and held briefly under the tongue before swallowing. The dosage then continues at the maintenance dose typically daily for 3 years, although precise regimens are in evolution, and, for seasonal allergens, many manufacturers now recommend 4–8 weeks of pre-seasonal, then co-seasonal, treatment repeated for 3 consecutive years. Local antigen-presenting cells in the lining of the mouth take up and process the allergen. Much greater quantities of the allergen (typically 10- to 100-fold higher than those in subcutaneous vaccines) are required for effectiveness, an issue which contributes to cost. Sublingual treatment is convenient for patients because it can be taken at home, in theory without supervision (there are, as yet, very few reported cases of significant systemic symptoms with sublingual treatment). Nevertheless, it is not devoid of unwanted effects; patients often experience oral itching and tongue and lip swelling, particularly in the early weeks of treatment, and sometimes even chronic oesophagitis. These symptoms are often alleviated by taking a regular antihistamine, but some patients find them intolerable. As mentioned, studies of the relative efficacy and duration of effect of subcutaneous and sublingual therapy are ongoing. Sublingual therapy also raises issues of compliance; there is a danger that patients may forget to take their therapy every day, especially if they have no current symptoms, and this should be anticipated and counselled.

A final word from the expert

In conclusion, effective diagnosis and management of concomitant allergic disease are an indispensible aspect of the management of asthma and rhinosinusitis. Allergy diagnosis and management should be incorporated into all asthma management regimens, whether these be hospital-based or 'in the field'. Astute allergy diagnosis requires very careful history-taking above all; carefully selected tests are used in a confirmatory, rather than predictive, fashion.

References

1. Royal College of Physicians. *Allergy: the unmet need. A blueprint for better patient care.* A report of the Royal College of Physicians Working Party on the provision of allergy services in the UK. London: Royal College of Physicians, 2003.
2. Bousquet J, Van Cauwenberge P, Khaltaev N. Allergic rhinitis and its impact on asthma. *J Allergy Clin Immunol* 2001;**108**(5 Suppl):S147–334.
3. Wilson DR, Lima MT, Durham SR. Sublingual immunotherapy for allergic rhinitis: systematic review and meta-analysis. *Allergy* 2005;**60**:4–12.
4. [No authors listed]. Allergen skin testing. Board of Directors. American Academy of Allergy and Immunology. *J Allergy Clin Immunol* 1993;**92**:636–7.
5. Dreborg S, Frew A. Position paper: allergen standardisation and skin tests. *Allergy* 1993;**48**(Suppl 14):49–82.
6. Starling-Schwanz R, Peake HL, Salome CM *et al.* Repeatability of peak nasal inspiratory flow measurements and utility for assessing the severity of rhinitis. *Allergy* 2005;**60**:795–800.
7. Ottaviano G, Scadding GK, Coles S, Lund VJ. Peak nasal inspiratory flow; normal range in adult population. *Rhinology* 2006;**44**:32–5.
8. Scadding G. Nitric oxide in the airways. *Curr Opin Otolaryngol Head Neck Surg* 2007;**15**:258–63.
9. Ortolani C, Ispano M, Pastorello E, Bigi A, Ansaloni R. The oral allergy syndrome. *Ann Allergy* 1988;**61**:47–52.
10. Valenta R, Twaroch T, Swoboda I. Component-resolved diagnosis to optimize allergen-specific immunotherapy in the Mediterranean area. *J Investig Allergol Clin Immunol.* 2007;**17**(Suppl 1):36–40.

11. Busse W, Corren J, Lanier BQ *et al*. Omalizumab, anti-IgE recombinant humanized monoclonal antibody, for the treatment of severe allergic asthma. *J Allergy Clin Immunol* 2001;**18**:254–61.
12. Humbert M, Beasley R, Ayres J *et al*. Benefits of omalizumab as add-on therapy in patients with severe persistent asthma who are inadequately controlled despite best available therapy (GINA 2002 step 4 treatment): INNOVATE. *Allergy* 2005:**60**:309–16.
13. Sheikh A, Hurwitz B. House dust mite avoidance measures for perennial allergic rhinitis. *Cochrane Database Syst Rev* 2001;**4**:CD001563.
14. Eggleston PA, Butz A, Rand C *et al*. Home environmental intervention in inner-city asthma: a randomized controlled clinical trial. *Ann Allergy Asthma Immunol* 2005;**95**:518–24.
15. Colloff MJ, Ayres J, Carswell F *et al*. The control of allergens of dust mites and domestic pets: a position paper. *Clin Exp Allergy* 1992;**22**(Suppl 2):1–28.
16. Joss JD, Craig TJ. Seasonal allergic conjunctivitis: overview and treatment update. *J Am Osteopath Assoc* 1999;**99**:S13–18.
17. Wilson AM, O'Byrne PM, Parameswaran K. Leukotriene receptor antagonists for allergic rhinitis: a systematic review and meta-analysis. *Am J Med* 2004;**116**:338–44.
18. Nayak AS, Schenkel E. Desloratadine reduces nasal congestion in patients with intermittent allergic rhinitis. *Allergy* 2001;**56**:1077–80.
19. Ciprandi G, Cosentino C, Milanese M, Mondino C, Canonica GW. Fexofenadine reduces nasal congestion in perennial allergic rhinitis. *Allergy* 2001;**56**:1068–70.
20. Ciprandi G, Cirillo I, Vizzaccaro A, Tosca MA. Levocetirizine improves nasal obstruction and modulates cytokine pattern in patients with seasonal allergic rhinitis: a pilot study. *Clin ExpAllergy* 2004;**34**:958–64.
21. Van SJ, Clement PA, Beel MH. Comparison of five new antihistamines (H1-receptor antagonists) in patients with allergic rhinitis using nasal provocation studies and skin tests. *Allergy* 2002;**57**:346–50.
22. Patou J, De SH, Van CP, Bachert C. Pathophysiology of nasal obstruction and meta-analysis of early and late effects of levocetirizine. *Clin Exp Allergy* 2006;**36**:972–81.
23. Canonica GW, Tarantini F, Compalati E, Penagos M. Efficacy of desloratadine in the treatment of allergic rhinitis: a meta-analysis of randomized, double-blind, controlled trials. *Allergy* 2007;**62**:359–66.
24. Bousquet J, Khaltaev N, Cruz AA *et al*. Allergic Rhinitis and its impact on Asthma (ARIA) 2008 update (in collaboration with the World Health Organization, GA(2)LEN and AllerGen). *Allergy* 2008;**63**(Suppl 86):8–160.
25. Simpson RJ. Budesonide and terfenadine, separately and in combination, in the treatment of hay fever. *Ann Allergy* 1994;**73**:497–502.
26. Ratner PH, van Bavel JH, Martin BG *et al*. A comparison of the efficacy of fluticasone propionate aqueous nasal spray and loratadine, alone and in combination, for the treatment of seasonal allergic rhinitis. *J Fam Pract* 1998;**47**:118–25.
27. Yanez A, Rodrigo GJ. Intranasal corticosteroids versus topical H1 receptor antagonists for the treatment of allergic rhinitis: a systematic review with meta-analysis. *Ann Allergy Asthma Immunol* 2002;**89**:479–84.
28. Weiner JM, Abramson MJ, Puy RM. Intranasal corticosteroids versus oral H1 receptor antagonists in allergic rhinitis: systematic review of randomised controlled trials. *BMJ* 1998;**317**:1624–9.
29. Fokkens WJ, Godthelp T, Holm AF, Klein-Jan A. Local corticosteroid treatment: the effect on cells and cytokines in nasal allergic inflammation. *Am J Rhinol* 1998;**12**:21–6.
30. Wood CC, Fireman P, Grossman J, Wecker M, MacGregor T. Product characteristics and pharmacokinetics of intranasal ipratropium bromide. *J Allergy Clin Immunol* 1995;**95**:1111–16.

31. Bronsky EA, Druce H, Findlay SR *et al.* A clinical trial of ipratropium bromide nasal spray in patients with perennial nonallergic rhinitis. *J Allergy Clin Immunol* 1995;**95**:1117–22.
32. Pras E, Stienlauf S, Pinkhas J, Sidi Y. Urinary retention associated with ipratropium bromide. *DICP* 1991;**25**:939–40.
33. Hall SK. Acute angle-closure glaucoma as a complication of combined beta-agonist and ipratropium bromide therapy in the emergency department. *Ann Emerg Med* 1994;**23**:884–7.
34. Storms WW. Pharmacologic approaches to daytime and nighttime symptoms of allergic rhinitis. *J Allergy Clin Immunol* 2004;**114**:S146–53.
35. Scadding GK. Rhinitis medicamentosa. *Clin Exp Allergy* 1995;**25**:391–4.
36. Malm L. Pharmacological background to decongesting and anti-inflammatory treatment of rhinitis and sinusitis. *Acta Otolaryngol* 1994;**515**(Suppl):53–5.
37. Naclerio RM. Optimizing treatment options. *Clin Exp Allergy* 1998;**28**(Suppl 6):54–9.
38. Ratner PH, Ehrlich PM, Fineman SM, Meltzer EO, Skoner DP. Use of intranasal cromolyn sodium for allergic rhinitis. *Mayo Clin Proc* 2002;**77**:350–4.
39. James IG, Campbell LM, Harrison JM, Fell PJ, Ellers-Lenz B, Petzold U. Comparison of the efficacy and tolerability of topically administered azelastine, sodium cromoglycate and placebo in the treatment of seasonal allergic conjunctivitis and rhino-conjunctivitis. *Curr Med Res Opin* 2003;**19**:313–20.
40. Meltzer EO. Efficacy and patient satisfaction with cromolyn sodium nasal solution in the treatment of seasonal allergic rhinitis: a placebo-controlled study. *Clin Ther* 2002;**24**:942–52.
41. Wilson AM, O'Byrne PM, Parameswaran K. Leukotriene receptor antagonists for allergic rhinitis: a systematic review and meta-analysis. *Am J Med* 2004;**116**:338–44.
42. Bousquet J, Lockey R, Malling HJ. Allergen immunotherapy: therapeutic vaccines for allergic diseases. A WHO position paper. *J Allergy Clin Immunol* 1998;**102**:558–62.
43. Durham SR, Walker SM, Varga EM *et al.* Long-term clinical efficacy of grass-pollen immunotherapy. *N Engl J Med* 1999;**341**:468–75.
44. Moller C, Dreborg S, Ferdousi HA *et al.* Pollen immunotherapy reduces the development of asthma in children with seasonal rhinoconjunctivitis (the PAT-study). *J Allergy Clin Immunol* 2002;**109**:251–6.
45. Passalacqua G, Durham SR. Allergic rhinitis and its impact on asthma update: allergen immunotherapy. *J Allergy Clin Immunol* 2007;**119**:881–91.
46. Alvarez-Cuesta O, Bousquet J, Canonica GW, Durham Malling HJ, Valovirta E. Standards for practical allergen-specific immunotherapy. *Allergy* 2006;**61**(Suppl 82):1–20
47. Durham SR, Yang WH, Pedersen MR, Johansen N, Rak S. Sublingual immunotherapy with once-daily grass allergen tablets: a randomized controlled trial in seasonal allergic rhinoconjunctivitis. *J Allergy Clin Immunol* 2006;**117**:802–9.

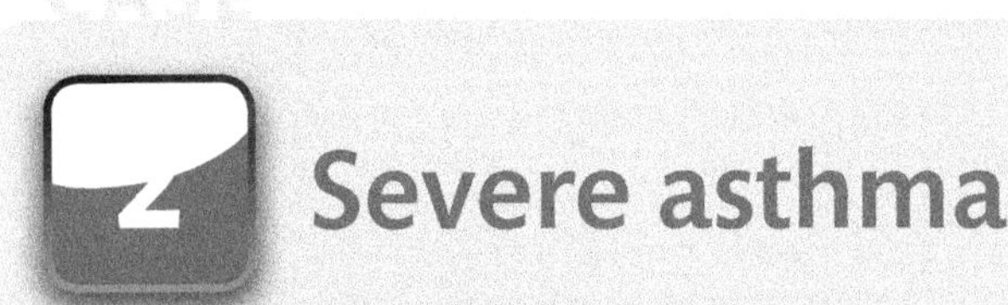

Severe asthma

Anand Shah

Expert commentary Andrew Menzies-Gow

Case history

A 25-year-old female presented to an outpatient respiratory clinic with a history of uncontrolled asthma. She had been diagnosed 16 years previously, following recurrent episodes of dyspnoea associated with wheeze, particularly worse nocturnally, and demonstrated improvement with corticosteroid inhaler use. She had a long history of eczema and atopic rhinosinusitis, but no significant family history of asthma. Her medications included inhaled budesonide 400 micrograms, inhaled salmeterol 50 micrograms, montelukast 10 mg at night, and inhaled salbutamol as required. She had previously been trialled on oral theophylline but stopped due to gastrointestinal intolerance. Over the preceding year, she had required six courses of oral prednisolone for exacerbations and had been hospitalized on two occasions for a short period. She had never required intensive care support during these admissions and had self-discharged on both occasions after 24 hours.

Expert comment

This patient has uncontrolled asthma, despite steps IV/V of the British Thoracic Society (BTS)/ Scottish Intercollegiate Guidelines Network (SIGN) guidelines. As well as considering adherence and efficacy of drug delivery, which are discussed in Learning box, p. 19, it is important to consider potential triggers. An occupational history should be taken to include whether the patient's symptoms are worse during the week and better at the weekend. A history of allergic triggers should also be sought and confirmed with skin prick tests to the common aero-allergens.

Patients with this level of asthma severity should always be referred to a specialist asthma service.

On examination, she appeared well, with no peripheral stigmata associated with chronic respiratory disease. Respiratory examination revealed mildly hyperexpanded lung fields, with a prolonged expiratory phase associated with mild polyphonic wheeze throughout. Cardiovascular and other examinations were unremarkable. Clinic investigations showed a reduced peak flow with evidence of airflow obstruction on spirometry, sputum eosinophilia with no bacterial growth, and mild peripheral blood eosinophilia (Table 2.1). A chest X-ray (CXR) performed in clinic showed mild bronchial wall thickening (Figure 2.1).

Table 2.1 Clinic investigations, including peak flow measurement, spirometry, sputum culture, haematology, and biochemistry

Peak expiratory flow rate	270 mL (67% predicted)
FEV_1	2.4 L (62% predicted)
FVC	3.6 L (94% predicted)
Sputum culture	No microbiological growth
Sputum cytology	10% eosinophils
Hb	12.5 g/dL
WCC	7.7×10^9/L
Neutrophils	4.7×10^9/L
Lymphocytes	2.1×10^9/L
Eosinophils	0.9×10^9/L
Platelets	210×10^9/L
UEs/LFTs	Normal
CRP	10

CRP, C-reactive protein; FEV_1, forced expiratory volume in 1 second; FVC, forced vital capacity; Hb, haemoglobin; LFTs, liver function tests; UEs, urea and electrolytes; WCC, white cell count.

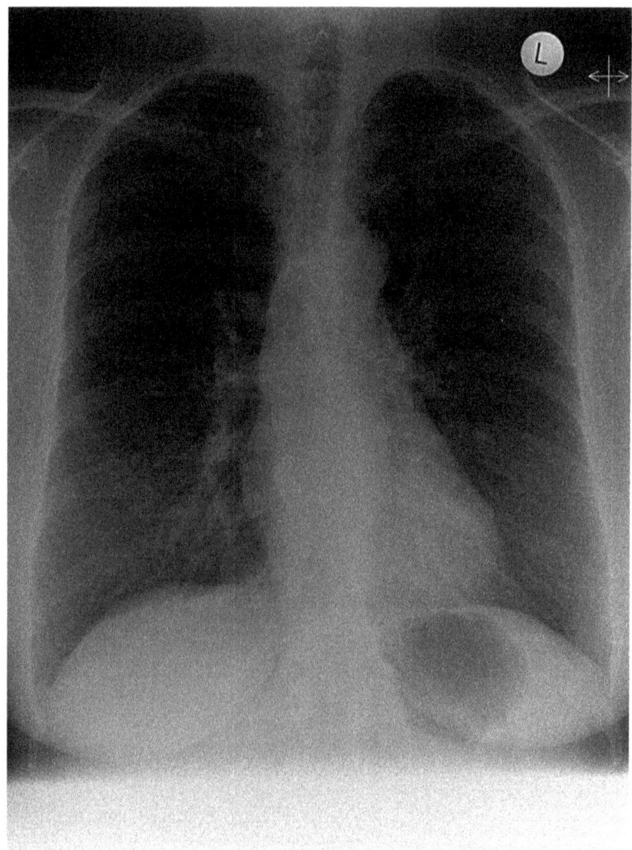

Figure 2.1 Chest radiograph showing mild bronchial wall thickening.

Learning point

Patients presenting with uncontrolled severe asthma should be assessed as to their probability of a diagnosis of asthma, given their history. In this case, according to BTS/SIGN guidelines, the diagnosis is highly likely, with a good initial response to treatment confirming the diagnosis. Given the presence of obstructive lung function (FEV_1/FVC ratio <0.7), a bronchodilator reversibility trial (>400 mL improvement in FEV_1, following either a beta-2 agonist or corticosteroid treatment) could additionally be used to confirm the diagnosis. In patients where the history is inconclusive and there is no obvious obstructive lung function abnormality, more detailed respiratory investigations are necessary such as formal lung function, including body plethysmography and carbon monoxide (CO) diffusion, serum total IgE, sputum eosinophilia, exhaled nitric oxide (NO), skin prick tests to the common aero-allergens, and measurement of airways hyperreactivity such as the histamine challenge test.

Patients with a confirmed diagnosis of asthma who are uncontrolled on maintenance medication should have a detailed history taken regarding their treatment compliance and have their inhaler technique assessed. Compliance with asthma treatment has been shown to be extremely poor in numerous studies [1–3], often related to poor understanding of asthma and the role of inhalers. Inhaler modification can dramatically improve compliance, with a resulting improvement of symptoms [4]. Psychological support may be necessary to improve symptoms of depression and anxiety which is related to poor compliance and increased mortality and morbidity [5–7]. A smoking history should additionally be assessed, as smoking cessation has been shown to reduce asthma severity if successful [8, 9]. A practical asthma self-management plan should be provided [10, 11].

Expert comment

Skin prick tests are extremely informative and easy to perform. Patients must withhold antihistamines for 72 hours prior to testing, but oral corticosteroids are not a contraindication. A positive test is defined as a wheal 3 mm greater in diameter than the negative control, read after 15 minutes.

The patient had reasonable compliance with medication but found the number of inhalers annoying. She was a non-smoker, with no passive exposure and no symptoms suggestive of an anxiety or depressive disorder. She was switched to a combination inhaler with budesonide 200 micrograms and formoterol 12 micrograms at two inhalations bd, alongside her regular oral montelukast treatment. Her inhaler technique was assessed and found to be good, and she was provided with a self-management plan and asked to keep a diary of her symptoms and rescue inhaler use over the next 4 weeks.

On return review, an asthma control questionnaire (ACQ-7) showed significant ongoing symptoms, suggestive of poor asthma control, with her diary recording good inhaler compliance but over four inhalations of rescue medication on most days. She additionally complained of significant rhinitis and nocturnal cough, with an ongoing daytime productive cough. She underwent further testing in the clinic, including total IgE which was raised at 680 and an *Aspergillus* radioallergosorbent test (RAST) which was positive (Table 2.2). A skin prick test showed positive reactions to *Aspergillus* and grass pollen (Figure 2.2).

Table 2.2 Further clinical investigations showing raised total IgE with positive *Aspergillus* RAST, raised exhaled NO, and sputum eosinophilia

Total IgE	680 IU/mL
Aspergillus RAST	15.5 IU/mL
ANCA	Negative
Sputum culture	Upper respiratory flora
Sputum cytology	20% eosinophils
Exhaled NO	Elevated

ANCA, anti-neutrophil cytoplasmic antibody; NO, nitric oxide; RAST, radioallergosorbent test.

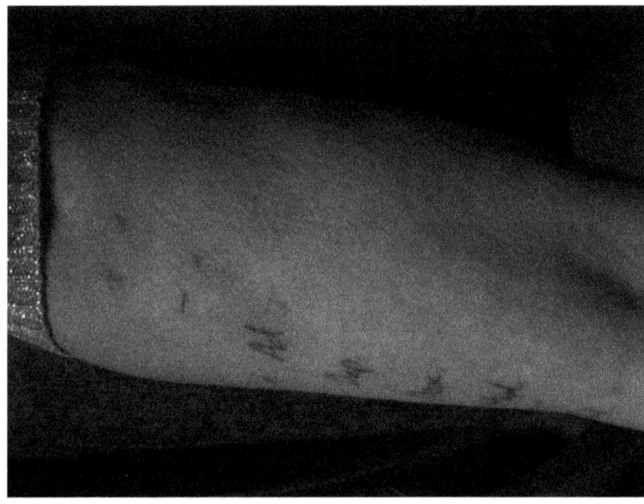

Figure 2.2 Skin prick test showing positive response to grass pollen and appropriate negative and positive controls.

Learning point

The asthma control questionnaire (ACQ) [12,13] is validated to measure asthma control in adults. It is completed in the clinic, asks patients to recall their experiences during the previous week, and includes a measure of FEV_1 % predicted. The ACQ has seven questions, and patients are asked to respond to the symptom and bronchodilator use questions on a 7-point scale (0 = no impairment, 6 = maximum impairment). Clinic staff scores the FEV_1 % predicted on a 7-point scale. The questions are equally weighted, and the ACQ score is the mean of the seven questions and therefore between 0 (totally controlled) and 6 (severely uncontrolled). On the 7-point scale of the ACQ, a change or difference in score of 0.5 is the smallest that can be considered clinically important. This means that changes of 0.5 or greater would justify a change in the patient's treatment (in the absence of undue side effects or excessive costs).

The patient was started on a regular intranasal corticosteroid and an oral antihistamine and was changed to an increased-strength corticosteroid inhaler (equivalent 2000 micrograms beclometasone), alongside an inhaled long-acting beta-2-agonist. A high-resolution computed tomography (CT) scan demonstrated bronchial wall thickening, but no evidence of bronchiectasis (Figure 2.3).

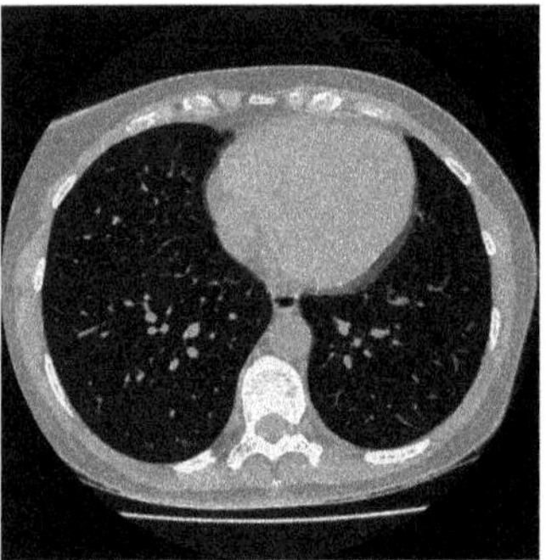

Figure 2.3 High-resolution CT scan showing evidence of bronchial wall thickening, without evidence of central bronchiectasis and no evidence of pulmonary interstitial infiltrates.

Clinical tip

Asthma severity has been shown to be associated with the presence of chronic rhinosinusitis [14]. The presence of Samter's triad (nasal polyposis, aspirin sensitivity, and asthma) has been recognized for many years and responds well to intranasal corticosteroids, alongside leukotriene antagonist therapy. This combination has additionally been shown to be effective for chronic rhinosinusitis associated with nasal polyposis [15]. Although, as yet, a definitive reduction in lower airway inflammation following treatment for rhinosinusitis has not been proven, patients with difficult-to-control symptoms of asthma should have a thorough ENT examination performed and evidence of rhinosinusitis actively treated [16].

Clinical tip

The use of sputum cell type has been used to 'phenotype' patients into those with significant eosinophilia (>2%) who are more likely to respond to high-dose inhaled corticosteroids and those without significant eosinophilia (<2%) where this may not be appropriate [17]. The use of exhaled NO has recently been used in a similar capacity in those who are not on regular oral corticosteroids, but data from studies are still conflicting, and further research is needed to determine its role in asthma management [18–20].

Despite regular use of high-dose inhaled corticosteroid therapy and optimization of the patient's rhinosinusitis, on repeat review 3 months later, she was still uncontrolled. She had had two further hospital admissions and was now on oral prednisolone 10 mg a day, with regular increases to achieve asthma symptom control. A repeat total IgE level was 680 IU/L. Spirometry revealed an FEV_1 of 2.51 (65% predicted). A medication diary and prescription check from the local pharmacy confirmed regular compliance with inhaled and oral therapy. A serum cortisol level was depressed, indicating oral corticosteroid compliance. Given the absence of central bronchiectasis on high-resolution CT imaging and a total IgE level of <1000, the patient did not fit the criteria for ABPA. However, given the positive skin tests to mould, alongside positive *Aspergillus*-specific IgE levels, mildly raised IgE, and severe asthma, she is suffering from severe asthma with fungal sensitization (SAFS) (Table 2.3). She was subsequently started on omalizumab (humanized monoclonal

Table 2.3 ABPA or SAFS? Table detailing the differences in diagnostic criteria of ABPA and SAFS

	Severe asthma with fungal sensitization (SAFS)	Allergic bronchopulmonary aspergillosis (ABPA)
Skin testing to fungal antigen or increase in fungus-specific IgE antibodies	Present	Present
Severe asthma	By definition, asthma is severe	Often severe
Total IgE levels	Mildly elevated (usually <500 IU/mL)	Grossly elevated (usually >1000 IU/mL)
Fungal precipitins	Usually not seen	Commonly present
Eosinophilia	Mildly raised (usually <10%)	Usually elevated (>10%)
Fleeting pulmonary opacities on chest radiograph	Absent	Seen in majority
Mucus plugs of fungal hyphae	Absent	Often seen (20%)
Central bronchiectasis	Absent	Seen in majority (80%)

anti-IgE antibody) therapy. Within 6 months, the patient had stopped oral corticosteroid therapy and was maintained on inhaled therapy alone. No antifungal therapy was started. A repeat ACQ showed significantly improved symptoms. The patient was able to return to regular studies and continues to do well.

Expert comment

The response to omalizumab is assessed after a 16-week treatment trial. In clinical practice, a response rate of up to 80% is seen in the type of patient described in this clinical vignette. The response is assessed by the respiratory physician on the basis of pre- and post-spirometry, exacerbation frequency, asthma quality of life and control questionnaires, bronchodilator use, and emergency health-care utilization.

Learning point Indications for omalizumab—BTS/SIGN guidelines and NICE guidance

Omalizumab is a humanized monoclonal antibody which binds to circulating IgE, markedly reducing the levels of free serum IgE. In adults and children over 6 years of age, it is licensed in the UK for patients on high-dose inhaled steroids and long-acting beta-2-agonists who have impaired lung function, are symptomatic with frequent exacerbations, and have allergy as an important cause of their asthma. Omalizumab is given as a subcutaneous injection every 2 or 4 weeks, depending on the dose. In adults and children >12 years, the licensed indication is IgE up to 1500 IU/mL. Current NICE guidance for the use of omalizumab is:

- omalizumab is an option for the treatment of severe persistent allergic (IgE-mediated) asthma as an add-on therapy to optimized standard therapy;
- optimized standard therapy is defined as a full trial of, and documented compliance with, inhaled high-dose corticosteroids and long-acting beta-2-agonists, in addition to leukotriene receptor antagonists, theophyllines, oral corticosteroids, and beta-2-agonist tablets, and smoking cessation where clinically appropriate;
- confirmation of IgE-mediated allergy to a perennial allergen by clinical history and allergy skin testing;
- either two or more severe exacerbations of asthma requiring hospital admission in the previous year, or three or more severe exacerbations of asthma within the previous year, at least one of which required admission to hospital and a further two which required treatment or monitoring in excess of the patient's usual regimen, in an A&E unit.

Evidence base Benefits of omalizumab as add-on therapy in patients with severe persistent asthma who are inadequately controlled despite best available therapy (GINA 2002 step 4 treatment): INNOVATE

The INNOVATE (INvestigatioN of Omalizumab in seVere Asthma TrEatment) study [21] was specifically designed to evaluate the efficacy and safety of add-on therapy with omalizumab in a difficult-to-treat moderate to severe asthma population (GINA step 3 or 4 clinical features despite step 4 therapy). The trial enrolled patients aged 12–75 years with severe persistent allergic asthma and reduced lung function and inadequate symptom control, despite therapy with a high dose of inhaled corticosteroids (ICS) (>1000 micrograms/day beclometasone dipropionate equivalent) and long-acting beta-agonist bronchodilators, with a recent history of clinically significant exacerbation. A total of 419 patients were included in the efficacy analyses (omalizumab, n = 209; placebo, n = 210). Treatment with omalizumab significantly reduced the rate of severe asthma exacerbations in comparison with placebo (0.24 vs 0.48; p = 0.002) and the rate of total emergency visits for asthma (0.24 vs 0.43; p = 0.038). Significantly greater improvements were obtained with omalizumab, compared with placebo, in quality of life scores, with a significantly greater proportion of patients receiving omalizumab achieving a clinically meaningful (>0.5 point) improvement from baseline, compared with placebo-treated patients (61% and 48%, respectively; p = 0.008).

Discussion

Asthma is a complex heterogenous disease with multiple clinical phenotypes, based on different patterns of airway inflammation involving numerous inflammatory cell types. In the majority of patients, good asthma control is possible with a combination of inhaled corticosteroids and beta-2-adrenoreceptor agonists. A small percentage, however, although compliant and receiving the best available inhaled treatments, remain symptomatic and inadequately controlled, thus having a poor quality of life [22,23].

The case illustrated is that of a severe atopic asthmatic with fungal sensitization that continued to have a poor quality of life with recurrent exacerbations despite standard medical therapy. We have described the stepwise approach to managing such patients in a real-life setting. Once compliance and the inhaler technique have been optimized, it is important to identify and treat any coexisting or additional disease processes that may be driving the patient's asthma. The development of ABPA is important to identify, as treatment with increased-dose corticosteroid is critical to gain initial control. The use of antifungal therapy in ABPA and SAFS and the role of anti-IgE therapy (omalizumab) are discussed in further text.

Exaggerated IgE responses to common environmental allergens are known to play a key role in the pathologic features and clinical manifestations of allergic asthma. Omalizumab is a recombinant humanized antibody comprising a human immunoglobulin G (IgG) framework, which embeds the complementarity-determining region obtained from an anti-IgE antibody raised in mice. By binding to IgE, omalizumab significantly reduces the level of circulating free IgE and prevents their interactions with high-affinity IgE receptors expressed by dendritic cells, mast cells, basophils, and eosinophils. As a consequence, IgE-dependent antigen presentation, mast cell/basophil degranulation, and eosinophil infiltration are inhibited. Anti-IgE therapy with omalizumab also results in decreased IgE receptor expression, resulting in a reduction of allergic airway inflammation, as well as of related asthma symptoms and exacerbations. The dosage of omalizumab is determined by serum baseline levels of total IgE and the patient's body weight. Utilization of omalizumab is currently approved only for allergic asthmatic patients with total plasma IgE levels ranging from 30 to 1500 IU/mL.

Omalizumab has been studied, in addition to stable treatment with inhaled corticosteroids and other anti-asthma drugs, with study results demonstrating fewer asthma exacerbations, improvements in asthma symptoms and quality of life, and decreased requirements for both inhaled corticosteroids and rescue bronchodilators in patients treated with omalizumab, compared with placebo. In comparison with placebo-treated asthmatics, omalizumab-treated patients had fewer hospitalizations, unscheduled outpatient visits, and emergency room visits. Overall, patients who benefited most from omalizumab treatment were those with the poorest lung function and receiving the highest inhaled corticosteroid doses [21,24].

One of the key questions for future research relates to the duration of omalizumab therapy. If discontinued after a few months, atopic patients return to their pre-treatment state due to a rapid rise in free serum IgE levels. This may suggest that treatment should be lifelong; however, recent research has shown that 6 years of treatment with omalizumab induced durable improvement in asthma symptoms and lung function, which was maintained in 14 of 18 patients for periods of 12–14 months after drug withdrawal [25]. Although the optimal duration of omalizumab treatment remains unclear, there is no doubt that the injections need to be continued for prolonged periods of time. Although this is costly, if omalizumab treatment is restricted to selected patients with severe persistent and uncontrolled allergic asthma who respond within 16 weeks with a marked improvement in disease control, it could be cost-effective [26].

More recently, there has been interest in mepolizumab, a monoclonal antibody to IL-5 which selectively inhibits eosinophilic inflammation and reduces the number of eosinophils in both sputum and circulating blood. This, in turn, should result in a reduction in the number of exacerbations and the use of high-dose oral corticosteroids. The MENSA study looked at the use of both intravenous (IV) and subcutaneous delivery of mepolizumab for 32 weeks in patients with severe asthma and peripheral blood eosinophilia and showed some promising results. While this is not yet in routine clinical use, it is clear that the future of difficult asthma management is likely to involve the modulation of specific immune cells.

Evidence base MENSA study (MEpolizumab as adjunctive therapy iN patients with Severe Asthma)

- Multicentre, randomized, double-blind, double-dummy, phase 3, placebo-controlled trial [27].
- Inclusion criteria: 12–80 years, clinical diagnosis asthma, FEV_1 <80% predicted or <90% predicted if <18 years, evidence of bronchodilator reversibility on objective testing, two exacerbations requiring oral corticosteroids in the previous year, maintenance of >880 micrograms/day of inhaled fluticasone or equivalent, and peripheral blood eosinophilia of >150 cells/microlitre at entrance or >300 cells/microlitre during the previous year.
- A total of 576 treated: 191 received placebo, 191 received 75 mg mepolizumab (IV), and 194 received 100 mg mepolizumab subcutaneously (SC).
- Primary outcome: number of exacerbations per year requiring oral steroids or hospital visit.
- 47% and 53% relative reduction in exacerbation rate, compared to placebo, for IV and SC treatment, respectively.
- Additional improvement in quality of life scores and asthma control.

ABPA is caused by allergy to the spores of *Aspergillus fumigatus* and is characterized by an intermittent or chronic colonization of the airways, associated with exacerbations of asthma and recurrent transient chest radiographic infiltrates. Patients with ABPA develop a hypersensitivity response, both a type 1 atopic response (associated with the formation of IgE) and a type 3 hypersensitivity response (associated with the formation of IgG) [28]. The reaction of IgE with *Aspergillus* antigens results in mast cell degranulation, with bronchoconstriction and increased capillary permeability. Immune complexes and inflammatory cells are then deposited within the mucous membranes of the airways, leading to necrosis and an eosinophilic infiltrate. The *Aspergillus* spores are not cleared, and proteolytic enzymes are released by the immune cells which, together with toxins released by the fungi, lead to central bronchiectasis and, with repeated episodes, if untreated, result in progressive pulmonary fibrosis often seen in the upper zones [29–31]. ABPA affects approximately 0.7–3.5% of asthmatic patients and 7–9% of patients with cystic fibrosis [32].

Although systemic corticosteroids remain the mainstay of ABPA treatment, the potential utility of systemic antifungal therapy for ABPA was first shown in the early 1990s, with placebo-controlled randomized studies demonstrating benefit from itraconazole treatment (200 mg bd initially) [33]. Outcome measures showed a reduction in corticosteroid oral dose, reduction in total IgE levels, decreased exacerbation frequency, increased exercise tolerance, and improved pulmonary function. Itraconazole levels should be monitored to optimize exposure, with low plasma levels requiring optimization of absorption (capsules should be taken on an empty stomach with an acidic fizzy drink) or a shift between capsules and oral solution to increase absorption and occasionally increasing the dose. Proton pump inhibitors (PPIs) and H2 blockers reduce absorption of itraconazole capsules, and different capsule formulations differ in bioavailability. Excessive itraconazole concentrations often result in adverse events, and dose reduction is advised. The duration of itraconazole therapy is not clear but should not be <6 months in those who tolerate it and might be extended safely, with benefit for years [34]. In patients who cannot tolerate itraconazole, newer azoles, such as voriconazole or posaconazole, may provide an alternative, although no large studies have been performed to date [35, 36]. There are a number of case series of patients reporting the benefit of omalizumab in the treatment of ABPA, but no randomized studies have been performed [37, 38].

The term severe asthma with fungal sensitization (SAFS) has been coined to illustrate the high rate of fungal sensitivity in patients with persistent severe asthma and possible improvement with antifungal treatment [39–41]. It is thought that some patients with SAFS may go on to develop ABPA due to increasing Th2 immune responses. Although the initial management of SAFS should be akin to that of severe asthma, as both are primarily immune-mediated, itraconazole has also been investigated for its use in SAFS in the recently published Fungal Asthma Sensitization Trial (FAST).

Evidence base Fast (Fungal Asthma Sensitization Trial)

- Randomized, placebo-controlled trial [39].
- 32 weeks' treatment with 200 mg itraconazole bd in patients with SAFS.
- Primary end point was improvement in Asthma Quality of Life Questionnaire (AQLQ) score.
- Significant improvement in AQLQ in the itraconazole group.
- Possible improvement due to the potentiating effect of itraconazole on inhaled steroids.
- Role of itraconazole requires further evaluation.

A final word from the expert

This clinical case clearly illustrates the complexity of severe asthma and the need for logical systematic assessment of these patients, which subsequently allows for therapy to be targeted to the clinical phenotype that is underlying the loss of asthma control.

There have been several important recent advances in the treatment of severe asthma, including the use of antifungals for SAFS and anti-IgE therapy for severe atopic asthma. Over the next decade, multiple new biological agents will become available that will benefit a larger number of patients with severe asthma and decrease their reliance on oral corticosteroids.

References

1. Jiang H, Han J, Zhu Z, Xu W, Zheng J, Zhu Y. Patient compliance with assessing and monitoring of asthma. *J Asthma* 2009;**46**:1027–31.
2. Starobin D, Bargutin M, Rosenberg I, Yarmolovsky A, Levi T, Fink G. Asthma control and compliance in a cohort of adult asthmatics: first survey in Israel. *Isr Med Assoc J* 2007;**9**:358–60.
3. Horne R. Compliance, adherence, and concordance: implications for asthma treatment. *Chest* 2006;**130**(1 Suppl):65S–72S.

4. Small M, Anderson P, Vickers A, Kay S, Fermer S. Importance of inhaler-device satisfaction in asthma treatment: real-world observations of physician-observed compliance and clinical/patient-reported outcomes. *Adv Ther* 2011;**28**:202–12.
5. Urrutia I, Aguirre U, Pascual S *et al.* Impact of anxiety and depression on disease control and quality of life in asthma patients. *J Asthma* 2012;**49**:201–8.
6. Lavoie KL, Boudreau M, Plourde A, Campbell TS, Bacon SL. Association between generalized anxiety disorder and asthma morbidity. *Psychosom Med* 2011;**73**:504–13.
7. Di Marco F, Santus P, Centanni S. Anxiety and depression in asthma. *Curr Opin Pulm Med* 2011;**17**:39–44.
8. Tan NC, Ngoh SH, Teo SS, Swah TS, Chen Z, Tai BC. Impact of cigarette smoking on symptoms and quality of life of adults with asthma managed in public primary care clinics in Singapore: a questionnaire study. *Prim Care Respir J* 2012;**21**:90–3.
9. McLeish AC, Zvolensky MJ. Asthma and cigarette smoking: a review of the empirical literature. *J Asthma* 2010;**47**:345–61.
10. Holt S, Masoli M, Beasley R. The use of the self-management plan system of care in adult asthma. *Primary Care Respir J* 2004;**13**:19–27.
11. Beasley R, Crane J. Reducing asthma mortality with the asthma self-management plan system of care. *Am J Respir Crit Care Med* 2001;**163**:3–4.
12. Juniper EF, O'Byrne PM, Ferrie PJ, King DR, Roberts JN. Measuring asthma control. Clinic questionnaire or daily diary? *Am J Respir Crit Care Med* 2000;**162**(4 Pt 1):1330–4.
13. Juniper EF, O'Byrne PM, Guyatt GH, Ferrie PJ, King DR. Development and validation of a questionnaire to measure asthma control. *Eur Respir J* 1999;**14**:902–7.
14. Lin DC, Chandra RK, Tan BK *et al.* Association between severity of asthma and degree of chronic rhinosinusitis. *Am J Rhinol Allergy* 2011;**25**:205–8.
15. Nonaka M, Sakanushi A, Kusama K, Ogihara N, Yagi T. One-year evaluation of combined treatment with an intranasal corticosteroid and montelukast for chronic rhinosinusitis associated with asthma. *J Nippon Med Sch* 2010;**77**:21–8.
16. Dixon AE. Rhinosinusitis and asthma: the missing link. *Curr Opin Pulm Med* 2009;**15**:19–24.
17. Petsky HL, Cates CJ, Lasserson TJ *et al.* A systematic review and meta-analysis: tailoring asthma treatment on eosinophilic markers (exhaled nitric oxide or sputum eosinophils). *Thorax* 2012;**67**:199–208.
18. Nair P, Kjarsgaard M, Armstrong S, Efthimiadis A, O'Byrne PM, Hargreave FE. Nitric oxide in exhaled breath is poorly correlated to sputum eosinophils in patients with prednisone-dependent asthma. *J Allergy Clin Immunol* 2010;**126**:404–6.
19. Perez-de-Llano LA, Carballada F, Castro Anon O *et al.* Exhaled nitric oxide predicts control in patients with difficult-to-treat asthma. *Eur Respir J* 2010;**35**:1221–7.
20. Gelb AF, Moridzadeh R, Singh DH, Fraser C, George SC. In moderate-to-severe asthma patients monitoring exhaled nitric oxide during exacerbation is not a good predictor of spirometric response to oral corticosteroid. *J Allergy Clin Immunol* 2012;**129**:1491–8.
21. Humbert M, Beasley R, Ayres J *et al.* Benefits of omalizumab as add-on therapy in patients with severe persistent asthma who are inadequately controlled despite best available therapy (GINA 2002 step 4 treatment): INNOVATE. *Allergy* 2005;**60**:309–16.
22. Blakey JD, Wardlaw AJ. What is severe asthma? *Clin Exp Allergy* 2012;**42**:617–24.
23. Poon AH, Eidelman DH, Martin JG, Laprise C, Hamid Q. Pathogenesis of severe asthma. *Clin Exp Allergy* 2012;**42**:625–37.
24. Sthoeger ZM, Eliraz A, Asher I, Berkman N, Elbirt D. The beneficial effects of Xolair (omalizumab) as add-on therapy in patients with severe persistent asthma who are inadequately controlled despite best available treatment (GINA 2002 step IV)-the Israeli arm of the INNOVATE study. *Isr Med Assoc J* 2007;**9**:472–5.
25. Nopp A, Johansson SG, Adédoyin J, Ankerst J, Palmqvist M, Oman H. After 6 years with Xolair; a 3-year withdrawal follow-up. *Allergy* 2010;**65**:56–60.
26. Curtiss FR. Selectivity and specificity are the keys to cost-effective use of omalizumab for allergic asthma. *J Manag Care Pharm* 2005;**11**:774–6.

27. Ortega HG, Liu MC, Pavord ID *et al.* Mepolizumab treatment in patients with severe eosinophilic asthma. *N Engl J Med* 2014;**371**:1198–207.
28. Patterson R, Roberts M. IgE and IgG antibodies against Aspergillus fumigatus in sera of patients with bronchopulmonary allergic aspergillosis. *Int Arch Allergy Appl Immunol* 1974;**46**:150–60.
29. Knutsen AP. Immunopathology and immunogenetics of allergic bronchopulmonary aspergillosis. *J Allergy* 2011;**2011**:785983.
30. Gibson PG. Allergic bronchopulmonary aspergillosis. *Semin Respir Crit Care Med* 2006;**27**:185–91.
31. McCarthy DS. Bronchiectasis in allergic bronchopulmonary aspergillosis. *Proc R Soc Med* 1968;**61**:503–6.
32. Moss RB. Allergic bronchopulmonary aspergillosis and Aspergillus infection in cystic fibrosis. *Curr Opin Pulm Med* 2010;**16**:598–603.
33. Denning DW, Van Wye JE, Lewiston NJ, Stevens DA. Adjunctive therapy of allergic bronchopulmonary aspergillosis with itraconazole. *Chest* 1991;**100**:813–19.
34. Hagihara M, Kasai H, Umemura T, Kato T, Hasegawa T, Mikamo H. Pharmacokinetic-pharmacodynamic study of itraconazole in patients with fungal infections in intensive care units. *J Infect Chemother* 2011;**17**:224–30.
35. Chishimba L, Niven RM, Cooley J, Denning DW. Voriconazole and posaconazole improve asthma severity in allergic bronchopulmonary aspergillosis and severe asthma with fungal sensitization. *J Asthma* 2012;**49**:423–33.
36. Glackin L, Leen G, Elnazir B, Greally P. Voriconazole in the treatment of allergic bronchopulmonary aspergillosis in cystic fibrosis. *Ir Med J* 2009;**102**:29.
37. Sastre I, Blanco J, Mata H, García F. A case of allergic bronchopulmonary aspergillosis treated with omalizumab. *J Investig Allergol Clin Immunol* 2012;**22**:145–7.
38. Tillie-Leblond I, Germaud P, Leroyer C *et al.* Allergic bronchopulmonary aspergillosis and omalizumab. *Allergy* 2011;**66**:1254–6.
39. Denning DW, O'Driscoll BR, Powell G *et al.* Randomized controlled trial of oral antifungal treatment for severe asthma with fungal sensitization: The Fungal Asthma Sensitization Trial (FAST) study. *Am J Respir Crit Care Med* 2009;**179**:11–18.
40. Khazeni N, Levitt JE. Does itraconazole improve quality of life in severe asthma with fungal sensitization? *Am J Respir Crit Care Med* 2009;**180**:191–2; author reply 192.
41. Agarwal R. Severe asthma with fungal sensitization. *Curr Allergy Asthma Rep* 2011;**11**:403–13.

CASE

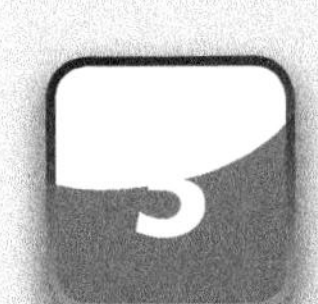

Bacterial lung infection

Simon Brill

Expert commentary Jeremy Brown

Case history

A 77-year-old woman presented to her GP complaining of a 3-week history of cough, breathlessness, and foul sputum production of approximately one cup per day. She admitted to night sweats, but there was no chest pain, haemoptysis, or weight loss. She was a lifelong smoker and had a previous medical history of treated hypertension and a single transient ischaemic attack. There was also a history of excessive alcohol use provided by her daughter, although exact details were unavailable. Her regular medications were aspirin 75 mg once daily (od) and bendroflumethiazide 2.5 mg od only.

On examination, she was alert and orientated, with a respiratory rate of 18 breaths/min, pulse of 90 beats/min, blood pressure of 125/82 mmHg, and temperature of 37.7 °C. Some fine crepitations were heard in the right upper zone on auscultation. The GP made a clinical diagnosis of community-acquired pneumonia (CAP) and prescribed a 7-day course of amoxicillin. In view of the smoking history, he also arranged a CXR and a review in 1 week with the result.

Clinical tip Defining pneumonia without radiology

Pneumonia is infection of the alveoli and presents as a clinical syndrome consistent with an acute lower respiratory tract infection, combined with new radiographic shadowing for which there is no other explanation. Where radiology is unavailable, community-acquired pneumonia (CAP) is defined [1] as the presence of:

- symptoms of an acute lower respiratory tract illness (new cough and at least one other lower respiratory tract symptom);
- **new** focal chest signs on examination (usually crepitations, occasionally pleural rub or bronchial breathing);
- at least one systemic feature (either a symptom complex of sweating, fevers, shivers, aches, and pains and/or a temperature of ≥38°C);
- no other explanation for the illness, which is treated as CAP with antibiotics.

Symptoms that specifically point to pneumonia are pleuritic chest pain and increased dyspnoea.

Expert comment

The patient has three important risk factors for pneumonia: her age, smoking, and alcohol abuse. However, CAP usually has a relatively short history of <10 days; a longer history (3 weeks in this case) should raise suspicion for an infection with an atypical pathogen such as *Mycoplasma pneumoniae* or *Chlamydophilia pneumoniae* or a more complex clinical problem. Foul sputum would be unusual for atypical pathogens, and the amount this patient is producing also suggests the situation is more complex; a cup per day suggests there is either bronchiectasis or marked pulmonary suppuration present. A CXR is vital for the proper assessment of the patient.

Learning point Risk stratification in CAP

Many different variables have been linked with mortality in pneumonia on univariate analysis. The most widely studied pneumonia-specific predictive model is the Pneumonia Severity Index [2], which uses a computed score based on 20 variables to identify those suitable for early hospital discharge. It is complex, however, and, in order to develop a user-friendly risk stratification system from information available at the point of hospital admission, in 2003, Lim and colleagues [3] combined data from three prospective studies of CAP (1068 patients) and used multiple regression analysis to identify prognostic variables; 30-day mortality was the primary end point. The result was the 'CURB-65' score, which scores one for each of **C**onfusion, **U**rea >7 mmol/L, **R**espiratory rate ≥30 breaths/min, **B**lood pressure (systolic <90 or diastolic ≤60 mmHg), or age ≥**65** years. Mortality was predicted as follows: score 0, 0.7%; score 1, 3.2%; score 2, 3%; score 3, 17%; score 4, 41.5%; and score 5, 57%. A subsequent study has validated this in over 12,000 patients, and the CRB-65 score (without urea) has similar validity and utility for primary care or where laboratory blood tests are unavailable. BTS guidance on pneumonia [1] recommends using these scoring systems in conjunction with appropriate clinical judgement; patients with a CURB-65 score of ≤1 (if seen in hospital) or a CRB-65 score of 0 (if seen in the community) are likely to be suitable for outpatient management if there are no other concerning features.

At the second appointment, her symptoms remained unchanged, despite antibiotic therapy, and she still had a productive cough, although the sputum volume had reduced. Her vital signs were similar to those at presentation, with a pulse of 90 beats/min, temperature of 37.4°C, respiratory rate of 20 breaths/min, and blood pressure of 124/75 mmHg. Her CXR is shown in Figure 3.1, with right upper lobe shadowing noted on the report seen by the GP. On the basis of this, she was referred for urgent assessment at the lung cancer clinic of her local hospital under the 2-week target referral pathway. Further antibiotic therapy was not given at this stage. Prior to this appointment, fibreoptic bronchoscopy and a CT thorax were arranged, and she attended first for bronchoscopy 2 weeks later.

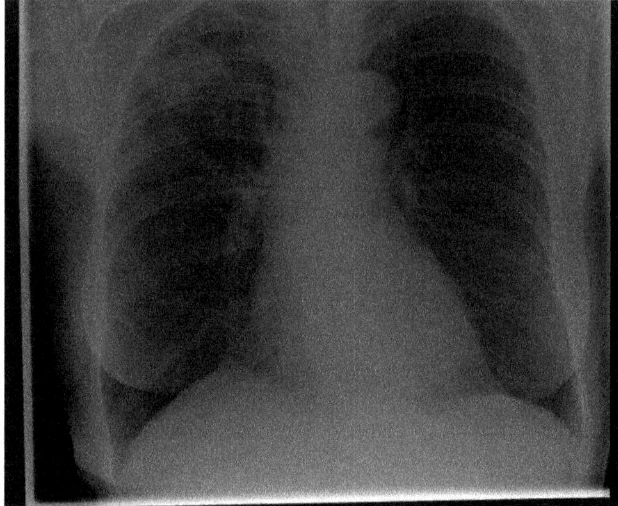

Figure 3.1 Chest radiograph (CXR) requested by the general practitioner at presentation.

Clinical tip Initial investigations of community-acquired pneumonia

The 2009 BTS guidelines [1] recommend that, in the community, low-risk (CRB-65 score of 0) uncomplicated CAP can be managed without further investigation in the first instance. Chest radiography is recommended only if there is doubt regarding the diagnosis, if the patient fails to improve, or if there is an underlying risk of lung cancer. Microbiological examination of the sputum is recommended if there is a clinical suspicion of tuberculosis (TB) or legionnaires' disease or if there is failure to respond to initial antibiotic therapy. Blood tests are not recommended for the majority of cases.

All hospitalized patients with suspected pneumonia should have a CXR within 4 hours to confirm the diagnosis and allow prompt antibiotic therapy to be given. Blood tests, including inflammatory markers, should also be arranged within this period, and blood cultures should be sent prior to the first dose of antibiotic (although this should not be delayed in an unwell patient). Microbiological examination (as detailed in Table 3.1) is recommended for all patients with moderate or high risk CAP (and low-risk CAP according to clinical judgement). Antibiotic therapy should be tailored to the pathogen(s) identified.

Learning point Spectrum of bacteria causing pneumonia

Although the microbial aetiology of CAP varies between studies, *Streptococcus pneumoniae* is consistently the most commonly isolated pathogen and accounts for around 40% of bacteriologically confirmed cases [1,4]. Other common pathogens causing CAP include the so-called atypical pathogens *M. pneumoniae* and *C. pneumoniae* (accounting for perhaps 25% of cases). Less common bacterial pathogens include *Haemophilus influenzae*, *Moraxella catarrhalis*, *Legionella pneumophila*, *Staphylococcus aureus*, Gram-negative enteric bacteria (including *Klebsiella* species), *Pseudomonas aeruginosa*, and other *Streptococcus* species. Around 10% of aetiologically confirmed cases of CAP are viral in origin [4], mainly influenza A. *M. pneumoniae* infections occur in outbreaks, approximately every 4 years in the UK [1], and prevalence varies accordingly. Mixed aetiologies are found in up to 15–20% of cases and is associated with higher mortality [4].

Empirical antibiotic therapy should be selected to provide a broad spectrum of activity against these common pathogens. Initial oral therapy should be with amoxicillin ± a macrolide for patients hospitalized with moderate-severity pneumonia; macrolide alone, doxycycline, moxifloxacin, or levofloxacin are oral alternatives if there is penicillin allergy [1]. If the pneumonia is severe, then treatment with IV combination of β-lactam/β-lactamase inhibitor (co-amoxiclav) and clarithromycin should be given immediately; a second- or third-generation cephalosporin can be used, instead of co-amoxiclav, if there is penicillin allergy.

Patients with CAP who are admitted from nursing homes or have complex medical backgrounds with frequent hospital admissions have been described as a separate clinical entity termed health care-associated pneumonia (HCAP). In some studies, HCAP is associated with a higher incidence of infections with resistant or Gram-negative organisms and higher mortality [5]. Guidance on HCAP was published by the American Thoracic Society (ATS)/Infectious Diseases Society of America (IDSA) in 2005 [6], with UK guidance issued in 2008 [7]. The recommendation is for empiric broad-spectrum antibiotic therapy with multiple agents to cover all suspected resistant organisms, particularly meticillin-resistant *S. aureus* (MRSA) and extended-spectrum β-lactamase (ESBL)-producing bacteria, where appropriate. However, there is growing evidence that resistant organisms are not as common as previously thought and that concordance with these guidelines may result in over-treatment with no effect on outcome [8]. At present, whether HCAP truly is a separate entity to CAP that requires different treatment remains controversial.

Evidence base Effect of procalcitonin-based guidelines vs standard guidelines on antibiotic use in lower respiratory tract infections: the ProHOSP trial

- Multicentre, non-inferiority, randomized controlled trial in Switzerland with an open intervention [9].
- A total of 1359 patients with mostly severe community-acquired lower respiratory tract infection (LRTI) treated in the emergency departments of participating hospitals; 925 had confirmed CAP.
- Randomized to either treatment according to a procalcitonin (PCT)-based algorithm with predefined values for starting or stopping antibiotics (PCT group, 687 patients) or standard treatment (control group, 694 patients).

(Continued)

- Primary end point was non-inferiority for a composite outcome of death, intensive care unit admission, disease-specific complications, or recurrent infection requiring antibiotic treatment within 30 days.
- The primary end point was met; the composite rate of overall adverse outcomes was similar in the PCT and control groups (15.4% [n = 103] vs 18.9 [n = 130], difference −3.5% [95% CI −7.6% to 0.4%]). Secondary outcomes also showed 34.8% lower mean antibiotic exposure in the PCT vs control group (5.7 vs 8.7 days, CI −40.3% to −28.7%) and less frequent antibiotic complications in the PCT group (19.8% [n = 133] vs 28.1% [n = 193], difference 8.2%, CI −12.7% to −3.7%). These results applied overall and also in analysis of all subgroups.
- This showed that the PCT-guided algorithm could be safely used to guide antibiotic therapy and appeared also to reduce mean antibiotic use and the incidence of antibiotic-related complications.

Clinical tip Hunting for pathogens

Investigation of suspected bacterial pneumonia consists of general investigations and, where appropriate, specific tests for certain pathogens. Table 3.1 summarizes some of the investigations that may be considered. The intensity of the investigation will be defined by the severity of the pneumonia, the response to initial antibiotic therapy, and the risk of unusual organisms. Invasive techniques (including bronchoalveolar lavage (BAL), thoracocentesis, and percutaneous fine needle aspiration) may need to be used when a specific microbiological diagnosis is important. This includes patients with severe pneumonia or HCAP, failure to respond to initial therapy, immunocompromise, or other specific risk factors (including, for example, recent travel or illness during a known disease outbreak).

Table 3.1 Specific investigations aimed at determining the aetiology of pulmonary infection

Test	Specimen	When to consider
Routine culture and sensitivity testing (with Gram stain if locally available)	Sputum/BAL Serum Pleural fluid (if present)	All patients with moderate to severe CAP plus selected other cases
Pneumococcal antigen test	Urine	All patients with moderate to severe CAP plus selected other cases
Legionella antigen test	Urine	All patients with severe CAP plus other cases at high risk
Specific culture for *Legionella* (prolonged)	Sputum/BAL	All patients with positive urinary antigen for *Legionella* All patients with severe CAP Suspected other cases, e.g. during a local outbreak
M. pneumoniae polymerase chain reaction (PCR) (if available)	Sputum/BAL Throat swab	During outbreaks Younger patients
M. pneumoniae serology	Serum	
C. pneumoniae serology	Serum	Younger patients
Respiratory viruses serology	Serum	During outbreaks
Respiratory viruses PCR	Throat swab	During outbreaks
Mycobacterial microscopy and culture	Sputum/BAL Pleural fluid (if present)	High-risk groups Suggestive history Other risk factors
HIV serology	Serum	All patients with CAP in regions with high rates of HIV infection Atypical presentations suggestive of unusual pathogens, e.g. *Pneumocystis jirovecii*
Pathogens of immunocompromised patients: • *Aspergillus* • *P. jirovecii* • Cytomegalovirus • *Nocardia*	BAL	At-risk groups (especially immunosuppressed patients)

Table 3.2 Blood test results on admission to hospital

Haemoglobin	12.5 g/dL	CRP	268 mg/dL
Total white cell count	20.3×10^9/L	Urea and electrolytes	Normal
Neutrophil count	17.4×10^9/L	Liver function tests	Normal
Platelet count	428×10^9/L	Coagulation screen	Normal

On arrival, she was noted to be unwell. Her respiratory rate was 22 breaths/min, pulse 100 beats/min, and oxygen saturations 93% on room air. It was deemed safe to proceed with bronchoscopy, which found an additional orifice that opened into a large cavity close to the right upper lobe bronchus. The cavity had obliterated the segmental bronchi of the right upper lobe and had a purulent and necrotic centre containing no obvious discrete lesion. Biopsies, brushings, and washings were taken and sent for histology, cytology, and standard and mycobacterial cultures with urgent microscopy.

She was admitted directly to the respiratory ward from the bronchoscopy suite for further investigations and treatment as an inpatient. She was initially placed in a side room with respiratory isolation precautions, pending the results of microscopy for mycobacteria. Blood tests are shown in Table 3.2.

A CT scan was arranged and performed the same day, and this is shown in Figure 3.2. A thick-walled right upper lobe cavity with no air–fluid level was confirmed, with visible communication into the right upper lobe bronchus; there was no significant mediastinal lymphadenopathy. These appearances clearly demonstrated rapid progression from the appearances on the plain radiograph 19 days earlier. Gram stain and microscopy for acid-fast bacilli were negative. In view of the clinical history, high inflammatory marker levels, and rapid radiological progression, the working diagnosis was a lung abscess complicating bacterial pneumonia.

Expert comment

Bacterial lung abscesses caused by conventional organisms are usually partially fluid-filled, thick-walled, and poorly defined (at least initially); dry cavities would suggest mycobacterial or fungal (*Aspergillus*) infection or another diagnosis such as squamous cell lung cancer or vasculitis. However, in this case, the abscess cavity has a direct communication with the bronchial tree, allowing the fluid to drain and preventing the formation of an air–fluid level. Direct access to an abscess cavity via an additional communication with the bronchus is very unusual and raises the suspicion that a neoplasm may be underlying the infective process.

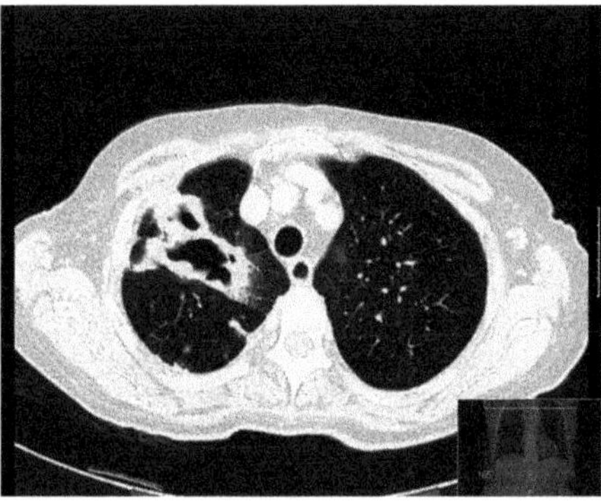
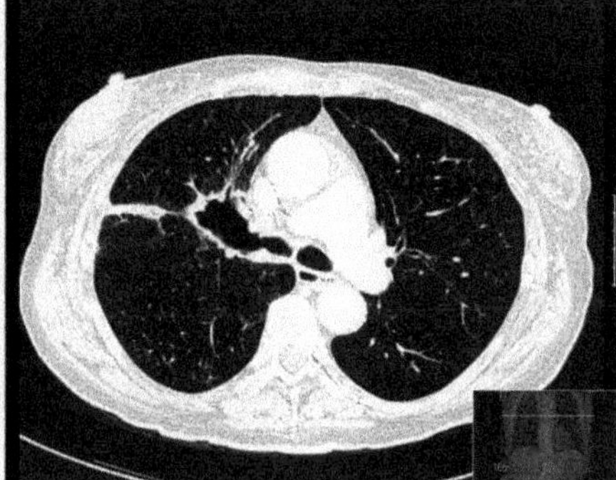

Figure 3.2 CT on admission to the respiratory ward.

Clinical tip Radiology of the lung abscess

A plain radiograph of a bacterial lung abscess classically shows a large, thick-walled cavity with an air–fluid interface contained within it. However, this finding may also be seen in other related conditions (e.g. TB, cavitatory lung cancer, infected bulla, pulmonary infarction, and vasculitis) and can often be difficult to differentiate from a hydropneumothorax, particularly if the lesion is in the lower lobes or there has been rupture into the pleural space. For this reason, CT has become standard for investigation of a suspected lung abscess. Characteristic CT findings are of a round, thick-walled cavity, with abrupt termination of the surrounding airways at the outer margin and an irregular inner border, often with multiple air–fluid levels seen within the abscess cavity [10]. CT may also show other diagnoses, such as pulmonary malignancy, and can clearly delineate the extent of lung involvement. There is also increasing interest in pleural ultrasound to identify a peripheral lung abscess [11], although again it can be difficult to differentiate this from pleural empyema [12].

Lung cavitation on imaging is often caused by conditions other than infection, and these should always be considered. Common differential diagnoses include:

- neoplasia (primary lung cancer or metastases);
- vasculitis (particularly Wegener's);
- cavitatory rheumatoid nodule;
- cavitatory pulmonary infarction;
- other structures (localized saccular bronchiectasis, infected bullus, air–fluid level in other viscus, e.g. oesophagus, stomach).

Empirical treatment was commenced on admission with IV piperacillin/tazobactam and teicoplanin to provide broad-spectrum and staphylococcal cover. Clinically, she remained symptomatic, although haemodynamically stable with some improvement in her parameters. Histology from the bronchoscopic biopsies showed chronic inflammation with some atypical features, but no evidence of malignancy. Cultures of the bronchial washings and the biopsy specimen after 48 hours were positive for *K. pneumoniae* and *M. catarrhalis*. Both organisms were sensitive to piperacillin/tazobactam and co-amoxiclav but resistant to amoxicillin. Blood anti-neutrophil and anti-neutrophil cytoplasmic antibodies were negative. Teicoplanin was stopped, and piperacillin/tazobactam continued for a total of 14 days.

The patient was discussed at the lung cancer multidisciplinary meeting on day 7 of her admission. The consensus opinion was that the presumptive diagnosis was likely to be correct, although an underlying cavitatory malignancy could not be excluded. The recommended course of action was to continue antibiotic therapy and repeat imaging at 6 weeks.

Learning point Antibiotic treatment of bacterial lung abscess

The mainstay of treatment for lung abscess is prolonged antimicrobial therapy. However, there is a lack of high-quality evidence regarding the best empirical antibiotic choice here. There should be broad-spectrum cover, including against anaerobes, although metronidazole lacks the aerobic cover also necessary and performs poorly in pulmonary infections [13]. Clindamycin has been shown superior to penicillin [14] and equivalent to ampicillin/sulbactam [15] and is accepted to be an effective treatment [16]. Combination β-lactam/β-lactamase inhibitors (e.g. co-amoxiclav) have efficacy against most isolated organisms causing lung abscesses and provide effective treatment [17]. Cephalosporins [18] and carbapenems [19] also appear to be effective in anaerobic lung infections, although there are no direct comparisons to other antibiotic classes. More recently, moxifloxacin has demonstrated similar efficacy to ampicillin/sulbactam [20] and appears to be effective as empirical therapy [21]. Other agents, including tigecycline and azithromycin, show *in vitro* anaerobic activity but lack clinical data [16].

(Continued)

Initial empirical treatment should therefore be with a combination β-lactam/β-lactamase inhibitor, carbapenem, or clindamycin, with additional cover for *S. aureus* if this is suspected clinically. Metronidazole monotherapy should be avoided, although it may have a role in combination with other broad-spectrum antibiotics. The optimum duration of antibiotic therapy is unclear, although most recommend a minimum treatment period of 3 weeks, often initially administered parenterally [22] and usually 6 weeks or longer, depending on clinical response [1].

Clinical tip Draining of lung abscess

Unlike abscess cavities elsewhere in the body, pulmonary abscesses rarely require surgical intervention. Drainage is often spontaneous via communication with the tracheobronchial tree, and the mainstay of treatment is antibiotic therapy. Where there is failure to improve, percutaneous CT-guided drainage of the abscess should be considered [10] and can avoid surgical intervention. Bronchoscopic drainage has previously been advocated but runs the risk of persistent fistula formation and seeding of infection to healthy parts of the lung. Surgical resection of the cavity is rarely necessary and usually reserved for cases where there is coexistent empyema.

On day 8 of her admission, she complained of palpitations and was noted to be tachycardic. She was examined by the ward senior house officer (SHO) who noted that she did not look markedly unwell and recorded a blood pressure of 112/72 mmHg and a heart rate of 120–130 beats/min. An ECG showed atrial fibrillation (AF) with a rapid ventricular response rate. She was given an IV bolus of 500 micrograms of digoxin, and, over the following 4 hours, her heart rate slowed to 90 beats/min, although it remained irregular. Oral digoxin was commenced and continued, with monitoring of her serum digoxin level.

Learning point Cardiac consequences in bacterial lung infections

Cardiac events, especially AF, are known to be strongly associated with acute infections and particularly pneumonia [23]. The aetiology of this is multifactorial. Pneumonia causes rapid release of pro-inflammatory cytokines, resulting in a heightened inflammatory state, which can persist after resolution of the pneumonia and is itself associated with cardiovascular events and mortality [24]. This causes increased myocardial oxygen requirements, which cannot be met due to impaired pulmonary gas exchange, hypoxia, and relative hypotension. Combined with a marked pro-thrombotic state and widespread endothelial dysfunction [25], this causes myocardial depression and microvascular infarction. As a consequence, there is an increase in myocardial infarction in the period following an episode of respiratory tract infection [26]. Other cardiac events are also common; a large cohort study of 50,119 patients (mean age 77.5) hospitalized with pneumonia in the United States (US) found a 90-day incidence of 9.5% for new arrhythmias, 10.2% for congestive cardiac failure, and 1.5% for myocardial infarction, the majority of which occurred during the initial hospitalization [27]. A smaller case series of patients with confirmed pneumococcal pneumonia [28] found that one or more cardiac events occurred in 19.4%, of patients, with AF in 4.1% and other events being mainly myocardial infarction (7.1%) and congestive heart failure (7.6%). AF is a poor prognostic marker and is associated with significantly increased mortality when it develops in medical inpatients [29]. Initial treatment should be with a rate control strategy until the infection resolves; if the arrhythmia persists, then anticoagulation and/or cardioversion may be appropriate in selected patients [23].

After a total of 2 weeks of IV piperacillin/tazobactam, the patient felt significantly better. The sputum purulence had resolved, and her C-reactive protein (CRP) had reduced to 120 mg/dL. She was therefore discharged home to complete a 6-week course of oral co-amoxiclav and to return for repeat imaging and clinic review.

Expert comment

Failure to improve in a smoker presenting with a diagnosis of lung infection should always raise the suspicion of an underlying cancer. In this case, it is difficult to know whether the tumour was causing obstruction, with distal abscess formation as a consequence, or whether a lung cancer cavity was secondarily infected and then fistulated into the bronchial tree.

At her clinic appointment, her systemic symptoms had resolved, but she remained lethargic and had significant weight loss. Repeat imaging showed persistence of the abscess cavity, with increased right hilar lymphadenopathy, and a second bronchoscopy was carried out. This confirmed a persistent cavity; biopsies from this again cultured *K. pneumoniae*, and histology this time showed a squamous cell carcinoma. Chemotherapy was not feasible due to her physical frailty (WHO performance status of 2–3) and ongoing infection. Her antibiotic treatment was continued, and appropriate ongoing palliative care organized.

She continued to lose weight and steadily declined. Two months later, she was readmitted as an emergency with worsening of her symptoms. A superimposed pneumonia was diagnosed, and, although there was an initial response to IV treatment with piperacillin/tazobactam and gentamicin, she subsequently worsened. When it became clear that this was a terminal deterioration, her antibiotics were stopped and symptomatic care prioritized; she passed away on the ward 4 months after her initial presentation.

Discussion

This case clearly demonstrates the potentially complicated course of anaerobic lung infection and the importance of being aware of potential differential diagnoses. Although the initial treatment was as for a standard bacterial CAP, with the benefit of hindsight, the history was typical for an anaerobic lung abscess with a gradual onset of pyrexia and putrid sputum production in a frail patient with a history of alcohol use.

Patients with pneumonia are prone to complications, and a failure to improve should prompt consideration of the reason. Table 3.3 shows some of the common reasons why patients may not improve with antibiotic therapy, and these will need to be treated accordingly (adapted from [1]).

Lung abscess refers to pulmonary infection causing necrosis of the lung parenchyma, with subsequent liquefaction and cavitation. Primary lung abscess is typically caused by aspiration of bacteria originating in the oral cavity [16]. Predisposing factors are therefore those leading to aspiration, especially alcohol abuse, decreased conscious level, and pre-existing dysphagia; poor oral hygiene and gum disease are often present. Lung cavitation can, however, be caused by conditions other than infection, and these may include neoplasia, vasculitis (especially Wegener's), cavitatory pulmonary infarction, cavitatory rheumatoid nodule, or other structures (localized saccular bronchiectasis, infected bullus, air–fluid level in other structures, e.g. oesophagus, stomach).

The bacteriology of lung abscess reflects the predominantly anaerobic oral flora and is often mixed flora, including *Peptostreptococcus*, *Prevotella*, *Bacteroides*, and *Fusobacterium* species [22]. Aerobic bacteria that can cause monobacterial lung abscess include *S. aureus*, Gram-negative bacilli (especially *K. pneumoniae*), and *Streptococcus milleri* (often isolated in conjunction with anaerobic bacteria and in patients with poor dental hygiene), and more rarely *Streptococcus pyogenes*, *Nocardia*, *Legionella*, and *Actinomyces*. Outbreaks of Panton-Valentine leukocidin-producing strains of *S. aureus* have been described, particularly in subjects living in conditions of close proximity, and can cause severe necrotizing pneumonia with cavitation. Mycobacteria are also important causes of lung abscess and must be considered in all cases.

Table 3.3 Potential reasons why patients may fail to improve following antibiotic therapy

Wrong diagnosis and/or complicating conditions	Pulmonary embolism/infarction Cardiac complications ± pulmonary oedema Bronchial carcinoma Bronchiectasis Pulmonary eosinophilia/eosinophilic pneumonia Cryptogenic organizing pneumonia Alveolar haemorrhage Foreign body Congenital abnormality, e.g. lobar sequestration
CAP with unusual pathogens	'Atypical' pathogens, usually penicillin-resistant 'Typical' pathogens may show unexpected resistance patterns; take local advice, and chase definitive cultures
Ineffective antibiotic therapy	Poor absorption Inadequate dose Poor compliance Hypersensitivity to antibiotics
Impaired host defences	Local, e.g. bronchiectasis, endobronchial obstruction Systemic, e.g. HIV (low threshold for testing for this)
Pulmonary complications	Parapneumonic effusion ± empyema Lung abscess Acute respiratory distress syndrome
Extrapulmonary complications	Phlebitis at cannula site and poor antibiotic delivery Metastatic infection Cardiac Septicaemia ± other organ dysfunction

P. aeruginosa, *Nocardia*, and fungi have a higher prevalence in immunocompromised hosts. Embolic infection may cause multiple lung abscesses; important specific causes are tricuspid valve endocarditis and Lemierre's syndrome (septic thrombophlebitis of the internal jugular vein, usually caused by *Fusobacterium necrophorum*). Other specific circumstances may predispose to infection with more unusual pathogens such as *Burkholderia pseudomallei*, an endemic soil contaminant that is prevalent in South East Asia but has also been associated with aspiration of saltwater [30]. Finally, as in this case, an obstructing pulmonary lesion, such as a tumour or foreign body, can be an underlying cause of lung abscess [22], and therefore follow-up imaging should always be arranged to ensure resolution. Diagnosis of an anaerobic lung abscess is hindered by the difficulty of obtaining specimens uncontaminated by oral flora. Transtracheal aspirate (as a means of bypassing the mouth) is now rarely performed, and diagnosis relies on cultures of blood and, where available, transthoracic aspirates of cavity contents and pleural fluid. Bronchoscopic access to the abscess cavity, as in this case, is unusual, and there is a risk of seeding infection to other areas of the lung. Cultures for anaerobic bacteria are very rarely informative once broad-spectrum antibiotic therapy has been given.

In conclusion, therefore, bacterial lung infection encompasses a wide range of potential pathogens and disease entities. A slow response or failure of initial therapy should always prompt reassessment and consideration of the original diagnosis, and further microbiological investigations should be organized as appropriate. Lung abscess is a complication which suggests a different aetiology to uncomplicated bacterial pneumonia, and thorough follow-up imaging is required to ensure resolution.

A final word from the expert

This unusual case of lung abscess related to an underlying bronchial carcinoma illustrates several important points about lung infection. These include: (a) the value of the history—the prolonged history and copious purulent sputum production in this patient indicating that a simple pneumonia was unlikely; (b) the necessity for early CXR if there are atypical features (especially in a smoker), even if the patient is not unwell enough to warrant immediate admission; (c) the often multiple pathogens associated with suppurative lung disease; (d) the need for invasive investigations (bronchoscopy) and cross-sectional imaging (CT scanning) for accurate evaluation of more complex cases of lung infection; and (e) the potential for lung infection to be the first presentation of an underlying lung carcinoma.

References

1. Lim WS, Baudouin SV, George RC *et al.* BTS guidelines for the management of community acquired pneumonia in adults: update 2009. *Thorax* 2009;**64**(Suppl 3):iii1–55.
2. Fine MJ, Auble TE, Yealy DM *et al.* A prediction rule to identify low-risk patients with community-acquired pneumonia. *N Engl J Med* 1997;**336**:243–50.
3. Lim WS, van der Eerden MM, Laing R *et al.* Defining community acquired pneumonia severity on presentation to hospital: an international derivation and validation study. *Thorax* 2003;**58**:377–82.
4. Cilloniz C, Ewig S, Polverino E *et al.* Microbial aetiology of community-acquired pneumonia and its relation to severity. *Thorax* 2011;**66**:340–6.
5. Kollef MH, Shorr A, Tabak YP, Gupta V, Liu LZ, Johannes RS. Epidemiology and outcomes of health-care-associated pneumonia: results from a large US database of culture-positive pneumonia. *Chest* 2005;**128**:3854–62.
6. American Thoracic Society; Infectious Diseases Society of America. Guidelines for the management of adults with hospital-acquired, ventilator-associated, and healthcare-associated pneumonia. *Am J Respir Crit Care Med* 2005;**171**:388–416.
7. Masterton RG, Galloway A, French G *et al.* Guidelines for the management of hospital-acquired pneumonia in the UK: report of the working party on hospital-acquired pneumonia of the British Society for Antimicrobial Chemotherapy. *J Antimicrob Chemother* 2008;**62**:5–34.
8. Ewig S, Welte T, Torres A. Is healthcare-associated pneumonia a distinct entity needing specific therapy? *Curr Opin Infect Dis* 2012;**25**:166–75.
9. Schuetz P, Christ-Crain M, Thomann R *et al.* Effect of procalcitonin-based guidelines vs standard guidelines on antibiotic use in lower respiratory tract infections: the ProHOSP randomized controlled trial. *JAMA* 2009;**302**:1059–66.
10. Yu H. Management of pleural effusion, empyema, and lung abscess. *Semin Intervent Radiol* 2011;**28**:75–86.
11. Chen HJ, Yu YH, Tu CY *et al.* Ultrasound in peripheral pulmonary air-fluid lesions. Color Doppler imaging as an aid in differentiating empyema and abscess. *Chest* 2009;**135**:1426–32.
12. Lin FC, Chou CW, Chang SC. Differentiating pyopneumothorax and peripheral lung abscess: chest ultrasonography. *Am J Med Sci* 2004;**327**:330–5.
13. Perlino CA. Metronidazole vs clindamycin treatment of anerobic pulmonary infection. Failure of metronidazole therapy. *Arch Intern Med* 1981;**141**:1424–7.
14. Gudiol F, Manresa F, Pallares R *et al.* Clindamycin vs penicillin for anaerobic lung infections. High rate of penicillin failures associated with penicillin-resistant Bacteroides melaninogenicus. *Arch Intern Med* 1990;**150**:2525–9.

15. Allewelt M, Schüler P, Bölcskei PL *et al.* Ampicillin + sulbactam vs clindamycin +/- cephalosporin for the treatment of aspiration pneumonia and primary lung abscess. *Clin Microbiol Infect* 2004;**10**:163–70.
16. Bartlett JG. Anaerobic bacterial infection of the lung. *Anaerobe* 2012;**18**:235–9.
17. Fernandez-Sabe N, Carratalà J, Dorca J *et al.* Efficacy and safety of sequential amoxicillin-clavulanate in the treatment of anaerobic lung infections. *Eur J Clin Microbiol Infect Dis* 2003;**22**:185–7.
18. Wang JL, Chen KY, Fang CT, Hsueh PR, Yang PC, Chang SC. Changing bacteriology of adult community-acquired lung abscess in Taiwan: Klebsiella pneumoniae versus anaerobes. *Clin Infect Dis* 2005;**40**:915–22.
19. Tokuyasu H, Harada T, Watanabe E *et al.* Effectiveness of meropenem for the treatment of aspiration pneumonia in elderly patients. *Intern Med* 2009;**48**:129–35.
20. Ott SR, Allewelt M, Lorenz J *et al.* Moxifloxacin vs ampicillin/sulbactam in aspiration pneumonia and primary lung abscess. *Infection* 2008;**36**:23–30.
21. Polenakovik H, Burdette SD, Polenakovik S. Moxifloxacin is efficacious for treatment of community-acquired lung abscesses in adults. *Clin Infect Dis* 2005;**41**:764–5.
22. Yazbeck MF, Dahdel M, Kalra A, Browne AS, Pratter MR. Lung abscess: update on microbiology and management. *Am J Ther* 2014;**21**:217–21.
23. National Institute for Health and Care Excellence (2014). *Atrial fibrillation: management.* NICE guidelines CG180. Available at: <https://www.nice.org.uk/guidance/cg180?unl id=81235962120166782425>
24. Yende S, D'Angelo G, Kellum JA *et al.* Inflammatory markers at hospital discharge predict subsequent mortality after pneumonia and sepsis. *Am J Respir Crit Care Med* 2008;**177**:1242–7.
25. Singanayagam A, Elder DH, Chalmers JD. Is community-acquired pneumonia an independent risk factor for cardiovascular disease? *Eur Respir J* 2012;**39**:187–96.
26. Smeeth L, Thomas SL, Hall AJ, Hubbard R, Farrington P, Vallance P. Risk of myocardial infarction and stroke after acute infection or vaccination. *N Engl J Med* 2004;**351**:2611–18.
27. Perry TW, Pugh MJ, Waterer GW *et al.* Incidence of cardiovascular events after hospital admission for pneumonia. *Am J Med* 2011;**124**:244–51.
28. Musher DM, Rueda AM, Kaka AS, Mapara SM. The association between pneumococcal pneumonia and acute cardiac events. *Clin Infect Dis* 2007;**45**:158–65.
29. Chen SX, Amir KA, Bobba RK, Arsura EL. New onset atrial fibrillation developing in medical inpatients. *Am J Med Sci* 2009;**337**:169–72.
30. Kongsaengdao S, Bunnag S, Siriwiwattnakul N. Treatment of survivors after the tsunami. *N Engl J Med* 2005;**352**:2654–5.

Non-surgical management of early-stage lung cancer

Jim Brown

Expert commentary Neal Navani

Case history

A 76-year-old lifelong smoker was monitored in the chest clinic for 2 years, having been referred when a cardiac magnetic resonance imaging (MRI) scan picked up an incidental 7-mm lung nodule. He has severe chronic obstructive pulmonary disease (COPD), with an FEV_1 of 1.2 (35% predicted, GOLD stage III), a transfer factor of the lung for carbon monoxide (TLCO) of 45%, and an exercise tolerance of 2–300 m, and suffers from frequent exacerbations. His co-morbid conditions include hypertension, ischaemic heart disease, and moderate aortic stenosis. Interval cross-sectional imaging initially showed a 7-mm nodule that was static over 2 years but, over the last 6 months, had rapidly increased in size to 19 mm. In addition, there was a corresponding change in morphology from original ground glass opacity (GGO) to something more solid in appearance. A positron emission tomography (PET)-CT scan was performed and demonstrated [18F]-fluorodeoxyglucose (FDG) avidity with a maximum standardized uptake value (SUVmax) of 3, but no distant disease.

A clinical diagnosis of lung cancer was made (stage T1aN0M0), and treatment options were discussed with the patient. The multidisciplinary team felt that a surgical resection would offer the best chance of cure; however, his fitness was a concern, as surgery would require a lobectomy or segmentectomy. The patient was keen to have definitive treatment but was uncertain about undergoing surgery, given his other medical problems. However, he agreed to proceed to preoperative consultation and assessment with the surgical and anaesthetic teams for further discussion.

At initial consultation in thoracic surgical outpatients, it was estimated that his post-operative FEV_1 may fall to below 30% predicted; he proceeded to have a myocardial perfusion scan which showed mild to moderate inducible ischaemia, and cardiopulmonary exercise testing (CPET) revealed a VO_2 max of 12 mL/kg/min.

When assessing surgical risk, the patient's age, baseline function, and co-morbidities must all be evaluated. Simple spirometry and crude assessment of physiological function can be carried out in clinic (6-minute walk test/stair assessment) and prompt further assessment of fitness. A baseline or predicted post-operative FEV_1 or TLCO <40% of the reference range or an inability to cover 400 m in 6 min should be followed by CPET, with a score of <15 mL/kg/min reflecting high risk. Other co-morbidities, in particular uncontrolled ischaemic heart disease, should be investigated preoperatively [1, 2].

Following a comprehensive preoperative assessment, the multidisciplinary team (MDT) felt he was at moderate to high risk of perioperative mortality or post-operative

Clinical tip Assessment of fitness for surgery

Features suggesting high surgical risk include:

- poor lung function (FEV_1 and/or TLCO <40% predicted);
- respiratory failure;
- age >70 years;
- poor exercise tolerance (6-minute walk test <400 m, VO_2 max <15 mL/kg/min, unable to climb two flights of stairs);
- cardiac disease.

Learning point BTS guidelines for assessing surgical risk

- Risk of perioperative death using a dedicated algorithm (e.g. THORACOSCORE).
- Risk of a peri-/post-operative cardiac event (American College of Cardiology/American Heart Association risk stratification).
- Risk of post-operative dyspnoea (dynamic lung function).

Once the assessment has been completed and modifiable factors adjusted, the patient and surgeon must agree that the risk and future impact on the quality of life are acceptable [3].

Learning point Criteria for radical radiotherapy

- All patients with early-stage non-small cell lung cancer who have an unacceptable surgical risk should be offered radical radiotherapy.
- Lung function of >40% predicted FEV_1 or TLCO.
- Lesion peripheral or located away from mediastinal structures.
- Lesion must be distant to any previous site of radical radiotherapy.

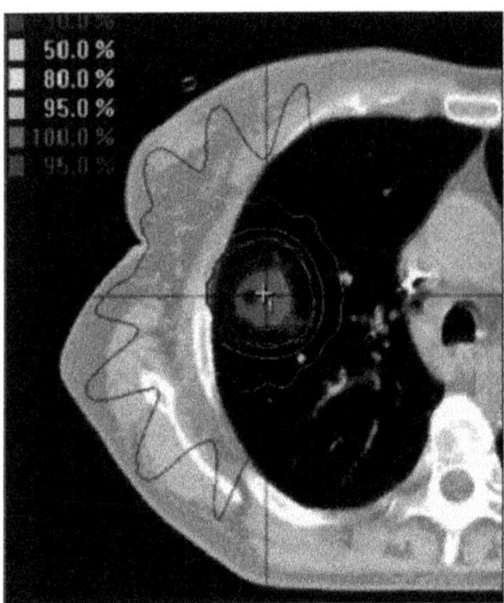

Figure 4.1 A typical SBRT field showing the zone of intensity of radiation delivered.

symptoms that would negatively affect his quality of life. In agreement with the patient, a decision was made to proceed with non-surgical management of his lung cancer. Due to his poor lung function, he was not a suitable candidate for radical radiotherapy, and so he was referred for consideration of stereotactic body radiotherapy (SBRT).

He underwent planning for SBRT (Figure 4.1) and proceeded to have 60 Gy over three fractions, with a good response. He suffered from minimal side effects and maintained a good performance status and quality of life. His lesion has remained stable over a 2-year follow-up period.

Discussion

This case highlights a common scenario in respiratory medicine; with an ageing population and the increasing use of cross-sectional imaging, solitary pulmonary nodules (SPNs) (defined as <3 cm and surrounded by lung parenchyma) are detected with increasing frequency and may require several years of follow-up in people with risk factors for lung cancer. The earlier lung cancer can be detected and treated, the better the prospect for cure, and surgery remains the gold standard treatment. However, up to 25% of patients with stage 1 disease may be ineligible on the grounds of severe co-morbidities [4].

There has been a push towards the screening of high-risk smokers with annual low-dose CT (LDCT) scans, since the National Lung Screening Trial (NLST) results were published in 2011 and showed a 20% reduction in lung cancer-specific mortality in the group undergoing CT surveillance [5]. In the NLST, being physiologically robust enough to withstand lung cancer surgery, if required, was one of the entry criteria for the study. However, in clinical practice, many patients who are kept under surveillance for SPN have other comorbidities associated with tobacco smoke exposure, including ischaemic heart disease and COPD, and may not be fit for surgery. Frequently, the lung cancer MDT must now consider the benefits of non-surgical alternatives for the treatment of early peripheral lung cancers.

Evidence base The National Lung Screening Trial (NLST)

This was the first randomized lung cancer screening study to show a mortality benefit and led to LDCT screening being recommended in North America for the same demographic included in the trial (ASCO 2012). The major features of the trial are listed below.

- Inclusion criteria:
  - 55–74 years;
  - >30 pack years;
  - current smoker or gave up within 15 years;
  - fit enough to have radical treatment;
  - three rounds of annual LDCT versus CXR follow-up.
- Results:
  - a total of 53,454 recruited;
  - 20% reduction in lung cancer-specific mortality with CT screening;
  - screen positivity in 24.2% with LDCT (96.4% false positive) and 6.9% with CXR (94.5% false positive).

Studies of the natural history of early-stage lung cancers in patients who have been untreated due to preference or comorbidities (medically inoperable) show that those with stage 1 tumours remain very likely to die from their disease, with a 5-year lung cancer-specific survival of only 16% and a median survival of 13 months. Adopting a wait-and-see approach will therefore be inappropriate for almost all patients. As local control is important prognostically for early-stage disease, it is imperative that treatment options be as inclusive as possible and those that are unable or unwilling to have surgery be offered alternative ablative therapies [6].

Surgical options

Current guidelines recommend lobectomy with lymph node sampling or en bloc dissection for the treatment of lung cancer; however, lung-sparing surgery (sublobectomy—wedge resection or anatomical segmentectomy) may be employed to preserve lung function in those less fit or if the lesion is small and peripheral [3]. The characteristics of the cancer on cross-sectional imaging also play a role; enlarging solid nodules are more suggestive of invasive cancer than opacities with a ground glass appearance (GGO) which are more likely to represent adenocarcinoma *in situ*, which has a lepidic pattern of growth (along intact alveolar septa) with no or minimal invasion. There is continuing controversy regarding the efficacy of lobectomy versus sublobectomy; a recent meta-analysis suggests that survival may be lower overall in the sublobectomy group; however, when considering lesions of ≤2 cm, there was no difference between lobectomy and anatomical segmentectomy [7]. Video-assisted thoracoscopic surgery (VATS) is often employed as a minimally invasive technique, compared to standard thoracotomy, and may be associated with lower morbidity and length of stay [8], but there is a current debate about the benefits of VATS, compared to conventional lobectomy. The VIOLET study has just started recruiting to compare the effectiveness of VATS to lobectomy on clinical outcomes and patient experience which will likely settle this. Lung cancer-specific 5-year survival was evaluated retrospectively by Okada *et al.* [9] in 1272 patients which showed that tumour size influenced outcome, with survival for pathological stage 1 tumours of ≤10 mm being 100% reducing to 56% for cancers of >30 mm, along with the choice of operation. Surgery remains the standard against which other minimally invasive and ablative interventions are measured.

Learning point Factors favouring long-term survival with lung-sparing surgery

- Lesion ≤2 cm.
- Peripheral location.
- Ground glass appearance.

Effect of cancer size and operative choice on 5-year cancer-specific survival in patients with pathological stage 1 disease is shown below:

	Lobectomy	Segmentectomy	Wedge resection
<20 mm	92.4%	96.7%	87.7%
21–30 mm	87.4%	84.6%	39.4%

The morbidity and mortality associated with surgery increase with age and comorbidities; more than two-thirds of operative procedures are carried out on patients over the age of 70. Damhuis *et al.* have evaluated the factors affecting outcome and shown that overall post-operative mortality in patients >80 years of age is 9.4% from a baseline of 1.7% in the under 60s [10]. Minimally invasive techniques and lung-sparing options may help to reduce morbidity but must be balanced against the likelihood of disease recurrence. If the risk is felt to outweigh the benefit, then other options should be explored.

Radiotherapy with curative intent

Radical radiotherapy has traditionally been the standard of care for patients with early-stage peripheral lung cancers who are inoperable on medical grounds or unwilling to have surgery. The regimen of choice is continuous hyperfractionated accelerated radiotherapy (CHART) where 56 Gy is delivered in 36 fractions over 12 consecutive days (three treatments per day). However, it is not universally available, and conventional radiation treatment is often substituted where approximately 60 Gy is delivered over a period of 6 weeks in 20–30 fractions. CHART offers prolonged survival, compared to conventional radiotherapy, with a 22% reduction in relative risk of death [11]. However, 5-year cancer-specific survival remains poor at 13–39% [12]. The commonest cause of relapse is local recurrence reported in up to 70% of patients, with 25% developing systemic metastases.

In the largest study of its kind to date, Smith *et al.* studied the patterns of treatment and survival in 1043 patients with early-stage lung cancer deemed medically inoperable (1996–2005). Only a third received radiotherapy with curative intent, with the remainder receiving palliative radiation or no treatment. The radically treated group had less comorbidities than the other groups, and cancer-specific 5-year survival was 20%, compared to 6% in both the palliative and no treatment groups. It was recognized that some patients were evaluated in the pre-PET era and may have been understaged by current standards [13].

Relapse rates increase with increasing size of the lesion, and higher total radiation dose is associated with prolonged progression-free survival [14]. Although patients may be inoperable on medical grounds, it is worth considering that only a minority of patients can be cured with conventional/radical radiotherapy when making treatment decisions, and any possibility of surgical excision should be explored.

Stereotactic body radiotherapy

The main cause of treatment failure with conventional radiotherapy is lack of durable local disease control which is proportional to the amount of radiotherapy delivered to the site of the tumour [12]. Patients who are considered unfit for surgery may also be turned down for radical radiotherapy on the basis of poor lung function due to the effect on neighbouring lung tissue. Therefore, techniques, such as SBRT, have been developed to enable highly targeted radiotherapy that is more efficacious, while also minimizing toxicity to local structures.

Clinical tip Selection of appropriate patients/lesions for SBRT

- Histological or clinical diagnosis of primary lung cancer.
- T1-3 (<5 cm) N0M0.
- Not suitable for surgery.
- WHO performance status 0–2.
- Peripheral lesion (>2 cm from the main bronchus).

SBRT involves the accurate delivery of multiple highly focussed non-coplanar radiation beams to a specific anatomical area, enabling a more potent dose per fraction with a steep dose gradient and low doses delivered to surrounding tissues. It is hypofractionated, meaning that a higher total treatment dose of tumour-specific radiation can be achieved in a shorter time (typically 60 Gy over 3–5 fractions), compared to radical/conventional radiotherapy (50–66 Gy over 20–33 fractions). Because of the intensity of the treatment, patient-specific highly conformal planning is required, including four-dimensional/cone beam CT (4DCT/CBCT) and gating for respiratory and tumour motion to minimize toxicity to off-target structures. This makes it an ideal choice for treating early peripheral lung cancers; however, caution is required when considering treatment of lesions that are either central or close to the spinal cord.

Current national guidelines do not include SBRT as a recommended treatment option for early lung cancers due to the lack of level 1 evidence from large, well-conducted randomized controlled trials (RCTs). There are a large number of published series predominantly from single institutions suggesting that SBRT is a safe and effective treatment for early lung cancers in the medically inoperable. Local disease control and overall survival at 3 years have been reported as 80–98% and 50–70%, respectively although up to a third may develop distant metastases [15]. Its efficacy for early disease, compared to surgery, is currently being investigated. A key benefit is the ability to treat patients whose poor lung function would have precluded radical radiotherapy and essentially left the patient at the mercy of the disease. Palma *et al.* have shown that patients with severe COPD (GOLD stages III–IV) have 1- and 3-year survival comparable to that in patients with matched lung function that undergo surgery [16]. The same group have also shown that the introduction of SBRT leads to a 16% increased use of radiotherapy in elderly patients with stage 1 lung cancer and an associated improvement in survival [17].

Deterioration in quality of life following surgery is a concern, given the loss of respiratory function and pain, particularly following thoracotomy. Handy *et al.* showed a significant reduction in quality of life 6 months after surgery [18] due to pain and loss of functional health status, although other papers have challenged this and shown no such effect [19]. It is suggested morbidity may be minimized with sublobar resection and a VATS approach. A study by Lagerwaard *et al.* demonstrated no impact on quality of life following SBRT, and lung function, including the diffusing capacity of the lungs for carbon monoxide (DLCO), is preserved following treatment, meaning even those with the poorest lung function can receive potentially curative treatment [20].

Evidence base Ongoing RCTs evaluating SBRT versus surgery

- JCOG 0403—results not yet reported.
- RTOG 0618—results not yet reported.
- STARS—closed early due to poor accrual.
- ACOSOG Z4099/Radiation Therapy Oncology Group (RTOG) 1021 study—closed early due to poor accrual.
- SABRTOOTH—due to start recruiting.

SBRT appears well tolerated, and toxicity is usually mild and self-limiting. In a prospective cohort of 245 patients, the development of toxicity of grade 2 or higher (National Cancer Institute Common Toxicity Criteria) for pneumonitis, oesophagitis, and dermatitis was 6.5%, 2%, and 1.2%, respectively, with a 0.8% incidence of rib fracture [21]. The location of the cancer is important, with higher toxicity reported for central tumours [22].

Radiofrequency ablation

This technique involves the insertion of a needle electrode percutaneously into the target lesion under CT image guidance, using local anaesthetic and conscious sedation; radiofrequency energy is then applied to heat the tip to cauterize the lesion with thermal injury, leading to coagulation and necrosis, including a surrounding cuff of normal tissue to ensure a clear margin and prevent local recurrence. It can be administered in single or multiple sessions and does not preclude the use of any other modality of treatment.

Radiofrequency ablation (RFA) has its strongest evidence base for the treatment of hepatic lesions but is increasingly used for the ablation of both primary and secondary tumours of the lung; in 2010, NICE issued an interventional procedure guidance document regarding RFA that confirmed efficacy for both indications [23]. Patient selection is important, as they must be physiologically robust enough to withstand a pneumothorax, a risk that increases if the needle tract traverses emphysematous lung. There are also areas that are anatomically difficult to access with RFA, including the lung apices and areas close to the diaphragm or behind the scapulae [24]; however, procedural success rates in experienced hands have been reported as up to 99% [25]. There has been an increasing number of published series in the literature examining the rate of local disease control and lung cancer-specific survival following RFA; however, few of the cohorts are mature enough yet to report 5-year survival figures. In a review of 17 recent publications, de Baere reported a median complete ablation rate of 90% (range 38–97%); the success is greater for tumours of <2 cm (78–96%) and reducing to 38% for lesion of >5 cm, suggesting tumour volume is key in determining outcome of local disease control. The median survival is reported as 29 months, with 3- and 5-year survival of 57% and 27%, respectively; however, the median survival for tumours of <3 cm is 50% [26]. These figures are similar to those from other publications [27].

Because it is an interventional procedure, the main concern is the associated mortality and morbidity, but there does not appear to be any sustained impact on lung function following RFA [28]. The causes of morbidity are pneumothorax which occurs in one-third of patients, with 4–16% requiring chest tube insertion, minor haemoptysis in 15%, and a major haemorrhage rate (haemothorax or haemoptysis) of around 2%. Alexander *et al.* have retrospectively reported a 13.5% radiological incidence of rib fracture following RFA in 163 patients; it was commoner if the ablation zone was close to the chest wall. However, only 9.1% were symptomatic, and no organ injury resulted [29]. A procedural mortality of up to 2.6% has been reported but predominantly in patients with a single lung [30].

The benefit of RFA is effective local disease control in the short term following a single treatment, and it is much more efficacious for smaller lesions, making patient selection vital. There is a significant risk of morbidity that must be balanced with potential benefits and also when considering this option, compared to other treatment modalities.

Conclusions

The options for patients with enlarging SPNs and borderline fitness for surgical intervention are increasing with thoracoscopic, lung-preserving surgical techniques and newer ablative therapies that have an expanding evidence base. It seems certain that there will be a solid evidence base for SBRT in the short to medium term. Whether SBRT may replace surgery in the management of early small parenchymal lung cancers is yet to be determined. RFA offers substantial benefit over conventional radiotherapy, with durable local control rates from a single treatment, and remains an alternative to wedge resection or SBRT. However, concern remains over the side effect profile, and further randomized data are required to determine its role in the treatment of early lung cancers. RFA is considerably less costly, and therefore health economic analysis of each intervention is required.

A final word from the expert

The management of patients with early-stage lung cancer is increasingly a key component of lung cancer MDT meetings. The promise of CT screening together with the increased use of CT imaging in secondary care has meant that more patients with early lung cancer are being detected. Surgery remains that best chance of cure in these patients and offers several clear advantages over non-surgical techniques. Not only does surgery provide a histological diagnosis, but it also allows for pathological nodal staging which may direct further adjuvant systemic therapy. In view of this, comorbidities in patients with early-stage lung cancer should be optimized as early as possible in the patient pathway. This often involves improving lung function and exercise capacity, and the role of 'pre-hab', i.e. preoperative pulmonary rehabilitation, is currently under investigation. The risks from surgery in patients with early-stage lung cancer should always be discussed and can be stratified into perioperative risk and longer-term post-operative comorbidities, particularly breathlessness. In some patients, sublobar resection offers a useful alternative to lobectomy, and trials are ongoing to establish the oncological outcomes from this approach.

Despite these considerations, surgery is often not possible or preferred by the patient. In these cases, the advent of non-surgical techniques for the management of early-stage disease represents a real advance for patients with lung cancer. Currently, SABR is preferred to RFA, in view of better efficacy and safety data. SABR can be employed in most patients, even in the context of severely impaired lung function, as long as the patient can lie flat and the tumour is located >2 cm from the main bronchi. An important consideration for the MDT when offering SABR or RFA is the hilar and mediastinal nodal staging. Since these techniques treat only the primary tumour, they do not offer pathological nodal staging and should not be undertaken when lymph nodes are involved. Recent data suggest that most recurrences after SABR occur in draining lymph nodes, and I would advocate nodal staging by PET-CT and endobronchial ultrasound prior to SABR or RFA.

The management of patients with early-stage lung cancer is increasingly complex. It is therefore critical that the respiratory physician, radiologist, thoracic surgeon, and clinical oncologist work together in MDT meetings to offer patients with early-stage lung cancer the best treatment options.

References

1. Brunelli A, Charloux A, Bolliger CT *et al.* ERS/ESTS clinical guidelines on fitness for radical therapy in lung cancer patients. *Eur Respir J* 2009;**34**:17–41.
2. Colice GL, Shafazand S, Griffin JP *et al.* Physiological evaluation of the patient with lung cancer being considered for resectional surgery: ACCP evidence-based clinical practice guidelines (2nd edition). *Chest* 2007;**132**:161–77.

3. Lim E, Baldwin D, Beckles M *et al*. Guidelines on the radical management of patients with lung cancer. *Thorax* 2010;**65** Suppl 3:iii1–27.
4. Donington JFerguson M, Mazzone P *et al*. American College of Chest Physicians and Society of Thoracic Surgeons consensus statement for the evaluation and management for high risk patients with stage I non-small-cell lung cancer. *Chest* 2012;**142**:1620–35.
5. National Lung Screening Trial Research Team. Reduced lung-cancer mortality with low-dose computed tomographic screening. *N Engl J Med* 2011;**365**:395–409.
6. Raz DJ, Zell JA, Ou SH *et al*. Natural history of stage 1 non-small cell lung cancer: implications for early detection. *Chest* 2007;**132**:193–9.
7. Fan J, Wang L, Jiang GN *et al*. Sublobectomy versus lobectomy for stage I non-small-cell lung cancer, a meta-analysis of published studies. *Ann Surg Oncol* 2012;**19**:661–8.
8. Paul S, Alkorki, Sheng S *et al*. Thoracoscopic lobectomy is associated with lower morbidity than open lobectomy: a propensity-matched analysis from the STS database. *J Thorac Cardiovasc Surg* 2010;**139**:366–78.
9. Okada M, Nisho W, Sakamoto T *et al*. Effect of tumor size on prognosis in patients with non-small cell lung cancer: the role of segmentectomy as a type of lesser resection. *J Thorac Cardiovasc Surg* 2005;**129**:87–93.
10. Damhuis R, Coonar A, Plaisier P *et al*. A case-mix model for monitoring of postoperative mortality after surgery for lung cancer. *Lung Cancer* 2006;**51**:123–9.
11. Saunders M, Dische S, Barrett A *et al*. Continuous, hyper-fractionated, accelerated radiotherapy (CHART) versus conventional radiotherapy in non-small cell lung cancer: mature data from the randomised multicentre trial. CHART steering Committee. *Radiother Oncol* 1999;**52**:137–48.
12. Rowell NP, Williams C. Radical radiotherapy for stage I/II non-small cell lung cancer in patients not sufficiently fit for or declining surgery (medically inoperable). *Thorax* 2001;**56**:628–38.
13. Smith SL, Palma D, Parhar *et al*. Inoperable early stage non-small cell lung cancer: comorbidity, patterns of care and survival. *Lung Cancer* 2011;**72**:39–44.
14. Qiao X, Tullgren O, Lax I *et al*. The role of radiotherapy in treatment of stage I non-small cell lung cancer. *Lung Cancer* 2003;**41**:1–11.
15. McCloskey P, Balduyck B, Van Shil PE *et al*. Radical treatment of non-small cell lung cancer during the last 5 years. *Eur J Cancer* 2013;**49**:1555–64.
16. Palma D, Lagerwaard F, Rodrigues G *et al*. Curative treatment of stage I non-small-cell lung cancer in patients with severe COPD: stereotactic radiotherapy outcomes and systematic review. *Int J Radiat Oncol Biol Phys* 2012;**82**:1149–56.
17. Palma D, Visser O, Lagerwaard FJ *et al*. Impact of introducing stereotactic lung radiotherapy for elderly patients with stage I non-small-cell lung cancer: a population-based time-trend analysis. *J Clin Oncol* 2012;**28**:5153–9.
18. Handy JR Jr, Asaph JW, Skokan L *et al*. What happens to patients undergoing lung cancer surgery? Outcomes and quality of life before and after surgery. *Chest* 2002;**122**:21–30.
19. Brunelli A, Socci L, Refai M *et al*. Quality of life before and after major lung resection for lung cancer: a prospective follow-up analysis. *Ann Thorac Surg* 2007;**84**:410–16.
20. Ohashi T, Takeda A, Shigematsu N *et al*. Differences in pulmonary function before vs. 1 year after hypofractionated stereotactic radiotherapy for small peripheral lung tumours. *Int J Radiot Oncol Biol Phys* 2005;**62**:1003–8.
21. Onishi H, Araki T, Shirato H *et al*. Stereotactic hypofractionated high-dose irradiation for stage I nonsmall cell lung carcinoma: clinical outcomes in 245 subjects in a Japanese multiinstitutional study. *Cancer* 2004;**101**:1623–31.
22. Timmerman R, McGarry R, Yiannoutsos C *et al*. Excessive toxicity when treating central tumours in a phase II study of stereotactic body radiation therapy for medically inoperable early-stage lung cancer. *J Clin Oncol* 2006;**24**:4833–9.

23. National Institute for Health and Care Excellence (2010). *Percutaneous radiofrequency ablation for primary or secondary lung cancers*. NICE interventional procedure guidance IPG372. Available at: <https://www.nice.org.uk/guidance/ipg372>.
24. Iguchi T, Hiraki T, Gobera H *et al*. Percutaneous radiofrequency ablation of lung tumours close to the heart or aorta: evaluation of the safety and effectiveness. *J Vasc Interv Radiol* 2007;**18**:733–40.
25. Lenconi R, Crocetti L, Cioni R *et al*. Response to radiofrequency ablation of pulmonary tumours: a prospective, intention-to-treat, multicentre clinical trial (the RAPTURE study). *Lancet Oncol* 2008;**9**:621–8.
26. De Baere T. Lung tumour radiofrequency ablation: where do we stand? *Cardiovasc Intervent Radiol* 2011;**34**:241–51.
27. Lanuti M, Sharma A, Willers H *et al*. Radiofrequency ablation for stage I non-small lung cancer: management of locoregional recurrence. *Ann Thorac Surg* 2012;**93**:921–8.
28. De Baere T, Palussiere J, Auperin A *et al*. Midterm local efficacy and survival after radiofrequency ablation of lung tumours with minimum follow-up of 1 year: prospective evaluation. *Radiology* 2006;**240**:587–96.
29. Alexander ES, Hankins CA, Machan JT *et al*. Rib fractures after percutaneous and microwave ablation of lung tumours: incidence and relevance. *Radiology* 2013;**266**:971–8.
30. Simon CJ, Dupuy DE, Dipetrillo TA *et al*. Pulmonary radiofrequency ablation: long-term safety and efficacy in 152 patients. *Radiology* 2007;**243**:268–75.

5 Central sleep apnoea

Marcus Pittman

Expert commentary Adrian Williams

Case history

A 72-year-old gentleman was referred to the sleep disorders clinic, having presented to his GP with a 6-month history of regular waking, unrefreshing sleep, and excessive daytime sleepiness. On closer questioning of him and his wife, they reported episodes of him waking, often associated with palpitations, and brief periods overnight when he appeared not to be breathing, during which she often felt the need to wake him to start him breathing again. He had been experiencing nocturia regularly for some years, although he had put this down to his age. He had also noticed some breathlessness on exertion, although he was able to walk an unrestricted distance on the flat.

There was a past medical history of hypertension and recently diagnosed type 2 diabetes mellitus (diet-controlled at this stage). He was taking bendroflumethiazide (2.5 mg od) and simvastatin (20 mg at night). He was an ex-smoker, having given up 30 years ago, and drank around 20 units of alcohol per week. The patient drove a car and had not had any problems or near misses relating to sleepiness while driving. He generally only drove short distances. He was a retired civil servant.

On examination in the clinic, he was obese with a body mass index (BMI) of 31. He was comfortable at rest. Pulse was 76 beats/minute with a regular rhythm; blood pressure was 152/86 mmHg; heart sounds were dual with no murmur, and auscultation of the lung fields revealed a few bibasal coarse inspiratory crackles. Minimal peripheral oedema was noted.

Epworth sleepiness scale (ESS) was completed to help quantify his daytime sleepiness, and he scored 17/24 (normal <11). Sleep apnoea was suspected, so overnight home oximetry (Figure 5.1) was performed, revealing a mean saturation of 90.5% and a 4% desaturation index of 67/hour. The oxygen trace appeared sinusoidal with desaturations of regular amplitude.

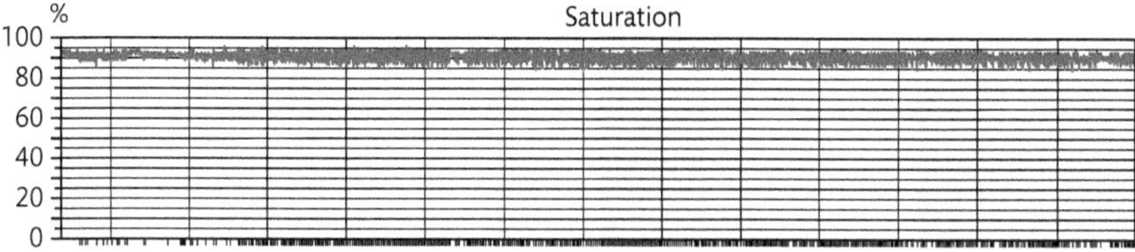

Figure 5.1 Overnight single-channel oximetry.

Expert comment

Although home oximetry alone cannot be used to rule out sleep apnoea, there is a second channel, i.e. pulse rate, which may show increased pulse rate variability consistent with arousals. In experienced hands, home oximetry can be used to determine if desaturations are due to central or obstructive apnoeas.

Clinical tip Driving and central sleep apnoea

Patients have a legal duty to inform the DVLA of any medical condition which can cause daytime sleepiness. If they fail to do this, they can be fined up to £1000, invalidate their insurance, and, if involved in an accident, be prosecuted. Driving can resume when satisfactory control of symptoms has been attained. Group 2 licence holders (those entitled to drive heavy goods vehicles) require an annual review to confirm ongoing compliance with treatment and that symptoms are controlled.

Learning point

Home oximetry is sometimes used as an easy-to-perform screening test to investigate the possibility of sleep apnoea. However, a false-negative rate of up to a third of patients has been demonstrated [1], and therefore oximetry alone cannot be used to rule out sleep apnoea and is not reliably able to determine if desaturations are due to central or obstructive apnoeas. Continuous positive airway pressure (CPAP) machines in diagnostic mode have also been used to diagnose sleep apnoea. However, they also have significant false-negative rates [2]. The American Academy of Sleep Medicine (AASM) recommends the use of full polysomnography (PSG) for the diagnosis of sleep apnoea [3]. However, encouraging results have been found using home portable monitoring equipment for the diagnosis of obstructive sleep apnoea, with a high degree of agreement with full PSG [4]. The AASM does not currently recommend the use of home monitoring equipment for the diagnosis of central sleep apnoea [3]. However, they are often used in the UK. Full PSG has the advantage of being able to determine if central apnoeas are associated with arousals from sleep and also to diagnose other primary sleep disorders, such as periodic limb movements of sleep, which may coexist.

A respiratory sleep study was performed, using portable equipment in the patient's home, to determine the nature of the desaturations. The study demonstrated predominantly central apnoeas and hypopnoeas, with an apnoea–hypopnoea index (AHI) of 75 events/hour of total time in bed, diagnostic of severe central sleep apnoea (CSA) in a pattern consistent with Cheyne–Stokes respiration (CSR) (Figure 5.2). The diagnosis was explained to the patient, and, as there was associated sleepiness, it was explained that he had a legal duty to inform the Driver and Vehicle Licensing Agency (DVLA) and that he would need to cease driving until he had started treatment and his symptoms were controlled.

Outpatient echocardiography, 24-hour ECG monitoring, and routine bloods, including urea and electrolytes, were performed. The patient was found to have systolic and diastolic left ventricular dysfunction, with an ejection fraction of 40%; mild mitral regurgitation was also noted. The 24-hour ECG showed periods of self-terminating AF with a rapid ventricular response. The routine blood tests were unremarkable, with no suggestion of renal failure. The patient was commenced on an

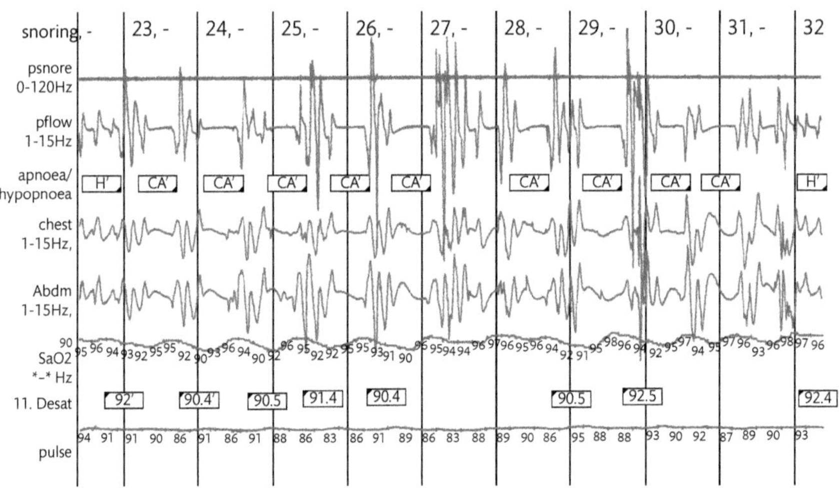

Figure 5.2 Respiratory sleep study showing central events.

angiotensin-converting enzyme inhibitor (ramipril 2.5 mg daily, with advice to the GP to consider titrating the dose and/or adding in a beta-blocker).

Learning point

CSA has a number of underlying physiological mechanisms, including hypoxia (for any reason) and raised left atrial pressure due to left ventricular failure or AF. Diurnal ventilation is increased, so that carbon dioxide (CO_2) is lowered below the apnoeic threshold during sleep. An apnoea results, during which the CO_2 rises again, eventually resulting in increased respiration. The apnoeic threshold changes with sleep stage. Cheyne–Stokes respiration is a form of CSA, with a regular pattern of waxing and waning ventilation, often ending in an apnoea. CSA is often associated with other medical conditions, including renal disease [5], diabetes [6], cardiac failure [7], and AF [8]. CSA is also commonly seen in patients using opioids [9]. Treatment of co-morbidities may improve associated CSA. For example, patients with end-stage renal disease commencing nocturnal haemodialysis have been demonstrated to have an improvement in central apnoeas [10]. Those with cardiac failure have shown improvement after optimization of their medication [11] or even treatment of associated anaemia [12].

The patient was admitted to the specialist ventilation unit to commence CPAP treatment. He was fitted with a nasal mask and started at a pressure of 5 cmH_2O. This was titrated up through the night, based on the oximetry trace and breathing pattern, as observed by the specialist nursing staff. By the end of the night, the pressure had been increased to 14 cmH_2O, and the oximetry trace showed resolution of the desaturations (Figure 5.3). The next day, the nursing staff checked that the patient was able to use the CPAP machine and was able to correctly put on and take off his mask. He was discharged home to be followed up in 4–6 weeks.

Evidence base The CANPAP trial

- RCT of fixed CPAP (n = 128) vs no CPAP (n = 130) in patients with heart failure (ejection fraction 24.5 ± 7.7%) and CSA (AHI 40 ± 16) followed up for 24 months [13].
- The CPAP group, compared to the control group, had greater reductions in AHI (−21 ± 16 vs −2 ± 18 events/hour).
- The CPAP group had greater increases in nocturnal oxygen saturations (1.6 ± 2.8% vs 0.4 ± 5.3%), ejection fraction (2.2 ± 5.4% vs 0.4 ± 5.3%), and 6MWD (20.0 ± 55 vs −0.8 ± 64.8 m).
- No significant differences in hospitalizations, quality of life, death, or heart transplantation between the two groups.
- Established CPAP can improve central apnoeas in heart failure patients but not alter prognosis.

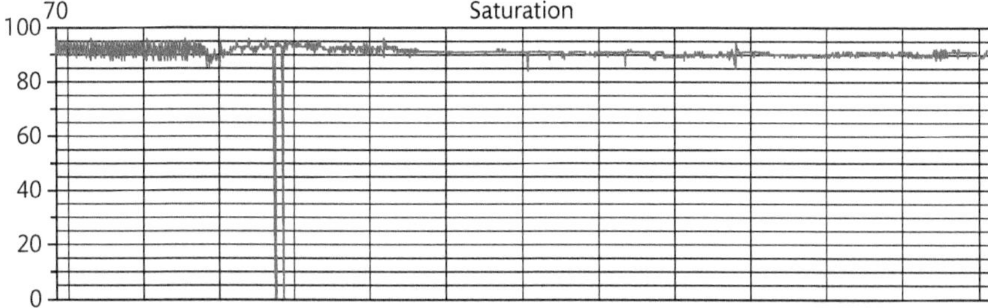

Figure 5.3 Overnight oximetry during titration of CPAP.

Expert comment

This study nicely illustrates the entity of CSA and, in particular, CSR which, if encountered, should raise first the question of heart failure as here (the other causes, i.e. 'brain failure' and 'lung failure' are less common)

Learning point

The AASM recommends titrating CPAP for CSA during full PSG, so that the sleep stage can be scored and any arousals noted and treated [14]. In practice, in the UK, CPAP is usually titrated either using pulse oximetry, with bedside observation, or using an autotitrating CPAP device which can be performed at home and has been shown to have similar outcomes, compared to PSG-guided titration in obstructive sleep apnoea [15].

Two weeks after commencing CPAP, the patient contacted the specialist nurses via their helpline. He had been having difficulties with his CPAP. His wife was aware of air leaking from his mouth, and he was still feeling sleepy. A chin strap was sent out to the patient to try to resolve the mouth leaks. At his follow-up appointment 2 weeks later, the patient reported still feeling sleepy, with an ESS of 16/24. In addition, although the mouth leaks had improved with the chin strap, they were still occurring. He was fitted with a full face mask, and follow-up was arranged with a telephone consultation and an outpatient visit, with overnight home oximetry to be performed the night before his appointment.

When contacted by telephone, the patient reported no further problems with mask leaks but that he still felt sleepy and that his wife had still noticed the occasional apnoea. His CPAP pressure was increased (the patient was guided through this over the telephone by the CPAP nurse specialist) to 16 cmH_2O. At his return visit, oximetry showed evidence of breakthrough apnoeas with a 4% desaturation index of 8/hour. The patient also reported ongoing unrefreshing sleep and excessive daytime sleepiness. A decision was made to initiate a trial of overnight oxygen.

The patient was admitted for initiation and titration of oxygen therapy. Oxygen delivered via nasal cannulae was gradually titrated overnight to a flow rate of 3 L/min, based on the oximetry trace. Arterial blood gases were performed the following morning to rule out CO_2 retention. He was discharged, with arrangements made for an oxygen concentrator to be delivered to his home. At his follow-up appointment, the patient stated he tolerated the oxygen well; indeed he found it less intrusive than CPAP. However, he still felt unrefreshed on waking and still suffered from excessive daytime sleepiness. The ESS was 16/24.

Learning point

Adaptive servo-ventilation (ASV) provides a background end-expiratory pressure with an adaptive degree of inspiratory pressure support which varies according to the patient's ventilation. If the patient's ventilation reduces, the degree of pressure support is increased, and vice versa, the target being the average ventilation. ASV has been shown to achieve better control of CSA, compared to oxygen [16] and, when compared to CPAP, achieves better control of breathing events, better compliance, and an increase in left ventricular ejection fraction (LVEF) [17]. See Evidence base, p. 56 for an update on using ASV in patients with symptomatic heart failure and an LVEF of ≤45%.

Evidence base CPAP versus ASV

- RCT of ASV (n = 12) versus CPAP (n = 13) in patients with stable heart failure and severe CSA followed up for 6 months [17].
- ASV induced greater improvement in AHI, quality of life, and ejection fraction, compared to CPAP.
- Compliance in the ASV group was significantly greater, compared to the CPAP group, at 6 months.
- ASV is more effective than CPAP in heart failure patients.

It was decided to switch the patient to adaptive servo-ventilation (ASV). He was admitted to the ward and familiarized with the new machine and fitted with an appropriate full face mask to minimize the chance of excessive air leak. The end-expiratory pressure was set at 5 cmH_2O, and the range of pressure support was set at between 3 and 15 cmH_2O. The patient was commenced on the ASV at bedtime and was observed for snoring, ongoing apnoeas, and desaturations. There was some snoring, so the minimum pressure support was increased by 2 cmH_2O which resolved this. At his follow-up appointment 6 weeks later, overnight oximetry was normal, with mean oxygen saturations of 93% and a 4% oxygen desaturation index of 3/hour. He reported feeling more refreshed on waking and less sleepy during the day. His ESS of 12 reflected this. A plan was made to continue the ASV and to review the patient in 6 months' time as an outpatient. The patient was advised that, as his symptoms were now controlled, he could request the DVLA that he resumed driving

Discussion

This case illustrates some of the dilemmas encountered when faced with a patient with CSA.

The initial decision to be made is which patients to treat. CSA is also commonly found in patients with AF, even in those with normal left ventricular systolic function [8]. CSA is common in patients with heart failure, with one series demonstrating 40% prevalence [18]. However, the majority of these patients did not have excessive daytime sleepiness. There is currently no evidence to suggest treatment of CSA in those with heart failure improves prognosis [19]. Therefore, treatment should be targeted at symptom control. In this group, the important symptoms to aim to control are symptoms associated with disrupted sleep (unrefreshing sleep and/or excessive daytime sleepiness), paroxysmal nocturnal dyspnoea, or nocturnal angina.

The next consideration is how to treat CSA. Management should initially be directed towards optimizing any underlying conditions. Treatment of heart failure itself has been shown to improve associated sleep apnoea. This can be achieved by optimizing medical therapy [11], cardiac resynchronization [20], or even cardiac transplantation [21]. Patients with renal failure and associated CSA have been demonstrated to have an improvement in breathing events with the introduction of nocturnal haemodialysis [22].

Clinical tip Complex sleep apnoea

Some patients with obstructive sleep apnoea, when commenced on CPAP, develop central apnoeas. This has been shown to occur in 13% of patients [23]. These central apnoeas are sometimes self-limiting with CPAP treatment; however, in some patients, it persists and may cause ongoing sleepiness. In such patients, bilevel non-invasive ventilation or ASV can be tried [24].

Specific treatment for central sleep apnoea

Respiratory stimulants have been investigated for the treatment of CSA. Acetazolamide [25] and theophylline [26] have both been shown to improve breathing events in those with CSA and heart failure, although both studies were short-term and the potential for side effects with these drugs is high and they are not used.

CSA is associated with changes in sleep stage, specifically sleep onset, and drugs which help consolidate sleep and reduce the number of sleep stage changes may be beneficial. An open-label study of zolpidem [27] demonstrated a reduction in AHI and arousals in patients with idiopathic CSA. Any potential benefit with using such drugs must be balanced with the risk of causing respiratory depression.

The use of CPAP in patients with CSA who have heart failure has been investigated in several trials and demonstrated to improve AHI [19]. The multicentre CANPAP trial, comparing CPAP with no treatment [13], demonstrated improvements in AHI, LVEF, and 6-minute walk distance (6MWD) with CPAP but failed to show a survival benefit. A subsequent post hoc analysis of the data suggested a survival benefit in those patients receiving CPAP who achieved an AHI of ≤15, when compared to the control group. A survival benefit has not been demonstrated in any other study, and use of CPAP to improve prognosis in this group cannot yet be supported. Those data also remind the physician of the importance of ensuring any treatment initiated is actually controlling the apnoeas. A meta-analysis of trials investigating the use of CPAP in this group has demonstrated an improvement in LVEF of 6% [19].

Oxygen may be considered in CSA. A meta-analysis has shown nocturnal oxygen improves AHI and LVEF in those with heart failure and CSA [19] but has not shown it to have a survival benefit. Interestingly, when oxygen was compared 'head to head' with CPAP [28], CPAP significantly reduced sleep efficiency, despite improving AHI to a similar degree, suggesting it is perhaps less well tolerated than oxygen, although this was a small study conducted over single nights.

Expert comment

The value of simple overnight oximetry is recognized and staged treatment properly encouraged, since some patients will obtain sufficient benefit with 'just' CPAP or oxygen.

ASV is a mode of ventilation allowing adjustment of the inspiratory pressure and backup rate to meet target minute ventilation. Several studies have demonstrated ASV significantly improves AHI, compared to baseline, in those with cardiac failure (see Evidence base, p. 54) and CSA and the improvement in AHI is significantly better, compared to CPAP [19]. However, this must be balanced against the considerable cost of ASV, compared to CPAP.

Evidence base

On 13 May 2015, a field safety notice was released due to early results from the RCT SERVE-HF which will change how CSA in patients with heart failure is treated. The SERVE-HF trial aimed to randomize 1200 patients with symptomatic chronic heart failure, LVEF of ≤45%, and moderate to severe CSA into either optimum medical management plus ASV or optimum medical management alone [29]. The primary end point was reduction in mortality and morbidity.

The early results demonstrate a 33.5% increased risk of cardiovascular death in patients treated with ASV, compared to controls (absolute annual risk of 10% in the ASV group, compared to 7.5% in controls). The study showed no statistically significant difference between the two groups for all-cause mortality or unplanned hospital admissions for worsening heart failure (based on a hazard ratio [HR] 1.136, 95% CI 0.974–1.325; p-value = 0.104).

The recommendations from the AASM are to:

- stop giving ASV to patients with symptomatic heart failure and LVEF of ≤45%;
- assess patients for heart failure before starting ASV;
- contact patients with symptomatic heart failure on ASV and discuss the risks. Alternative options of treatment will need to be on a case-by-case basis and may include CPAP or oxygen therapy.

Expert comment

The *New England Journal of Medicine* published the trial data in September 2015 [30] providing the data supporting the moratorium on ASV in symptomatic heart failure, although a plausible mechanism for this unexpected result has yet to be agreed, so advice may change in the future. However, this study plus the very specific advice given by the ASSM and the two main manufacturers of ASV devices must be considered, and no patients fitting the criteria should be started on ASV, while those already on ASV should have a frank discussion with the medical team as to whether to stop or continue.

Following the field safety notice, the sleep clinic database was reviewed for patients with CSA and heart failure treated with ASV. The patient was contacted with regard to his treatment with ASV, as he had an ejection fraction of 40%. He was informed of the concerns regarding his increased risk of cardiovascular death. The patient was reluctant to change his treatment, but a joint decision was made to stop the ASV and return to using overnight oxygen, despite the increased symptom burden. He will be reviewed in clinic in 6 months to discuss his treatment and symptoms.

Conclusions

Central sleep apnoea is common in patients with AF, heart failure and renal failure and is often asymptomatic. Prognostic benefit has not been demonstrated by treating CSA; therefore treatment should be aimed at symptom control. The most robust evidence is for the use of CPAP, nocturnal oxygen and ASV (with the recent exception of avoiding ASV in patients with heart failure), however respiratory stimulants may also be considered. Treatment of any underlying medical condition, particularly heart failure, is paramount.

It can be challenging to change treatments as new evidence emerges and keeping an up to date database is vital to allow identification of patients.

A final word from the expert

CSA, although a distinct form of sleep-disordered breathing, coexists on many occasions with the far commoner obstructive sleep apnoea, with central events (post-arousal or heart failure- or brain failure-driven) ending in, or degenerating into, obstruction.

The caution now shown to using ASV when heart failure is present will make CPAP a commoner initial treatment modality, and perhaps a logical one, with no current evidence for worse outcome in the setting of heart failure.

References

1. Douglas NJ, Thomas S, Jan MA. Clinical value of polysomnography. *Lancet* 1992;**339**:347–50.
2. Mayer P, Meurice JC, Philip-Joet F *et al.* Simultaneous laboratory-based comparison of ResMed Autoset with polysomnography in the diagnosis of sleep apnoea/hypopnoea syndrome. *Eur Respir J* 1998;**12**:770–5.
3. Collop NA, Anderson WM, Boehlecke B *et al.* Clinical guidelines for the use of unattended portable monitors in the diagnosis of obstructive sleep apnoea in adult patients. *J Clin Sleep Med* 2007;**3**:738–47.
4. Santos-Silva R, Sartori DE, Truksinas V *et al.* Validation of a portable monitoring system for the diagnosis of obstructive sleep apnoea syndrome. *Sleep* 2009;**32**:629–36.
5. Perl J, Unruh ML, Chan CT. Sleep disorders in end stage renal disease: 'Markers of inadequate dialysis'? *Kidney Int* 2006;70:1687–93.
6. Sanders MH, Givelber R. Sleep disordered breathing may not be an independent risk factor for diabetes but diabetes may contribute to the occurrence of periodic breathing in sleep. *Sleep Med* 2003;4:349–50.
7. Tremel F, Pepin JL, Veale D *et al.* High prevalence and persistence of sleep apnoea in patients referred for acute left ventricular failure and medically treated over 2 months. *Eur Heart J* 1999;**20**:1201–9.
8. Bitter T, Langer C, Vogt J *et al.* Sleep disordered breathing in patients with atrial fibrillation and normal left ventricular function. *Dtsch Arztebl Int* 2009;**106**:164–17.
9. Walker JM, Farney RJ, Rhondeau SM *et al.* Chronic opioid use is a risk factor for the development of central sleep apnoea and ataxic breathing. *J Clin Sleep Med* 2007;**3**:455–61.
10. Chan CT, Hanly P, Gabor J *et al.* Impact of nocturnal hemodialysis on the variability of heart rate and duration of hypoxemia during sleep. *Kidney Int* 2004;**65**:661–5.
11. Walsh JT, Andrews R, Starling R *et al.* Effects of captopril and oxygen on sleep apnoea in patients with mild to moderate congestive cardiac failure. *Br Heart J* 1995;**73**:237–41.
12. Zilberman M, Silverberg DS, Bits I *et al.* Improvement of anaemia with erythropoietin and intravenous iron reduces sleep related breathing disorders and improves daytime sleepiness in anaemic patients with congestive heart failure. *Am Heart J* 2007;**154**:870–6.

13. Bradley TD, Logan AG, Kimoff RJ *et al.* Continuous positive airway pressure for central sleep apnoea and heart failure. *N Eng J Med* 2005;**353**:2025–33.
14. Morgenthaler TI, Aurora RN, Brown T *et al.* Practice parameters for the use of auto titrating continuous positive airway pressure devices for titrating pressures and treating adult patients with obstructive sleep apnoea syndrome: an update for 2007. An American Academy of Sleep Medicine report. *Sleep* 2008;**31**:141–7.
15. Drummond F, Doelken P, Ahmed QA *et al.* Empiric auto-titrating CPAP in people with suspected obstructive sleep apnea. *J Clin Sleep Med* 2010;**6**:140–5.
16. Campbell AJ, Ferrier K, Neill AM. Effect of oxygen versus adaptive pressure support servo-ventilation in patients with central sleep apnoea-Cheyne Stokes respiration and congestive heart failure. *Intern Med* 2012;**42**:1130–6.
17. Philippe C, Stoica-Herman M, Drouot X *et al.* Compliance with and effectiveness of adaptive servoventilation versus continuous positive airway pressure in the treatment of Cheyne-Stokes respiration in heart failure over a six month period. *Heart* 2006;**92**:337–42.
18. Javaheri S, Parker TJ, Liming JD *et al.* Sleep apnea in 81 ambulatory male patients with stable heart failure. Types and their prevalences, consequences and presentations. *Circulation* 1998;**97**:2154–9.
19. Aurora RN, Chowdhuri S, Ramar K *et al.* The treatment of central sleep apnea syndromes in adults: practice parameters with an evidence-based literature review and meta-analyses. *Sleep* 2012;**35**:17–40.
20. Sinha AM, Skobel EC, Breithardt OA *et al.* Cardiac resynchronization therapy improves central sleep apnea and Cheyne-Stokes respiration in patients with chronic heart failure. *J Am Coll Cardiol* 2004;**44**:68–71.
21. Mansfield DR, Solin P, Roebuck T *et al.* The effect of successful heart transplant treatment of heart failure on central sleep apnea. *Chest* 2003;**124**:1675–81.
22. Hanly PJ, Pierratos A. Improvement of sleep apnea in patients with chronic renal failure who undergo nocturnal hemodialysis. *N Eng J Med* 2001;**344**:102–7.
23. Lehman S, Antic NA, Thompson C *et al.* Central sleep apnea on commencement of continuous positive airway pressure in patients with a primary diagnosis of obstructive sleep apnea-hypopnea. *J Clin Sleep Med* 2007;**3**:462–6.
24. Gilmartin GS, Daly RW, Thomas RJ. Recognition and management of complex sleep-disordered breathing. *Curr Opin Pulm Med* 2005;**11**:485–93.
25. Javaheri S. Acetazolamide improves central sleep apnea in heart failure: a double blind prospective study. *Am J Respir Crit Care Med* 2006;**173**:234–7.
26. Javaheri S, Parker TJ, Wexler L *et al.* Effect of theophylline on sleep-disordered breathing in heart failure. *N Engl J Med* 1996;**335**:562–7.
27. Quadri S, Drake C, Hudgel DW. Improvement of idiopathic central sleep apnoea with zolpidem. *J Clin Sleep Med* 2009;**5**:122–9.
28. Krachman SL, D'Alonzo GE, Berger TJ, Eisen HJ. Comparison of oxygen therapy with nasal continuous positive airway pressure on Cheyne-Stokes respiration during sleep in congestive heart failure. *Chest* 1999;**116**:1550–7.
29. Cowie MR, Woehrle H, Wegscheider K *et al.* Rationale and design of the SERVE-HF study: treatment of sleep-disordered breathing with predominant central. *Eur J Heart Fail* 2013;**15**:937–43.
30. Cowie MR, Woehrle H, Wegscheider K *et al.* Adaptive ServoVentilation for Central Sleep Apnea in Systolic Heart Failure. *N Engl J Med* 2015;**373**:1095–1105.

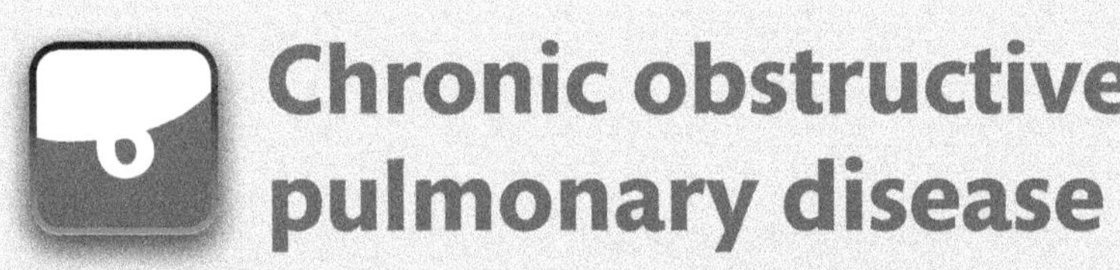

Chronic obstructive pulmonary disease

Amina Jaffer and Anant Patel

Expert commentary John Hurst

Case history

A 70-year-old man presented to the emergency department (ED) of his local hospital with a 3-day history of increased breathlessness, wheeze, and a cough productive of yellow sputum. This was preceded by a few days of coryzal symptoms. He had no chest pain, haemoptysis, fevers, or weight loss. His sleep had been interrupted by his symptoms for the last three nights, and he felt generally fatigued. His normal exercise tolerance was 200 m on the flat, and he had to walk more slowly on an incline or the stairs. For the past 2 days, he had to stop to catch his breath every 30 m when walking outside and, for the first time, had become breathless during his normal activities of daily living.

He had no known past history of lung disease but had experienced, for the last few years, episodes of winter colds 'going to his chest' with increased cough, wheeze, and breathlessness. He had not previously sought medical attention for these episodes, as they had self-resolved, although each time his baseline level of function had declined slightly.

His other past medical history was hypertension and AF. His medications included atenolol 50 mg od and warfarin as per the international normalized ratio (INR).

He was a current smoker of ten cigarettes per day and had previously smoked 20 cigarettes per day from the age of 16, giving him a 50–60 pack year smoking history. He drank 6 units of alcohol per week. He lived alone and was normally independent with his activities of daily living.

He was assessed by the ED doctor and was found to have minor use of the accessory muscles, bilateral air entry, and widespread wheeze. Initial investigations were performed (Table 6.1).

A CXR demonstrated hyperinflated lung fields, with a possible band of atelectasis in the right upper zone, but no focal consolidation, no effusion, and a normal cardiac silhouette (Figure 6.1).

He was given a presumed diagnosis of COPD and treated with systemic corticosteroids (prednisolone 30 mg), nebulized salbutamol and ipratropium, controlled oxygen therapy, and doxycycline orally (PO) (local antibiotic choice for an infective exacerbation of COPD). He was referred to the medical registrar and admitted for further observation and management.

Table 6.1 Observations, routine investigations, and results in the ED

Observations		Bloods		Arterial blood gas	On 28% oxygen Venturi mask
Blood pressure	145/95	Hb (g/dL)	15.2	pH	7.36
Pulse	92, irregular	Haematocrit	0.48	$PaCO_2$ (kPa)	5.98
Respiratory rate	28/min	WCC ($\times 10^9$/L)	15.3	PaO_2 (kPa)	9.34
O_2 sats (air)	87%	Neutrophils ($\times 10^9$/L)	13.2	HCO_3 units	25.0
O_2 sats (28% O_2)	92%	Eosinophils ($\times 10^9$/L)	0.1	Base excess	+1.4
Temperature	36.5°C	Platelets ($\times 10^9$/L)	320		
		INR	1.0		
		Na (mmol/L)	140	ECG	AF, 90/min, no ischaemia
		K (mmol/L)	4.3		
		Urea (mmol/L)	6.8		
		Creatinine (micromol/L)	70		
		CRP (mg/L)	56		
		Troponin (normal <0.032 units)	0.042		

Expert opinion

The diagnosis of COPD can only be made with spirometry, but this is rarely helpful at exacerbation, as patients find the test difficult with breathlessness, and it will not give a true picture of the degree of underlying airflow obstruction. Spirometry should be arranged following recovery to confirm the diagnosis and assess the severity of airflow obstruction. Note that exacerbation of COPD is a clinical diagnosis of exclusion. There is no confirmatory diagnostic test. A clinician needs to consider and, where appropriate, exclude with investigations other conditions that may cause symptom changes in a patient with COPD, e.g. pneumothorax, pulmonary embolism (PE), heart failure, and pneumonia.

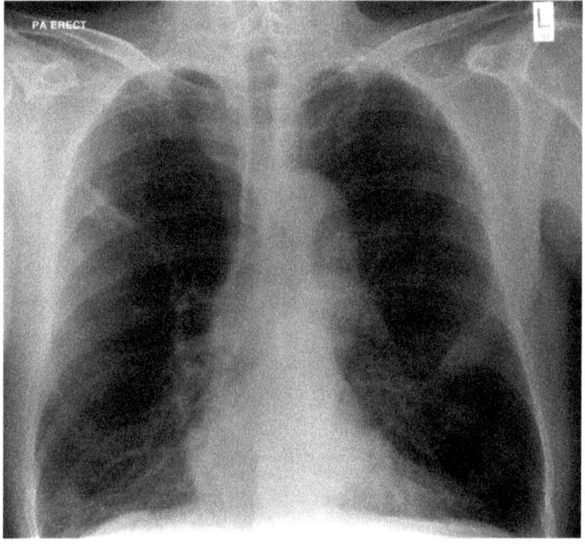

Figure 6.1 Admission CXR.

Learning point Confirming a diagnosis of COPD and assessing severity

This should be done when in steady state, and not during an acute exacerbation.

There must be:

- evidence of airflow obstruction, with post-bronchodilator spirometry showing FEV_1/FVC ratio of 0.70 or lower;
- if FEV_1 is >80% predicted, then a diagnosis of COPD must only be made when respiratory symptoms, such as shortness of breath and cough, are present [1].

Other features include:

- a history of chronic lower respiratory tract symptoms which start or intensify in mid to later life onwards;
- a history of exposure to a known noxious trigger that causes an abnormal inflammatory response, most commonly cigarette smoke but can be biomass fumes.

The traditional GOLD classification of severity was based on spirometry only. More recently, this has been further subdivided into four groups A, B, C, and D, based on symptoms and exacerbation frequency, as well as measured FEV_1 [2].

Classical measurement of severity by spirometry only

In patients with FEV_1/FVC <70%:

- GOLD 1: mild, FEV_1 >80%;
- GOLD 2: moderate, FEV_1 50–80%;
- GOLD 3: severe, FEV_1 30–50%;
- GOLD 4: very severe, FEV_1 <30%.

GOLD ABCD severity scoring

Superimposed on the spirometric severity are the:

1. CAT (COPD assessment test) score of symptoms (<http://www.catestonline.org>). Score ranges from 0 to 40, with over 10 indicating significant symptoms;
2. mMRC (modified Medical Research Council) dyspnoea score (range 0–4; 0 = I only get breathless with strenuous exercise, 1 = I get short of breath when hurrying on level ground or walking up a slight hill, 2 = On level ground, I walk slower than people of the same age because of breathlessness, or I have to stop for breath when walking at my own pace, 3 = I stop for breath after walking about 100 yards or after a few minutes on level ground, 4 = I am too breathless to leave the house, or I am breathless when dressing;
3. exacerbation frequency and severity.

   A: GOLD 1 or 2 spirometry, 1 or less exacerbation, no hospital admission, CAT <10, mMRC score 0 or 1.
   B: GOLD 1 or 2 spirometry, 1 or less exacerbation, no hospital admission, but CAT ≥10, mMRC ≥2.
   C: GOLD 3 or 4 spirometry OR ≥2 exacerbations/one requiring hospital admission, but CAT <10 and mMRC 0 or 1.
   D: GOLD 3 or 4 OR ≥2 exacerbations/one requiring hospital admission and CAT ≥10 and mMRC ≥2.

If there is a discrepancy between spirometric severity and exacerbation frequency, then whichever is the more severe is used to allocate the patient. For example, if a patient has an FEV_1 of 55% predicted but had three exacerbations in the last year and had a CAT score of 15 and an mMRC score of 3, then they would be classified in group D, even though their spirometry was only classified as GOLD 2.

There is evidence that severity measurement by spirometry alone does not correlate strongly with other measured parameters in COPD such as health-related quality of life (HRQoL), respiratory-specific questionnaires such as St George's Respiratory Questionnaire (SGRQ), Medical Research Council (MRC) dyspnoea score, exacerbation frequency, and exercise capacity (often measured by 6-minute walk distance). It is increasingly recognized that there are different phenotypes of COPD patients, and their risk may not depend simply on the severity of the airflow obstruction. There is a lack of strong correlation between the degree of airflow obstruction and other measured variables [3].

(Continued)

Figure 6.2 demonstrates that, although there is a relationship between FEV_1 values and other measured parameters of breathlessness, exacerbation frequency, HRQoL, and walk distance, these relationships are not strongly correlative, and hence using primary end points in trials of change in FEV_1 will not necessarily correspond to an increase in exercise tolerance or improvement in symptoms.

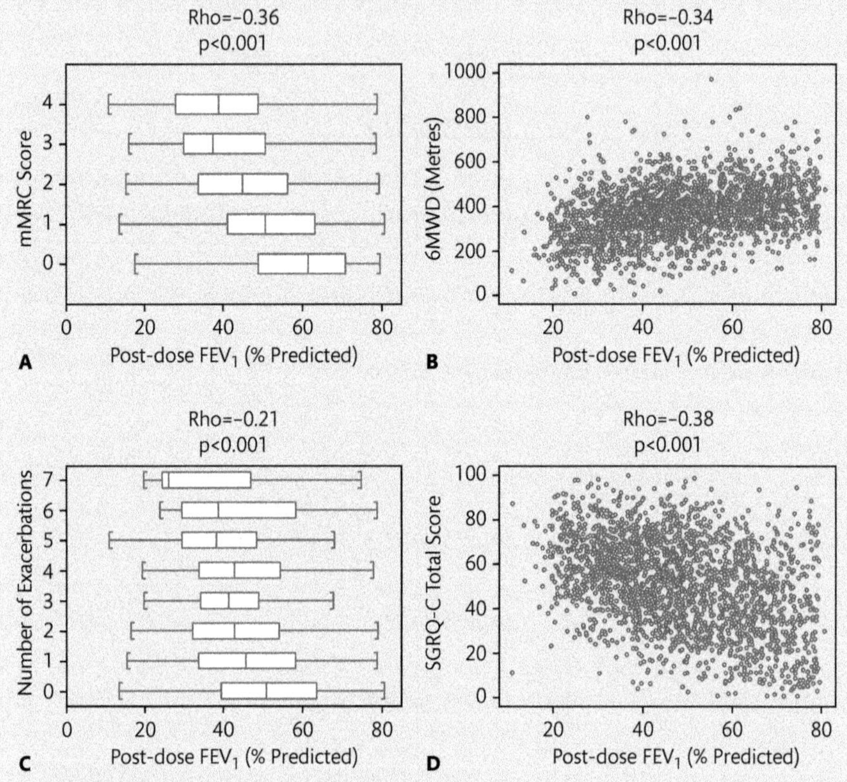

Figure 6.2 Relationship between the severity of airflow limitation and breathlessness as assessed by the mMRC questionnaire (A), exercise capacity as assessed by the 6-minute walk distance (6MWD) (B), reported exacerbations in the year before inclusion in the study (C), and health status as assessed by SGRQ-C (D).

It has also been demonstrated that exacerbation frequency is best predicted by a patient's own history, and there may be a frequent exacerbator phenotype, independent of disease severity [4].

A number of studies have suggested that more comprehensive assessments of health, such as the BODE index comprising measures of BMI, airflow obstruction (FEV_1 % predicted), dyspnoea (mMRC score), and exercise tolerance (6-minute walking distance), may be better predictors of mortality, but it may not be practical to assess this in all clinical settings.

Expert opinion

There is no single assessment of COPD severity. Current approaches combine spirometric impairment with symptoms and exacerbation frequency. Comorbidities are an important driver of outcomes and therefore also an important component of a holistic assessment. Disease severity should be distinguished from disease activity—the speed of progression of disease. This is difficult to assess in clinical practice but may be apparent by frequent exacerbations or an accelerated decline in FEV_1. Note that the severity of a COPD exacerbation is a composite outcome, reflecting both the severity of the underlying COPD and of the exacerbation insult.

The patient returned to clinic 6 weeks post-discharge and reported that he was still more short of breath than his pre-admission baseline but that his cough, wheeze, and sputum production had settled. His MRC dyspnoea score was 3, and he had been using his salbutamol inhaler 4–5 times a day. This was his first exacerbation in the last year. His saturations were 95% on air, and his chest examination was unremarkable.

His **post-bronchodilator** lung function showed the following:

- FEV_1 = 0.72L, 21% predicted;
- FVC = 2.66L, 56.8% predicted;
- FEV_1/FVC = 0.47;
- TLCO = 38.2% predicted;
- KCO = 58.7% predicted;
- RV = 6.93L, 257.1% predicted;
- RV/TLC = 0.715, 178.5% predicted.

There was no significant reversibility with bronchodilation.

Clinical tip Inhaled therapy

Most symptomatic patients are rapidly initiated on inhaled therapy and are often on 'triple therapy' comprising a long-acting muscarinic antagonist (LAMA) and a combination long-acting beta-agonist (LABA) and inhaled corticosteroid (ICS) inhaler. The latest guidelines [1, 2] have tried to review the evidence and give improved guidance as to which inhalers to prescribe.

Patients who are symptomatic, despite short-acting inhaler use, or with significantly impaired lung function (i.e. FEV_1 <50% predicted) should be initiated on treatment.

- FEV_1 >50%: LAMA or LABA single inhaler.
- FEV_1 <50%: combination LABA/ICS or LAMA inhaler is suggested.
- Frequent exacerbator and not controlled on LAMA only: then a LABA only inhaler or a LABA/ICS combination inhaler should be added, irrespective of FEV_1 value.

Much of the evidence for benefits for different inhaler regimens is based on post hoc and subgroup analysis of trials, and there are few trials directly comparing different inhaled therapies, in particular in the less severe COPD patients.

Evidence base Towards a revolution in COPD health (TORCH) 2007

- Randomized, double-blind, controlled trial in 444 centres in 42 countries [5]
- Comparing salmeterol at a dose of 50 micrograms plus fluticasone propionate at a dose of 500 micrograms bd (combination regimen) administered with a single inhaler (N = 1533), with placebo (N = 1524), salmeterol alone (N = 1521), or fluticasone propionate alone (N = 1534) for a period of 3 years.
- Primary end point: all-cause 3-year mortality. Secondary end points: exacerbation frequency, health status (measured by SGRQ), and spirometry.
- Mean post-bronchodilator FEV_1 for all groups = 44% predicted.
- Trend towards reduced mortality in combination inhaler, compared to placebo, but did not reach clinical significance (p = 0.052).
- Significant reduction in exacerbation frequency, improvement in health status, and improvement in spirometry with combined inhaler versus placebo (p <0.001 for all).
- The rate of pneumonia was significantly higher in both groups where inhaled therapy contained fluticasone (combination group and fluticasone only group), compared to placebo (p <0.001).

Evidence base Understanding potential Long-Term Impacts on Function with Tiotropium (UPLIFT) 2008

- Randomized, double-blinded, controlled trial in 490 centres in 37 countries [6].
- Comparing once-a-day inhaled tiotropium (N = 2987) to placebo (N = 3006) over 4 years.
- Mean post-bronchodilation FEV_1 = 44% predicted in both groups.
- All other respiratory medications, including LABA or LABA/steroid combinations, were allowed to be continued. Other anticholinergic inhaled medications were prohibited.
- Co-primary end points were rate of decline in the mean FEV_1 before and after bronchodilation, beginning on day 30.
- Secondary end points included measures of FVC, changes in response on SGRQ, exacerbations of COPD, and mortality.
- No significant difference in the rate of decline in FEV_1 pre- or post-bronchodilation in the tiotropium versus placebo group.
- The absolute FEV_1 values at each time point from 30 days onwards were significantly higher in the tiotropium versus placebo group.
- The SGRQ was significantly lower (better health status) at each time point in the tiotropium versus placebo group.
- Significantly lower incidence of exacerbations per patient year in the tiotropium, compared to placebo, group ($p < 0.001$), although not in exacerbations requiring hospital admission ($p = 0.34$).
- There was no significant difference in all-cause mortality at the end of the study between the tiotropium and placebo groups ($p = 0.09$).

Our patient was initiated on a LAMA inhaler and referred for smoking cessation advice and pulmonary rehabilitation. On review a few months later, he was still breathless and had experienced one further exacerbation requiring steroids and antibiotics from his GP. A combination LABA and ICS inhaler was started, in addition to his LAMA. His saturations remained at 95% on air.

Learning point Pulmonary rehabilitation

Pulmonary rehabilitation programmes vary widely in contents, but the core components include:

- disease education;
- exercise training;
- smoking cessation;
- nutritional advice.

There is grade A evidence for statistically significant improvement in the factors listed below in pulmonary rehabilitation groups versus usual care, when available evidence was analysed in a Cochrane review in 2015 [7]:

- total scores in HRQoL, as measured by chronic respiratory questionnaire (CRQ) and SGRQ. There were clinically significant improvements in domains for dyspnoea, fatigue, and emotional function;
- functional and maximal exercise capacity.

Early referral to pulmonary rehabilitation has now been incorporated into many 'COPD discharge bundles' [8] which are filled out in conjunction with the patient prior to hospital discharge. NICE guidelines recommend that pulmonary rehabilitation should be offered to all of those who consider themselves functionally impaired by their COPD (usually MRC score of 2 or above), including those who have recently had an exacerbation [1].

Our patient continued to symptomatically progress with frequent exacerbations and a gradually reducing baseline exercise tolerance. Despite attending smoking cessation services, he continued to smoke, but, at every clinic visit, he was encouraged to stop smoking.

Learning point Smoking cessation

There is a wealth of evidence to support the overall, as well as respiratory, health benefits of smoking cessation. The Lung Health Study in 1994 [9] showed a significantly reduced rate of decline of FEV_1 in the smoking cessation intervention groups, compared to controls. Most patients were young and earlier in their disease trajectory, and this highlights the importance of intervening early to prevent irreversible lung damage.

Programmes include psychological (such as cognitive behavioural therapy) and pharmacological interventions (such as nicotine replacement therapy or bupropion). A Cochrane review [10] of available evidence found that programmes containing psychological and pharmacological interventions were superior to no intervention and to psychological only interventions in achieving smoking cessation. There was insufficient evidence to know the effect of psychological only interventions versus no intervention, as there were no good-quality RCTs.

Due to worsening symptoms he had a CT scan of his chest that showed predominantly upper zone emphysema (Figure 6.3).

He continued to be very symptomatic with worsening breathlessness and reduced exercise capacity, despite LAMA and LABA/ICS inhalers and completing pulmonary rehabilitation. Given the heterogenous nature of his disease, lung volume reduction surgery (LVRS) was considered.

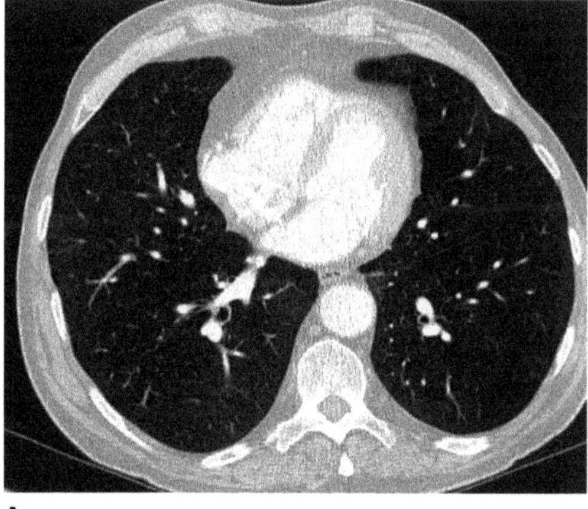

A

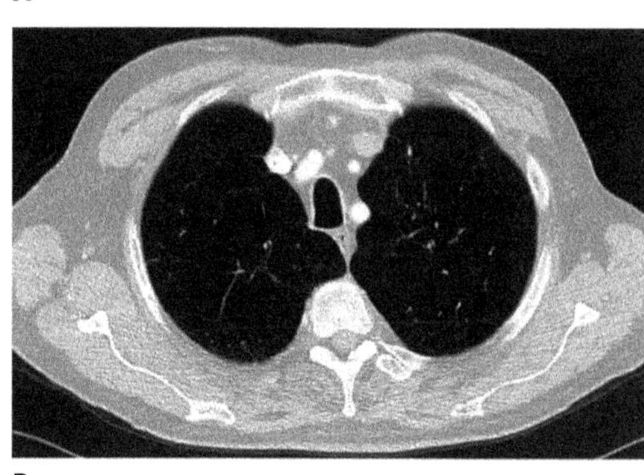

B

Figure 6.3 CT scan demonstrating relative preservation of the lower zone (A), with predominantly upper zone emphysema (B).

Evidence base The National Emphysema Treatment Trial (NETT) 2011

- Randomized, controlled, multicentre trial in the US: LVRS (N = 608) versus medical management (N = 610) [11].
- Primary end points were survival and maximal exercise performance.
- Secondary end points of lung function, patient symptoms, and quality of life.
- Inclusion: bilateral emphysema with pre-rehabilitation post-bronchodilator TLC >100% and RV >150% predicted, 15% ≤ FEV_1 ≤ 45%, BMI <32, $PaCO_2$ ≤60 mmHg/8 kPa and PaO_2 on air ≥49 mmHg/5.9 kPa, smoking abstinence ≥4 months.
- Exclusion: diffuse emphysema, bulla >30% of lung volume; previous LVRS, lobectomy, or sternotomy; pulmonary hypertension, 6MWD ≤140 m post-rehabilitation; >20 mg prednisolone/day; significant cardiac co-morbidities.
- Subgroup of high-risk patients FEV_1 ≤20% or TLCO ≤20% or homogenous emphysema stopped 2001 as 30-day mortality 16%. LVRS not recommended for this high-risk group.
- In non-high-risk patients, 30-day mortality rate was 2.2% with LVRS and 0.2% with medical treatment ($p < 0.001$). The 90-day mortality rate was 5.2% with LVRS and 1.5% with medical treatment ($p < 0.001$). The 5- and 8-year follow-up mortality figures showed no significant difference between the groups.
- The commonest adverse event post-surgery was prolonged air leak.
- Improvements in 6MWD, maximal exercise capacity, FEV_1 % predicted, and quality of life (disease-specific and general) were more likely to occur after LVRS, compared with medical treatment ($p < 0.001$ for each comparison).
- Subgroup patients with upper lobe-predominant emphysema and low preoperative exercise capacity appeared to gain most benefit.

Evidence base Bronchoscopic lung volume reduction with endobronchial valves for patients with heterogeneous emphysema and intact interlobar fissures (the BeLieVeR-HIFi study)

- Single-centre, double-blind, sham-controlled trial in 50 patients with both heterogeneous emphysema and a target lobe with intact interlobar fissures on CT of the thorax (hence no collateral ventilation) [12].
- Stable outpatients with COPD who had an FEV_1 of <50% predicted, significant hyperinflation (TLC >100% and RV >150%), a restricted exercise capacity (6MWD <450 m), and substantial breathlessness (MRC dyspnoea score ≥3).
- Participants were randomized (1:1) by computer-generated sequence to receive either valves placed to achieve unilateral lobar occlusion (bronchoscopic lung volume reduction, BLVR) or a bronchoscopy with sham valve placement (control).
- Powered to detect 15% change in primary end point (FEV_1 3 months after procedure).
- Results in the BLVR group were highly skewed, so median results and non-parametric statistical analysis were used. Median (interquartile range, IQR) FEV_1 changes at 3 months were 8.77% (2.27–35.85) in the BLVR group and 2.88% (0–8.51) in controls (Mann–Whitney $p = 0.0326$). There was also a statistically significant increase in gas transfer results in the treatment group, compared to control, but again with a high degree of variability amongst participants.
- The BLVR group had a statistically significant increase in 6MWD: median 25 m (IQR 7–64) in the treatment group, compared to 3 m (IQR −14 to 20) in the control group ($p = 0.0119$).
- There was an improvement in quality of life measures, such as CAT and SGRQ, in the treatment group, compared to the control, but this did not reach statistical significance.
- The mean number of valves per patient was three in the 3-month follow-up period.
- In the BLVR group, eight patients were scored as having 'complete collapse' of the target lobe, five 'a band of atelectasis', two 'some volume loss', and eight 'no change'. This may explain the high degree of variability in the results.
- Two deaths in the treatment group (one from underlying COPD and one with tension pneumothorax occurring after valve removal at 49 days) and one dropout from the control group due to pneumothorax with persistent air leak.

Although our patient had severe airflow obstruction and was only just above the high-risk group, according to the criteria listed in Evidence base, p. 66, he did go on to have LVRS, with a very good clinical outcome with reduced breathlessness and improved exercise capacity.

His post-operative lung function showed the following:

- FEV_1 = 1.28 L, 35.7% predicted (preoperative 0.72 L);
- FVC = 4.16 L, 88.9% predicted (preoperative 2.66 L);
- FEV_1/FVC = 0.31.

Clinical tip Consider referral for LVRS if very symptomatic despite medical therapy and pulmonary rehabilitation and:

- FEV_1 >20% predicted;
- upper lobe-predominant emphysema;
- TLCO >20% predicted.

Other surgical options can include bullectomy and lung transplantation (single or double).

As yet, the referral criteria and pathway for BLVR are not clear and need further research.

Discussion

COPD is a very common condition affecting hundreds of millions of people worldwide and, according to the WHO, directly caused 6% of all world deaths in 2012 [13]. It is managed by a wide range of doctors (GPs, acute and general medical hospital physicians, respiratory physicians), as well as allied health professionals.

The existing management of COPD as a chronic disease includes a number of evidence-based management interventions—pharmacological and non-pharmacological. The latter includes smoking cessation and pulmonary rehabilitation. There may be missed opportunities to treat people and offer smoking cessation earlier in patients' disease trajectories and prevent further decline in lung function and performance status.

It is increasingly recognized that we should adjust our management based not only on lung function, but also on increased symptomatology and exacerbation frequency. The definition of an exacerbation is a debated topic, but most would agree that there should be a new onset or worsening of symptoms, including cough, shortness of breath, sputum production, fever, and wheeze. These symptoms should last several days and be beyond day-to-day variability, and they may require healthcare contact and additional treatment.

COPD patients have varied phenotypes that depend not only on classical measures of severity such as lung function. Increased exacerbation frequency is associated with increased hospitalizations, poorer quality of life, and worsened prognosis [14]. The 'frequent exacerbator' phenotype has been described in a number of studies [4, 15]. Disease severity, as measured by lung function, is of course a significant factor in identifying those likely to have frequent and serious exacerbations, but it is also clear that those with only moderately impaired lung function can still be frequent exacerbators. In an analysis of data from the Evaluation of COPD Longitudinally to Identify Predictive Surrogate Endpoints (ECLIPSE) observational study [4], it was found that previous high exacerbation frequency in itself was the strongest predictor of ongoing frequent exacerbations, independent of the severity of lung function impairment. A post hoc analysis of data from the 1-year Prevention of Exacerbations with Tiotropium in COPD (POET-COPD) study [16] demonstrated that the frequent exacerbator group (two or more exacerbations) accounted for 56.6% of exacerbation-related hospital admissions, despite only representing 13.6% of the study group. Increased hospital admission rate was predictably related to increased mortality. We have some evidence that inhaled therapy can reduce exacerbation frequency [5, 6]. However, most evidence is based on post hoc analysis, and exacerbation frequency has not been the primary measured end point in these studies. There is also a lack of evidence to apply to patients with less severe lung function impairment. The current guidelines [1, 2] recommend an escalation of inhaled therapy if a patient continues to have frequent exacerbations, irrespective of the degree of lung function impairment. More studies are required to explore the causality of the frequent exacerbator phenotype and how the disease management should vary in these patients.

Inhaled therapy and pulmonary rehabilitation may improve symptoms but are not able to reverse the structural damage that exists in the lungs. Hyperinflation caused by emphysema has a significant impact on respiratory mechanics, including chest wall movement and increased breathlessness. It also adversely impacts on attempts at ventilation and prolongs ventilator weaning [17]. It has also been shown that hyperinflation negatively affects cardiac function, reducing venous return and left ventricular filling [18].

LVRS can be performed via median sternotomy or VATS for bilateral surgery or via open thoracotomy or VATS for unilateral surgery. The intention is to remove the worst affected emphysematous lung (usually 20–30%) to allow improved respiratory muscle, diaphragm, and chest wall function and expansion of the remaining less diseased lung to improve gas exchange, and decrease ventilation–perfusion (V/Q) mismatch. It is not a curative procedure but is performed with the intention of improving symptoms and quality of life.

LVRS should clearly not be undertaken lightly, as there is a significant early mortality associated with the surgery. However, it has been demonstrated that, in carefully selected patients with heterogeneously distributed predominantly upper lobe emphysema with poor preoperative exercise capacity despite pulmonary rehabilitation, there can be good outcomes with improved quality of life and exercise capacity [11]. A small study by Jorgensen *et al.* [19] has also shown that LVRS can improve left ventricular filling and function. Endobronchial approaches to lung volume reduction are in the process of being evaluated and may offer a lower-risk alternative. The BeLieVer-HIFi study [12], discussed in Evidence base, p. 66, has shown that these less invasive techniques can have successful outcomes but are in themselves not without risk. There are thus far no trials comparing bronchoscopic techniques to surgical LVRS. It is not clear whether the referral criteria for the two should be the same or different and whether bronchoscopic techniques should be tried earlier or are appropriate for those not fit for surgery. A concern with the latter approach is that there is a risk of pneumothorax with the bronchoscopic procedure, and the ability to tolerate this complication should be considered prior to the procedure.

Further surgical techniques for selected patients include bullectomy and lung transplantation. Bullectomy should be considered in symptomatic patients with a single large bulla on a CT scan and an FEV_1 <50% predicted [1]. This should be thought particularly about in patients with complications from the bulla such as recurrent pneumothoraces. The exact criteria for transplantation referral in COPD varies, but it is generally considered as an option in patients with severe disease with an FEV_1 <20% predicted (without reversibility) and/or $PaCO_2$ over 55 mmHg (7.3 kPa) and/or elevated pulmonary artery pressures with progressive deterioration. Age cut-off varies between centres but usually is only considered in those <65 years. The patient must not be a current smoker and must undergo a number of tests to assess their clinical co-morbidities, as well as their psychological and emotional fitness. The risk:benefit ratio of transplantation and its sequelae must be carefully considered on an individual patient basis.

In summary, this chapter has highlighted the diagnosis and stepwise management of a COPD patient, as well as explored the evidence behind our pharmacological and non-pharmacological treatment options. We have discussed the concept of different phenotypes within COPD patients and how this may influence our management and future research. It has also been demonstrated that, in selected patients, surgical options can have good outcomes and should be considered if symptoms are not well controlled with good medical management.

A final word from the expert

COPD is a prevalent condition, but each patient presents a unique set of challenges. Only by addressing each of these in an evidence-based way can we hope to change outcomes in this debilitating disease.

References

1. National Institute for Health and Care Excellence (2010). *Chronic obstructive pulmonary disease in over 16s: diagnosis and management*. NICE guideline CG101. Available at: <http://www.nice.org.uk/guidance/cg101/evidence>.
2. Global Initiative for Chronic Obstructive Lung Disease (2015). *Pocket guide to COPD diagnosis, management, and prevention. A guide for health care professionals*. Available at: <http://www.goldcopd.it/materiale/2015/GOLD_Pocket_2015.pdf>.
3. Agusti A, Calverley PM, Celli B *et al*. Characterisation of COPD heterogeneity in the ECLIPSE cohort. *Respir Res* 2010;**11**:122.
4. Hurst JR, Vestbo J, Anzueto A *et al*. Susceptibility to exacerbation in chronic obstructive pulmonary disease. *N Engl J Med* 2010;**363**:1128–38.
5. Calverley PM, Anderson JA, Celli B *et al*. Salmeterol and fluticasone propionate and survival in chronic obstructive pulmonary disease. *N Engl J Med* 2007;**356**:775–89.
6. Tashkin DP, Celli B, Senn S *et al*. A 4-year trial of tiotropium in chronic obstructive pulmonary disease. *N Engl J Med* 2008;**359**:1543–54.
7. McCarthy B, Casey D, Devane D, Murphy K, Murphy E, Lacasse Y. Pulmonary rehabilitation for chronic obstructive pulmonary disease. *Cochrane Database Syst Rev* 2015;**2**:CD003793.
8. Hopkinson NS, Englebretsen C, Cooley N *et al*. Designing and implementing a COPD discharge care bundle. *Thorax* 2012;**67**:90–2.
9. Anthonisen NR, Connett JE, Kiley JP *et al*. Effects of smoking intervention and the use of an inhaled anticholinergic bronchodilator on the rate of decline of FEV1. The Lung Health Study. *JAMA* 1994;**272**:1497–505.
10. van der Meer RM, Wagena EJ, Ostelo RW, Jacobs JE, van Schayck CP. Smoking cessation for chronic obstructive pulmonary disease. *Cochrane Database Syst Rev* 2003;**2**:CD002999.
11. Criner GJ, Cordova F, Sternberg AL, Martinez FJ. The National Emphysema Treatment Trial (NETT) Part II: Lessons learned about lung volume reduction surgery. *Am J Respir Crit Care Med* 2011;**184**:881–93.
12. Davey C, Zoumot Z, Jordan S *et al*. Bronchoscopic lung volume reduction with endobronchial valves for patients with heterogeneous emphysema and intact interlobar fissures (the BeLieVeR-HIFi study): a randomised controlled trial. *Lancet* 2015;**386**:1066–73.
13. World Health Organization (2015). *Chronic obstructive pulmonary disease (COPD)*. Available at: <http://www.who.int/mediacentre/factsheets/fs315/en/>.
14. Lange P, Marott JL, Vestbo J *et al*. Prediction of the clinical course of chronic obstructive pulmonary disease, using the new GOLD classification: a study of the general population. *Am J Respir Crit Care Med* 2012;**186**:975–81.

15. Han MK, Agusti A, Calverley PM *et al.* Chronic obstructive pulmonary disease phenotypes: the future of COPD. *Am J Respir Crit Care Med* 2010;**182**:598–604.
16. Beeh KM, Glaab T, Stowasser S *et al.* Characterisation of exacerbation risk and exacerbator phenotypes in the POET-COPD trial. *Respir Res* 2013;**14**:116.
17. Alvisi V, Romanello A, Badet M, Gaillard S, Philit F, Guerin C. Time course of expiratory flow limitation in COPD patients during acute respiratory failure requiring mechanical ventilation. *Chest* 2003;**123**:1625–32.
18. Watz H, Waschki B, Meyer T *et al.* Decreasing cardiac chamber sizes and associated heart dysfunction in COPD: role of hyperinflation. *Chest* 2010;**138**:32–8.
19. Jorgensen K, Houltz E, Westfelt U, Nilsson F, Schersten H, Ricksten SE. Effects of lung volume reduction surgery on left ventricular diastolic filling and dimensions in patients with severe emphysema. *Chest* 2003;**124**:1863–70.

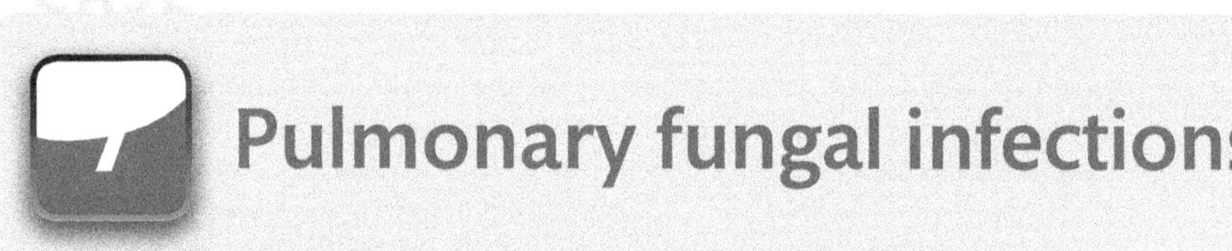

Pulmonary fungal infections

Georgia Tunnicliffe

Expert commentary Matthew Wise

Case history 1

A 43-year-old male presented to the A&E department with a 4-day history of increasing breathlessness, dry cough, general malaise, and fever. He had a history of Crohn's disease since the age of 22 and had been on oral prednisolone intermittently for the last 5 years. He had been started on infliximab (a monoclonal antibody against tumour necrosis factor alpha (TNF-α)) infusions 2 months previously for fistulating Crohn's disease.

On examination, he was breathless at rest but able to speak in full sentences. His temperature was 38.2°C. Oxygen saturations were 86% on room air, and his respiratory rate was 24 breaths/minute. Blood pressure was 90/60 mmHg, with a heart rate of 120 beats/minute. Auscultation of heart sounds was normal, and occasional crackles were heard throughout both lung fields.

Routine investigations revealed normal renal and liver function, and a full blood count was unremarkable, except for an elevated platelet count of 755 × 10^3/mL. The ECG demonstrated sinus tachycardia, and a plain CXR showed patchy airspace opacification throughout the lungs. Arterial blood gas (ABG) analysis revealed a PaO_2 of 6.5 kPa, $PaCO_2$ of 2.9 kPa, HCO_3 of 20 mEq/L, and pH 7.38. On high-flow oxygen, his oxygenation improved slightly, with saturations of 90% and a PaO_2 of 9.1 kPa. He was transferred to the intensive care unit (ICU) for respiratory support and was commenced on IV co-amoxiclav and clarithromycin for presumed bacterial pneumonia.

Clinical tip Biological agents and fungal infection

- Biological agents, including blockade of TNF-α, have emerged as a useful therapy for several diseases, including collagen vascular diseases and inflammatory bowel disease.
- With increasing use of these agents, there has been a rise in infections caused by a wide spectrum of pathogens, including bacteria, viruses, protozoa, and fungi.
- The risk of TB is sufficiently high that it is recommended that all patients have skin testing before initiation of infliximab treatment [1].
- A review of reported cases of fungal Infections complicating TNF-α blockade found 281 cases of invasive fungal infections [2].
- The most prevalent were histoplasmosis (30%), candidiasis (23%), and aspergillosis (23%).
- Pneumonia was the commonest pattern of infection.
- 80% were associated with infliximab, 16% with etanercept, and 4% with adalimumab.

Expert comment

Although biological agents, such as infliximab, are recognized as increasing the risk of fungal infection, this patient had also received corticosteroids. The latter are not only immunosuppressive but can augment the growth of fungi *in vitro*. Corticosteroids alone may place otherwise healthy individuals at risk of fungal infection of the upper airways or lung, especially if exposed to a large number of spores.

In 2010, the ATS published a statement on the treatment of fungal infections in adult pulmonary and critical care patients [3]. This recognized that, in recent years, there has been a rise in the number of patients with immunocompromise due to disease, e.g. HIV and malignancy, or immunosuppressive drugs, which has led to a significant increase in the incidence and clinical severity of pulmonary fungal infections. There has also been an increase in definitive diagnosis with improved diagnostic methods. The statement covers the commonest fungi responsible for pulmonary infections in the critical care setting, endemic mycoses, and finally rare fungi. Table 7.1 illustrates the key points for the common fungi encountered in the critical care setting, i.e. species of *Candida*, *Cryptococcus*, *Aspergillus*, and *Pneumocystis jirovecii*.

Blood cultures were negative, and the patient did not improve on antibiotic therapy. A CT of the thorax was performed (Figure 7.1). This illustrates a cavitating nodule surrounded by a halo of ground glass opacification, which is consistent

Table 7.1 Summary of the ATS statement for treatment of fungal infections

Organism and disorder	At-risk groups and features	Diagnosis	Treatment	Remarks
Candida species Candidiasis Candida pneumonia (rare)	In ICU, at high risk if central venous line for >4 days and two of: (i) total parenteral nutrition on days 1–4; (ii) dialysis days 1–4; (iii) pancreatitis in 7 days prior to ICU; (iv) systemic steroids in 7 days prior to ICU; (v) neutropenia [4, 5]	Positive blood culture	**Candidaemia confirmed:** remove all existing central venous catheters **Clinically stable:** commence either fluconazole, caspofungin or micafungin or anidulafungin **If clinically unstable/ unknown species:** amphotericin or caspofungin, micafungin, anidulafungin, voriconazole	Ocular candidiasis can result in blindness—need formal ophthalmologic examination
Cryptococcus neoformans + *Cryptococcus gatti* Cryptococcosis	**Commonest manifestation** is meningitis **Secondary sites** include skin, prostate, eye, and bone **Common respiratory symptoms:** cough, dyspnoea, fever [6] **Multiple manifestations:** pneumonitis/consolidation/ pulmonary nodules and effusions	Visualization and culture Serum/cerebrospinal fluid cryptococcal antigen Lumbar puncture should be considered (with India ink staining)	**Mild localized:** fluconazole or itraconazole **Central nervous system/disseminated:** amphotericin for 6 weeks or fluconazole for 2 weeks, followed by fluconazole or itraconazole **Immunocompromise:** initial treatment also with flucytosine Manage intracranial pressure	Colonization is common and does not require treatment Pulmonary involvement in up to 39% of patients with AIDS and cryptococcosis [7] In HIV, if CD4 <200, maintain fluconazole
Aspergillus species Invasive aspergillosis	**Radiology:** pulmonary macronodules typically surrounded by a halo of GGO 'Air crescent' sign (haemorrhagic infarction)	Difficult—up to 70% of immunocompromised with confirmed invasive pulmonary aspergillosis have negative culture ↑ galactomannan in serum and BAL, and follow level	First line: voriconazole Second line: liposomal amphotericin Salvage therapy with caspofungin or posaconazole Prolonged therapy required Reverse immune suppression	Groups traditionally not considered to be at risk emerging, e.g. ICU population, COPD, post-operative, alcohol excess

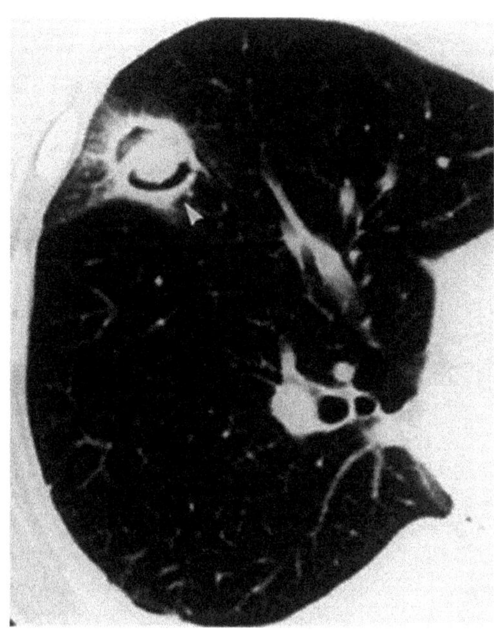

Figure 7.1 CT thorax showing the air crescent and halo signs.

with both the 'air crescent' and 'halo' signs. These lesions represent foci of fungal infection, with each halo representing a perimeter of haemorrhage associated with alveolar invasion [8]. A diagnosis of invasive pulmonary aspergillosis (IPA) was made, and voriconazole was commenced. In recent years, the probable importance of monitoring voriconazole levels has emerged, although this remains controversial [9, 10].

Our patient recovered with treatment. However, mortality rates in IPA are very high, even if therapy is instituted early [11].

Evidence base Randomized study of monitoring of voriconazole levels in patients with invasive fungal infections 2012

- Randomized, assessor-blinded, single-centre study to evaluate the clinical utility of routine therapeutic drug monitoring (TDM) of voriconazole in invasive fungal infections [9].
- Total of 110 adult patients randomly assigned to TDM (where voriconazole dose was adjusted to target range of 1.0–5.5 mg/L, according to serum trough levels) or non-TDM (fixed dose) groups.
- The proportion of voriconazole discontinuation due to adverse events was significantly lower in the TDM group (4% versus 17%; $p = 0.2$).
- A complete or partial response was observed in 81% of those in the TDM group, compared to 57% in the non-TDM group ($p = 0.4$).

Had the patient presented with the same clinical features and a history of foreign travel, the differential diagnosis would need to broaden to include endemic mycosis. If a patient of a similar age, who was not immunosuppressed, presented with symptoms of night sweats, fever, weight loss, and cough and had recently returned from an ornithology holiday bordering Lake Michigan, then endemic fungal infections would need to be included in the list of differential diagnoses. Features of endemic mycosis are described in Table 7.2.

Expert comment

The halo sign is typically observed in the early phase of disease but is less likely to occur if the patient is not neutropenic, while an air crescent sign occurs later as a result of necrosis. The halo sign may occur with neoplastic or inflammatory pathologies, but its occurrence in an immunocompromised patient with fever should prompt initiation of antifungal therapy if there is no alternative diagnosis such as pneumonia caused by *Staphylococcus aureus* or *Klebsiella pneumoniae*.

Expert comment

Other fungi—*Fusarium*, *Scedosporium*, and mucoraceous mould—will give the same picture and are more 'frequent' in the UK than endemic fungi. Endemic fungi are Category 3 pathogens, and the laboratory should be warned before cultures are sent.

Table 7.2 Features of endemic mycoses

Organism and infection	At-risk areas/activities	Presentation/radiology	Comments
Histoplasma capsulatum Histoplasmosis	Mississippi and Ohio River basin Less common Europe, Asia Central, and South America Chicken coops Bat caves	Spectrum from malaise to acute respiratory distress syndrome (ARDS) Commonly fever, cough, chills, and chest pain Extrapulmonary: erythema nodosum, pericarditis, myalgias, and arthralgias **Radiology:** localized or diffuse infiltrates, nodular disease, or cavitatory lesions. Mediastinal granulomas and fibrosis are rare	Over 90% are subclinical/ mild However, with heavy exposure, more than half of patients develop symptomatic disease [12–14]
Blastomyces dermatitidis Blastomycosis	As above and also Midwestern states, Canada bordering the Great Lakes and bordering St Lawrence River, including New York Exposure to woodland/soil associated with animals [12]	Similar to acute pneumonia Also subacute pneumonic process with associated symptoms of fever, night sweats and weight loss Small proportion with infection, leading to ARDS Cutaneous lesions in 50% (painless, crusted nodules or plaques) **Radiology:** alveolar mass-like infiltrates or (less common) reticulonodular pattern. Cavities rare	Immune suppression does not predispose to acquiring blastomycosis, but immunosuppressed may have more severe disease [15]
Coccidioides immitis and *Coccidioides posadasii* Coccidioidomycosis	Semi-arid and arid areas of South West USA and northern Mexico Follows earthquakes/wind-driven storms, archaeological digs	Many are subclinical 'Flu-like' symptoms with fever and cough **Radiology:** pulmonary infiltrates 1–3 weeks after exposure Nodular lesions may cavitate	Disseminated disease, in immunocompromised and pregnant women, especially in the third trimester [16]
Sporothrix schenckii Sporotrichosis	Worldwide, although most cases reported in the Americas [17]	Cutaneous lesions, fever, cough, night sweats, weight loss, and haemoptysis **Radiology:** nodular lesions or cavities. Can mimic TB/other fungal infections	Pulmonary disease commoner in alcohol abuse, COPD, diabetes, and steroid use [18]

Learning point Endemic mycoses: key features

- As international travel becomes commoner, clinical suspicion for endemic mycoses should increase. These are a heterogeneous group of diseases due to specific fungi which are endemic to North America.
- Disease can occur in otherwise healthy hosts who are exposed to these pathogens.
- Severity of infection is dependent on the individual's immune status and the degree of exposure.
- These fungi exist in the mould or mycelial phase in the environment at room temperatures and are usually found in the soil. They change to the yeast phase at body temperatures (temperature dimorphism).
- The route of infection is inhalation, except for sporotrichosis which occurs after cutaneous inoculation of the organism.
- Diagnosis is by culture or microscopic visualization.
- Antigen-based tests are becoming available and are useful in histoplasmosis. Serology is helpful for coccidioidomycosis
- Treatment is usually with an oral azole, such as fluconazole or itraconazole, although, for severe cases and in pregnancy, amphotericin is still used. Full guidance has been issued by the IDSA in 2007–2008 [19–22].

Case history 2

A 69-year-old gentleman was referred to the chest clinic via his GP with an abnormal CXR. He attended his annual review at the practice for COPD and was noted to have lost 11 kg in weight since his last appointment 1 year ago. He complained of feeling generally unwell for the last 6 months and of progressive breathlessness, with productive cough and haemoptysis. Past medical history included COPD diagnosed 9 years previously and diet-controlled diabetes mellitus identified 5 years earlier. His medications were tiotropium 18 micrograms (od), a combination inhaler of salmeterol 50 mg/fluticasone 500 micrograms (one activation bd), and inhaled salbutamol as required. He was a retired factory worker living with his wife. He was an ex-smoker of 5 years standing, with a 43 pack-year history. His CXR showed apical cavities with adjacent pleural thickening.

> **Expert comment**
> A lung neoplasm would be top of the differential diagnosis in a smoker with weight loss and haemoptysis.

He underwent cross-sectional imaging with a CT scan, fibreoptic bronchoscopy with BAL, and a battery of blood tests. IgG precipitating antibodies against *Aspergillus* antigens were positive, and both total IgE and *Aspergillus*-specific IgE (RAST) levels were elevated. The BAL fluid cultured *Aspergillus fumigatus*, and a diagnosis of chronic cavitatory pulmonary aspergillosis was made. The patient was commenced on itraconazole therapy.

> **Clinical tip** Semi-invasive ***Aspergillus***
>
> - It is important to recognize the potential overlap between colonization, hypersensitivity, and invasive syndromes.
> - Several chronic forms of *Aspergillus* infection with overlapping clinico-radiological characteristics exist and are challenging to define, such as chronic necrotizing pulmonary aspergillosis (CNPA) and also chronic fibrosing pulmonary aspergillosis (CFPA) which refers to respiratory failure caused by chronic pulmonary aspergillosis and complete opacification of one lung or both upper lobes [23]. In CFPA, the fibrosis leads to major loss of lung function.
> - Although able to destroy lung tissue, CNPA can also remain indolent for quite some time without causing vascular invasion. It is most commonly encountered in those with chronic or debilitating systemic illnesses [24].
> - The main differential diagnosis for CNPA is chronic cavitatory pulmonary aspergillosis (CCPA), a disease notable for the formation of multiple pulmonary cavities that do not invariably contain fungal masses.
> - Unlike in aspergilloma, such cavities may arise directly as a result of fungal tissue infiltration, although some cases also occur in individuals with prior TB lung disease. There can be overlap between these syndromes.
> - Patients with CNPA and CCPA may report considerable constitutional disturbance before a final diagnosis is secured.
> - IgG precipitating antibodies against *Aspergillus* antigens are positive in the majority of patients; successful culture of *Aspergillus* in the sputum or BAL fluid or histological confirmation of fungal tissue invasion help to establish the diagnosis.
> - The mainstay of treatment of these conditions is high-dose systemic antifungal therapy. Oral triazole compounds, exemplified by itraconazole and voriconazole, have superseded amphotericin, although the latter is still used for severe disease [3].
> - Surgical intervention is rarely undertaken due to high risk of complications and poor physiological reserve of affected individuals.
> - Other fungi, such as histoplasmosis, can cause a similar chronic pulmonary disease, and the differential diagnosis includes TB, actinomycosis, and malignancy.

He was lost to follow-up due to relocation but, 1 year later, attended the A&E department at his local hospital with large-volume haemoptysis. As part of his investigations, he had a CT chest which showed a mobile mass has developed in one of the apical cavities. An aspergilloma was diagnosed.

> **Expert comment**
> Demonstrating a mobile mass on supine and prone CT scans is pathognomonic of an aspergilloma.

Clinical tip Management of aspergilloma

- Optimal treatment for indolent or mildly symptomatic aspergilloma is unknown.
- Systemic antifungal therapy does not effectively alter the disease course in such cases due to its poor penetration into mycetomal cavities [26].
- Intra-cavitatory instillation of antifungals has previously been used, with variable clinical response [27, 28].
- Selective embolization of bronchial and non-bronchial arteries offers only a temporizing effect until surgical treatment can be undertaken [29].

Expert comment

Both arterial embolization and instillation of antifungal drugs may provide short-term control of haemoptysis, but recurrence is common. Intrapulmonary instillation may also be complicated by pneumothorax. Pulmonary resection is the optimal surgical procedure; however, cavernostomy may be used in older patients with limited physiological reserve and peripheral pulmonary aspergilloma.

Clinical tip Diagnosis of aspergilloma

- Pulmonary mycetoma refers to a fungal ball within a pre-existing cavity in the lung.
- Mycetoma formation occurs in up to 50% of cases of CCPA.
- Most mycetoma are due to *Aspergillus* and are called aspergilloma.
- The most frequent symptom is haemoptysis, usually mild but can be severe and even life-threatening in a small number of cases [25].
- On plain radiography, an aspergilloma typically appears as an ovoid or round opacity located within a lung cavity. Localized pleural thickening may occasionally be apparent; this sign is more sensitively appreciated on CT.
- Examination of the sputum, BAL fluid, and surgically resected material may reveal the presence of *Aspergillus* hyphae.
- Elevated titres of serum *Aspergillus*-specific IgG precipitins may be detected, particularly in corticosteroid-naïve patients.

The patient was transferred to a specialist centre for bronchial artery embolization followed by resection of the right upper lobe. Figure 7.2 shows an aspergilloma in an explanted lung. Unfortunately, he developed a broncho-pleural fistula and empyema and died 1 week later. Surgery can offer definitive treatment for this condition, provided that cases are well selected.

Evidence base Surgical outcome of pulmonary aspergilloma 2008

- Prospective study of patients admitted between 2001 and 2008 for resection for pulmonary aspergilloma [30].
- Patients with invasive aspergillosis, ABPA, and active TB were excluded.
- Two groups: group A (simple aspergilloma) and group B (complex aspergilloma).
- A total of 42 patients (28 males, 14 females) with a mean age of 44 (± 11 years).
- Haemoptysis was the commonest presentation and indication for surgery (83.5%).
- A total of 36 patients underwent lobectomy; two patients in group B had a pneumonectomy; one patient in group A had a segmentectomy; two patients had a bilobectomy (group B), and one had a palliative cavernostomy.
- One patient died (group B) 7 days following cavernostomy from respiratory failure.
- Non-fatal complications occurred in 12 patients (three in group A, nine in group B) which were most commonly empyema (three patients), prolonged air leak (three patients), and bleeding (two patients).

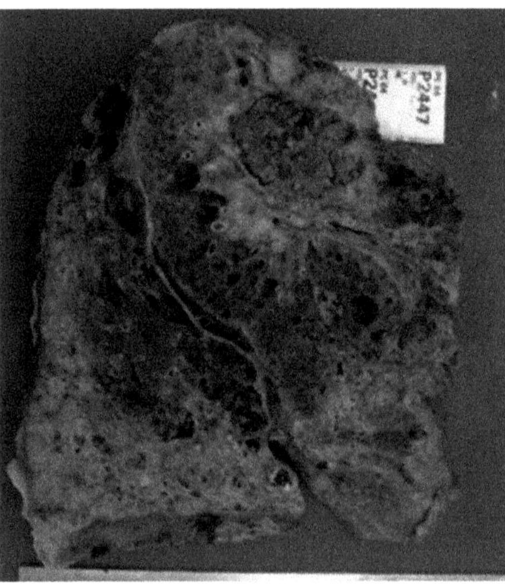

Figure 7.2 Aspergilloma in an explanted lung.

Discussion

These cases illustrate the spectrum of diseases which can be caused by fungi. Making a diagnosis of fungal disease may be difficult, as symptoms and signs are often non-specific. Consequently, a high index of suspicion is required when considering fungal infection. The diagnosis may be more obvious in groups such as the returning traveller (for endemic mycoses) or bone marrow transplant recipients who have symptoms consistent with invasive disease. However, new groups are being recognized as being at risk such as those with COPD or diabetes mellitus.

One of the challenges when making a diagnosis of invasive and semi-invasive fungal diseases is determining whether the presence of positive cultures represents colonization or true infection. Often cultures can be negative, even where there is invasive disease. In invasive aspergillosis, up to 70% of immunocompromised individuals with confirmed IPA have negative culture results. Aids to improve diagnosis have improved in recent years, and several new laboratory tests, such as assays of antigens like galactomannan for *Aspergillus* in serum and BAL or β-glucan, are commercially available. Radiology is often a crucial diagnostic tool.

Although some fungal infections respond well to treatment and new modalities offer the clinician more choice, there is still controversy about optimal management. Trials in the treatment of fungal diseases often do not include large numbers of patients. Invasive fungal diseases often occur in vulnerable hosts, and treatment with antifungal agents, such as amphotericin, may be limited by toxicity and severe side effects. Newer antifungal agents are less toxic, and there is now better guidance regarding the optimal treatment of invasive fungal lung diseases since the publication of the ATS guidelines in 2010. However, some invasive fungal infections are still associated with a high mortality. Semi-invasive fungal disorders and mycetoma usually occur in hosts who already have damaged lungs. This complicates treatment, which often needs to be prolonged. Surgical intervention for chronic semi-invasive disease is rarely undertaken due to the high risk of complications and the high level of comorbidity in affected individuals. In aspergilloma, surgical morbidity may be substantial and include intraoperative haemorrhage, persistent air leaks, and infection of the residual space.

In conclusion, the diagnosis and treatment of fungal lung diseases still offer the clinician and their patients a number of challenges which are likely to remain for some time.

A final word from the expert

Fungi are relatively rare causes of pulmonary infection and usually represent an opportunistic infection in an immunocompromised individual. The exception is endemic mycosis which should be considered in returning travellers. Patients with haematological malignancy or bone marrow transplantation who remain neutropenic represent the archetypal risk group for pulmonary fungal disease. In these patients, if respiratory symptoms and fever are present with prolonged neutropenia and no clinical improvement on antibacterial agents, fungal disease should be considered. Diagnostically driven strategies incorporating radiology, antigen testing, and molecular diagnostic techniques are replacing broad empiric antifungal therapy.

It must be remembered, however, that 50% of IPA now occurs in critically ill patients in intensive care where immune dysregulation is common, though often unrecognized. Mortality amongst the critically ill is extremely high and probably reflects both the underlying critical illness and delays in diagnosis and initiation of appropriate therapy. Many patients in critical care are not neutropenic and have a lower fungal load. Rather than the angioinvasion, thrombosis, and haemorrhage that characterize neutropenic patients, in the critically ill patient with normal neutrophil function, there is minimal angioinvasion and a predominance of endobronchial disease with low fungal burden. Haemorrhagic necrosis is driven by neutrophil infiltrates; consequently, 'classic' radiological signs on CT, such as nodules with a halo or the air crescent sign, are less common, and standard microbiological detection techniques are unreliable. Detection of the fungal cell wall antigen galactomannan on BAL may be useful in non-neutropenic critically ill patients, with a low fungal load as a diagnostic (but not screening) tool. However, the presence of neutropenia, corticosteroids, renal or liver failure, surgery, parenteral nutrition, and intravascular lines all increase the risk of invasive infection, and this should be taken into account when considering the aetiology of potential infections.

Hypersensitivity syndromes also contribute to the burden of fungal lung disease. Immune dysregulation also plays a role here, and chronic pulmonary damage may progress to semi-invasive disease. Distinguishing between fungal colonization, hypersensitivity, and true invasive disease can be problematic.

A number of polymorphisms in immune response genes have been identified as being associated with invasive fungal disease. Species-specific molecular tests for fungal pathogens are also being developed and optimized. It is likely that, in the future, these molecular tests for fungi and immune response genes may facilitate risk stratification and the diagnosis of pulmonary fungal infections.

References

1. Keane J, Gershon S, Wise RP *et al*. Tuberculosis associated with infliximab, a tumor necrosis factor alpha-neutralizing agent. *N Engl J Med* 2001;**345**:1098–104.
2. Tsiodras S, Samonis G, Boumpas DT, Kontoyiannis DP. Fungal infections complicating tumor necrosis factor alpha blockade therapy. *Mayo Clin Proc* 2008;**83**:181–94.
3. Limper AH, Knox KS, Sarosi GA *et al*. An official American Thoracic Society statement: Treatment of fungal infections in adult pulmonary and critical care patients. *Am J Respir Crit Care Med* 2011;**183**:96–128.
4. Pappas PG, Kauffman CA, Andes D *et al*. Clinical practice guidelines for the management of candidiasis: 2009 update by the Infectious Diseases Society of America. *Clin Infect Dis* 2009;**48**:503–35.
5. Ostrosky-Zeichner L, Pappas PG. Invasive candidiasis in the intensive care unit. *Crit Care Med* 2006;**34**:857–63.
6. Baddley JW, Perfect JR, Oster RA *et al*. Pulmonary cryptococcosis in patients without HIV infection: factors associated with disseminated disease. *Eur J Clin Microbiol Infect Dis* 2008;**27**:937–43.
7. Sider L, Westcott MA. Pulmonary manifestations of cryptococcosis in patients with AIDS: CT features. *J Thorac Imaging* 1994;**9**:78–84.
8. Franquet T, Müller NL, Giménez A, Guembe P, de La Torre J, Bagué S. Spectrum of pulmonary aspergillosis: histologic, clinical, and radiologic findings. *Radiographics* 2001;**21**:825–37.
9. Park WB, Kim NH, Kim KH. The effect of therapeutic drug monitoring on safety and efficacy of voriconazole in invasive fungal infections: a randomized controlled trial. *Clin Infect Dis* 2012;**55**:1080–7.

10. Racil Z, Winterova J, Kouba M, *et al*. Monitoring trough voriconazole plasma concentrations in haematological patients: real life multicentre experience. *Mycoses* 2012;**55**:483–92.
11. Denning DW. Therapeutic outcome in invasive aspergillosis. *Clin Infect Dis* 1996;**23**:608–15.
12. Vyas K, Bariola JR, Bradsher RW, Jr. Treatment of endemic mycoses. *Expert Rev Respir Med* 2010;**4**:85–95.
13. Cano MV, Hajjeh RA. The epidemiology of histoplasmosis: a review. *Semin Respir Infect* 2001;**16**:109–18.
14. Wheat J. Histoplasmosis. Experience during outbreaks in Indianapolis and review of the literature. *Medicine (Baltimore)* 1997;**76**:339–54.
15. Eggimann P, Garbino J, Pittet D. Management of Candida species infections in critically ill patients. *Lancet Infect Dis* 2003;**3**:772–85.
16. Peterson CM, Schuppert K, Kelly PC, Pappagianis D. Coccidioidomycosis and pregnancy. *Obstet Gynecol Surv* 1993;**48**:149–56.
17. Pappas PG, Tellez I, Deep AE, Nolasco D, Holgado W, Bustamante B. Sporotrichosis in Peru: description of an area of hyperendemicity. *Clin Infect Dis* 2000;**30**:65–70.
18. Pluss JL, Opal SM. Pulmonary sporotrichosis: review of treatment and outcome. *Medicine (Baltimore)* 1986;**65**:143–53.
19. Hage CA, Wheat LJ. Diagnosis of pulmonary histoplasmosis using antigen detection in the bronchoalveolar lavage. *Expert Rev Respir Med* 2010;**4**:427–9.
20. Wheat LJ, Freifeld AG, Kleiman MB, *et al*. Clinical practice guidelines for the management of patients with histoplasmosis: 2007 update by the Infectious Diseases Society of America. *Clin Infect Dis* 2007;**45**:807–25.
21. Kauffman CA. Histoplasmosis: a clinical and laboratory update. *Clin Microbiol Rev* 2007;**20**:115–32.
22. Chapman SW, Dismukes WE, Proia LA *et al*. Clinical practice guidelines for the management of blastomycosis: 2008 update by the Infectious Diseases Society of America. *Clin Infect Dis* 2008;**46**:1801–12.
23. Denning DW, Riniotis K, Dobrashian R, Sambatakou H. Chronic cavitary and fibrosing pulmonary and pleural aspergillosis: case series, proposed nomenclature change, and review. *Clin Infect Dis* 2003;**37**(Suppl 3): S265–80.
24. Binder RE, Faling LJ, Pugatch RD, Mahasaen C, Snider GL. Chronic necrotizing pulmonary aspergillosis: a discrete clinical entity. *Medicine (Baltimore)* 1982;**61**:109–24.
25. Jewkes J, Kay PH, Paneth M, Citron KM. Pulmonary aspergilloma: analysis of prognosis in relation to haemoptysis and survey of treatment. *Thorax* 1983;**38**:572–8.
26. Glimp RA, Bayer AS. Pulmonary aspergilloma. Diagnostic and therapeutic considerations. *Arch Intern Med* 1983;**143**:303–8.
27. Guleria R, Gupta D, Jindal SK. Treatment of pulmonary aspergilloma by endoscopic intracavitary instillation of ketoconazole. *Chest* 1993;**103**:1301–2.
28. Lee KS, Kim HT, Kim YH, Choe KO. Treatment of hemoptysis in patients with cavitary aspergilloma of the lung: value of percutaneous instillation of amphotericin B. *AJR Am J Roentgenol* 1993;**161**:727–31.
29. Chun JY, Belli AM. Immediate and long-term outcomes of bronchial and non-bronchial systemic artery embolisation for the management of haemoptysis. *Eur Radiol* 2010;**20**:558–65.
30. Brik A, Salem AM, Kamal AR *et al*. Surgical outcome of pulmonary aspergilloma. *Eur J Cardiothorac Surg* 2008;**34**:882–5.

Additional useful information

The Aspergillus Website. Available at: <http://www.aspergillus.org.uk/>.

HIV-related lung disease

Dami Collier

Expert commentary Robert F Miller

Case history

A 40-year-old male presented to the ED with a 3-week history of progressive shortness of breath and non-productive cough. He gave a 1-week history of night sweats, fatigue, poor appetite, and weight loss.

He was a man who had sex with men (MSM), and his past medical history included a diagnosis of HIV infection made 3 years previously, but he had been lost to follow-up in the HIV clinic. He had not commenced antiretroviral treatment (ART) and was not taking prophylaxis against *Pneumocystis* pneumonia (PCP). He had been treated for rectal *Chlamydia* and herpes simplex virus-2 perianal ulcers 3 weeks prior to this presentation. He had no recent travel, was a smoker with a 25 pack-year history, and had no known TB contacts.

On arrival in the ED, he was short of breath on minimal exertion and was unable to complete full sentences. His vital signs revealed a temperature of 38.2°C, blood pressure of 155/84 mmHg. He was tachycardic, with a heart rate of 110 beats/minute, and tachypnoeic with a respiratory rate of 28 breaths/minute, and oxygen saturations were 80% on air. On examination of the chest, he had bilateral vesicular sounds with no added sounds. Auscultation of the heart was normal. His abdomen was soft and non-tender; there was no organomegaly. His chest radiograph is shown in Figure 8.1.

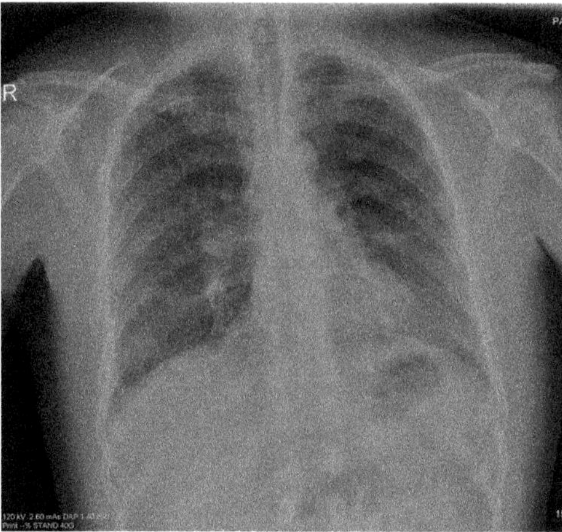

Figure 8.1 Chest radiograph showing diffuse interstitial shadowing in both lung fields.

Learning point Clinical examination and chest radiography

There are no pathognomonic clinical features of PCP, hence it is important to consider a diagnosis of PCP in any HIV-positive patient presenting with respiratory symptoms.

Oxygen desaturation on exercise is highly suggestive of PCP in those with a normal chest radiograph and normal resting oxygen saturations, and those who have never previously had PCP [1].

The classical radiological finding in PCP is diffuse bilateral pulmonary infiltrates extending from the perihilar region, with peripheral sparing [2].

Although the clinical features and radiological findings may be highly suggestive, neither are specific enough for a diagnosis of PCP, and laboratory confirmation is needed.

Expert opinion

HIV-infected persons are at greatest risk of developing PCP if they have low CD4 counts (<200 cells/microlitre) and are not in receipt of prophylaxis and ART. However, approximately 5% of HIV-associated PCP occurs in patients who have CD4 counts of >300 cells/microlitre. If the CD4 count is not known/available, the clinician may be able to recognize stigmata, including oral hairy leukoplakia, extragenital molluscum contagiosum, seborrhoeic dermatitis, and cutaneous ± palatal Kaposi's sarcoma which identify that the patient is profoundly immune-deficient. A diagnosis of TB should be excluded in any HIV-infected individual with subacute respiratory symptoms, regardless of their CD4 count and the chest radiographic appearances.

His arterial blood gas on air showed a pH of 7.51, PCO_2 of 4.6, PO_2 of 5.31, lactate of 1.9, HCO_3 of 28.6, and a base excess of 4.6. Blood investigations revealed haemoglobin of 145 g/L, white cell count of 7.46 × 10^9/L, with a normal differential, platelets of 375 × 10^9/L, and normal values for urea and electrolytes, liver function tests (LFTs), and CRP. A CD4 count was 110 cells/microlitre.

An assessment was made of probable severe PCP, as defined by the British HIV Association (BHIVA) opportunistic infection guidelines (Table 8.1), and he was commenced on treatment with intravenous trimethoprim–sulfamethoxazole (TMP-SMX, co-trimoxazole) at a dose of 120 mg/kg/day, with adjuvant prednisolone for 21 days, following US and UK recommendations for treatment of moderate to severe HIV-associated PCP (Table 8.2) [3].

Table 8.1 Severity of PCP

	Mild	Moderate	Severe
Clinical features	Dyspnoea on exertion ± cough and sweats	Dyspnoea on minimal exertion, cough ± sweats	Dyspnoea and tachycardia at rest, cough
Oxygen saturation on air (%)	>96	91–96	<91
PaO_2 on air (kPa)	>11.0	8.1–11.0	≤8.0
Chest radiograph	Normal or minor perihilar shadowing	Diffuse interstitial shadowing	Extensive shadowing ± diffuse alveolar shadowing

Nelson, M., et al., British HIV Association and British Infection Association guidelines for the treatment of opportunistic infection in HIV-seropositive individuals 2011. HIV Med, 2011. 12 Suppl 2: p. 1–140.

Table 8.2 Treatment of PCP

	Mild	Moderate/severe
First line	Oral TMP-SMX 1920 mg three times daily (tds), or 90 mg/kg/day tds	High-dose TMP-SMX intravenously 120 mg/kg/day for 3 days, then reduce to 90 mg/kg/day for 18 days; given in three or four divided daily doses AND Oral prednisolone 40 mg bd for days 1–5, 40 mg od for days 6–10, and 20 mg od for days 11–21 Or intravenous methylprednisolone at 75% of above doses
Second line	Trimethoprim 20 mg/kg/day orally in divided doses and dapsone 100 mg od orally OR Atovaquone liquid suspension 750 mg bd orally for 21 days	Clindamycin 600–900 mg four times daily (qds) intravenously or 300–450 mg qds orally and primaquine 15–30 mg od orally OR Pentamidine 4 mg/kg od intravenously for 21 days

Nelson, M., et al., British HIV Association and British Infection Association guidelines for the treatment of opportunistic infection in HIV-seropositive individuals 2011. HIV Med, 2011. 12 Suppl 2: p. 1–140.

Expert opinion

Assessment of the severity of PCP enables the clinician to choose treatment. Some treatment options are unproven or have been shown to be ineffective in patients with severe PCP. TMP-SMX is the treatment of first choice for PCP of any grade of severity. Adjunctive steroids should be given to those with moderate and severe PCP (PaO_2 <9.3 kPa or alveolar to arterial (A–a) oxygen gradient of >4.7 kPa). Corticosteroid treatment should begin at the same time that specific anti-*Pneumocystis* treatment is started; in some patients, they will be started empirically, pending confirmation of the diagnosis.

In the ED, despite high-flow oxygen, his respiratory function deteriorated rapidly, and he was commenced on non-invasive ventilation (NIV) with CPAP. He was transferred to the high dependency unit (HDU) for ongoing care. By day 4 of admission, his pressure support and oxygen requirements were weaned down, and he was able to tolerate further investigation with high-resolution CT (HRCT) (Figure 8.2) confirming emphysema with perihilar ground glass shadowing.

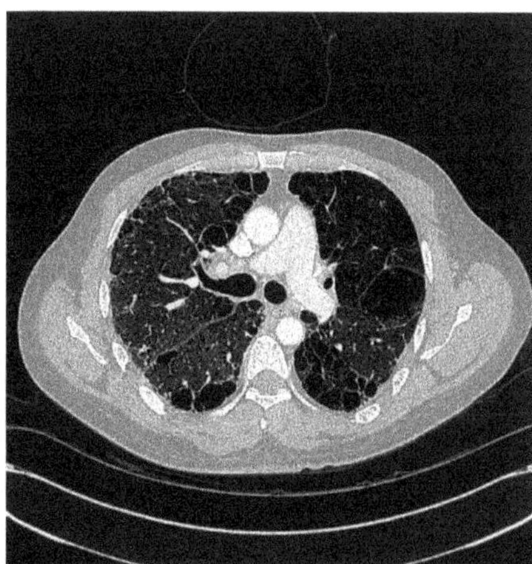

Figure 8.2 CT images showing emphysematous changes with diffuse ground glass changes in perihilar distribution, predominantly in the upper and middle lobes.

Clinical tip Need for ventilatory support

Early intervention with CPAP should be considered in patients with suspected or confirmed PCP who are hypoxic. It may prevent deterioration and the need for mechanical ventilation [4].

Clinical tip Bronchoscopy versus induced sputum

If bronchoscopy and BAL is not available, an induced sputum specimen may be obtained. This has a diagnostic sensitivity of up to 67%.

Expert opinion

In the era of ART, the mortality of PCP is 10–12% in studies from the US and the UK. Several factors present at admission to hospital, or soon afterwards, are associated with a poor outcome. These include increasing patient age, lack of knowledge of HIV serostatus, injection drug use, recurrent PCP, low haemoglobin or serum albumin, poor oxygenation (low PaO_2 or widened A–a oxygen gradient), marked chest radiographic abnormalities, and peripheral blood leucocytosis. Other 'poor prognosis' factors identified following investigation include identification of a viral, e.g. cytomegalovirus (CMV), or bacterial co-pathogen, or >5% neutrophilia in BAL fluid, elevated blood lactate dehydrogenase (LDH) enzyme levels that do not fall in response to treatment, and the presence of co-morbidity, such as pregnancy or intercurrent malignancy, or of pulmonary Kaposi's sarcoma. Additionally, the need for admission to the ICU, a high APACHE II score, the need for mechanical ventilation, and the development of a pneumothorax are all associated with poor outcome from PCP. Improved outcome from severe PCP cases admitted to the ICU is probably due to improved ICU care, including 'protective' (low tidal volume) ventilator strategies, rather than to improved treatment of PCP per se or to early institution of ART on the ICU.

After 7 days in the HDU, the patient was stable enough to be 'stepped down' to a medical ward. He no longer required NIV and remained on 1 L of oxygen via nasal cannulae. On day 8, a bronchoscopy with BAL was done. Cytological examination of BAL fluid using Grocott–Gomori's methenamine silver stain revealed inflammatory cells and proteinaceous alveolar casts containing the cystic form of *Pneumocystis jirovecii*.

Expert opinion

Patients with PCP rarely have a productive cough. *Pneumocystis* can be identified in induced sputum obtained by inhalation of a hypertonic saline aerosol. Some patients experience marked desaturation during sputum induction, and so oxygen saturations should be monitored during, and immediately after, this procedure. The yield is lower than that from bronchoscopy and BAL and varies considerably from centre to centre. If *Pneumocystis* is not identified in induced sputum, then BAL should be performed. The yield for PCP from BAL remains high for up to 2 weeks, after starting specific anti-*Pneumocystis* therapy.

The patient continued to show clinical improvement on the ward but, 9 days after commencing treatment with TMP-SMX, developed a widespread macular rash on the torso, limbs, and face. This was associated with a new fever, but no mucosal, conjunctival, or genital involvement. This was clinically recognized as an adverse drug reaction associated with TMP-SMX. The patient was commenced on oral prednisolone 30 mg od for 5 days, and the TMP-SMX was switched to a second-line agent with a combination of oral primaquine 15 mg od and clindamycin 600 mg qds. He subsequently made a full recovery and was started on ART with a combination of efavirenz and Truvada® on day 21 of admission. On follow-up, he remains well, was compliant with ART, and has a sustained CD4 count response.

Clinical tip Risk of adverse drug reactions

Check glucose-6-phosphate dehydrogenase (G6PD) level, as a deficiency may result in a risk of haemolysis following primaquine or dapsone.

Discussion

PCP is a fungal infection of humans that occurs particularly in immunosuppressed individuals. It is caused by *P. jirovecii*, formerly known as *Pneumocystis carinii*. It is a common opportunistic infection among HIV-infected patients who have a CD4

T-cell count of <200 cells/microlitre (or a CD4 T-cell percentage of <14%) and an unsuppressed HIV viral load [5].

Pneumocystis is a ubiquitous yeast-like fungal organism that infects a wide array of mammalian hosts. Direct airborne transmission has been demonstrated in animal models. The reservoir for human infection is not completely understood, but the organism is also thought to be spread from person to person, and PCP is most likely the result of recent acquisition of *Pneumocystis*, rather than reactivation of a latent infection [6]. The incubation period from inhalation to presentation is thought to be between 4 and 8 weeks.

A review of post-mortem studies in Africa found PCP was accountable for 5.3% of death due to respiratory infections in adults and 17.9% of children. PCP in adults was found exclusively in HIV-infected persons and was 10-fold commoner in HIV-infected children than HIV-uninfected children [7]. It is increasingly being recognized as a cause of morbidity amongst HIV-infected persons in the developing world [8]. The HIV outpatient study cohort of 8070 patients in the US found that the incidence of PCP in this cohort decreased from 29.9 per 1000 person-years in the pre-ART era to 3.9 per 1000 person-years in the contemporary ART era [9].

In Europe, amongst 6578 patients diagnosed with AIDS across 17 countries, PCP was the commonest AIDS-defining illness in the pre-ART era (38.5%) [10]. In the UK, a review of routinely collected data, including hospital episode statistics, death certification, HIV surveillance data, and routine laboratory reporting, found that, although the number of cases of PCP amongst HIV-infected persons in the UK has decreased at a rate of 7% per year from 2000 to 2010, the number overall rose in the same time period and was accounted for by increasing diagnoses in transplant recipients and patients with haematological cancers [11].

The clinical features of PCP are non-specific and include progressive dyspnoea, fever, and non-productive cough [2]. The presentation in HIV-infected persons tends to be more indolent, when compared to non-HIV infected persons [12].

The diagnosis of PCP is made by visualizing the organism in an appropriately obtained microbiological specimen, either with a histochemical stain, such as Grocott–Gomori's methenamine silver stain, or an immunofluorescent stain. An induced sputum specimen (obtained by inhalation of nebulized hypertonic saline) has a diagnostic yield of between 55% and 67%, when compared to bronchoscopy and BAL [13]. Bronchoscopy with BAL has a high diagnostic yield of >90% [14]; transbronchial biopsy is rarely performed, as it adds little to diagnosis and is associated with complications, including haemorrhage and pneumothorax.

Detection of *Pneumocystis* DNA in BAL fluid or induced sputum using polymerase chain reaction (PCR) is better than histochemical staining for the diagnosis of PCP. Unfortunately, the specificity and clinical interpretation of finding *Pneumocystis* DNA in BAL fluid or induced sputum is reduced by the observation that *Pneumocystis* DNA can also be found in asymptomatic HIV-infected persons with low CD4 counts and in symptomatic patients who do not have PCP but instead have confirmed alternative diagnoses; in these situations, the detectable *Pneumocystis* DNA reflects colonization [15].

1,3-beta-D-glucan is a major cell wall component present in most pathogenic fungi, including *P. jirovecii*. Its concentration in serum has been used as an adjunctive test for invasive fungal disease, including PCP. It has a high sensitivity and specificity for the diagnosis of PCP [16, 17]. Caution is advised because false-positive results may occur due to beta-lactam antibiotic use and exposure to cellulose membranes/filters during haemodialysis, and in those who have recently received intravenous immunoglobulin [18]. Serial measurements of 1,3-beta-D-glucan cannot be used to monitor treatment response in PCP, as reductions in titre are unpredictable and sometimes delayed, despite clinical recovery.

TMP-SMX (co-trimoxazole) for 21 days is the first-line treatment for PCP [19–21]. TMP-SMX is effective in 70–80% of patients. Adverse reactions are common and are usually first evident after 7–10 days of treatment; anaemia and neutropenia occurring in approximately 40%, fever in approximately 30%, rash in approximately 25%, and abnormal LFTs in approximately 10% are the most commonly described. Adverse reactions are severe enough to warrant a change of treatment in approximately 15–17%. Co-administration of folic or folinic acid does not reduce the frequency of haematological toxicity. Treatment failure, defined as persistent fever and worsening hypoxia and/or radiographic deterioration, occurring after ≥4 full days of first-line or second-line therapy, occurs in approximately 7%. The overall prognosis of PCP is largely unchanged if TMP-SMX is stopped and second-line therapy is started because of toxicity. By contrast, if treatment is changed because of failure, the outcome is poor.

Before ascribing clinical deterioration to treatment failure, it is important to exclude pulmonary oedema caused by intravenous fluid overload when giving TMP-SMX, anaemia secondary to TMP-SMX, methaemoglobinaemia secondary to dapsone or primaquine, inadequate therapy, i.e. the wrong dosage is being administered, post-bronchoscopy deterioration due to sedation or pneumothorax, pneumothorax occurring spontaneously or associated with CPAP or mechanical ventilation, untreated pulmonary co-disease, e.g. Kaposi's sarcoma, PE, or bacterial infection, and consideration given to performing bronchoscopy if the diagnosis of PCP has been made empirically and the correct diagnosis is another disease. The choice of treatment with a second-line regimen is based on tolerance and toxicity, as the evidence base does not identify one regimen as being unequivocally superior to another [3, 22, 23].

Early initiation of ART (at 2 weeks) following the diagnosis of PCP is recommended by both US and UK treatment guidelines [3]. The optimal timing is not known. Clinicians need to balance the risk of an acute inflammatory response (immune reconstitution inflammatory syndrome) if ART is commenced early versus the benefit of ART in reducing mortality, when making treatment decisions. Some clinicians commence ART immediately following the diagnosis of PCP; others wait until there is an objective clinical response to PCP treatment. In patients with severe PCP who are admitted to the ICU, many clinicians wait until the patient has been extubated and has reducing oxygen requirements before starting ART.

Primary prophylaxis to prevent PCP is recommended for HIV-infected patients with a CD4 cell count of <200 cells/microlitre or a CD4 cell/total lymphocyte count ratio of <1:5 or <14% and for those with unexplained constitutional symptoms, oral *Candida*, or another AIDS-defining diagnosis, e.g. Kaposi's sarcoma, regardless of their CD4 count [24]. Secondary prophylaxis is given to patients after an episode of PCP to prevent recurrence, until the patient has shown a sustained CD4 count response after starting ART. The preferred regimen is one double-strength TMP-SMX tablet (960 mg) or one 480 mg tablet od. The 480 mg dose is associated with fewer side effects. Other drug regimens may be used if toxicity prevents the use of TMP-SMX (Table 8.3). Prophylaxis of PCP with TMP-SMX may also protect against toxoplasmosis and other bacterial infections [25].

Table 8.3 Primary and secondary prophylaxis for PCP

Drug	Dose
Trimethoprim-sulfamethoxazole (co-trimoxazole, TMP-SMX)	960 mg od or 480 mg od, orally
Dapsone	100 mg od orally or 50–200 mg od orally, together with pyrimethamine 75 mg and folinic acid 25 mg, both orally once a week
Pentamidine	300 mg nebulized every 4 weeks, given via a Respirgard II nebulizer (once every 2 weeks if CD4 count <50 cells/microlitre)
Atovaquone	750 mg bd orally, with or without pyrimethamine 75 mg and folinic acid 25 mg orally od

Nelson, M., et al., British HIV Association and British Infection Association guidelines for the treatment of opportunistic infection in HIV-seropositive individuals 2011. HIV Med, 2011. 12 Suppl 2: p. 1–140.

Evidence base Early Antiretroviral therapy trial in opportunistic infections

- A total of 282 patients randomized to either early ART (2 weeks after diagnosis) or deferred ART (6 weeks after diagnosis) [26].
- Opportunistic infections included PCP, cryptococcal meningitis, and bacterial infections.
- Early ART was associated with a significant reduction in HIV disease progression/mortality, but with no increased risk of immune reconstitution inflammatory syndrome.
- While there is evidence for starting early ART in mild to moderate PCP, the optimal timing in severe PCP remains to be determined.

Evidence base Consensus statement on the use of corticosteroids as adjunctive therapy for *Pneumocystis* pneumonia in acquired immune deficiency syndrome

- Assessed five RCTs including a total of 406 patients [27].
- Three of five studies showed reduced short-term mortality when adjunctive corticosteroids were used.
- Two studies showed stabilization of oxygenation when corticosteroids were initiated in conjunction with anti-*Pneumocystis* therapy.
- Final recommendation was to start adjunctive corticosteroid therapy simultaneously with anti-*Pneumocystis* therapy and definitely within 72 hours.
- Presumptive treatment should be started, while a definitive diagnosis is awaited.

A final word from the expert

In the UK and the US, PCP caused by the yeast-like fungus *P. jirovecii* continues to be a common presentation among HIV-infected persons unaware of their serostatus or who are unable to access, or are intolerant of, prophylaxis and/or ART. PCP is increasingly recognized in tropical and low- and middle-income countries. The 'gold standard' diagnostic test for PCP is bronchoscopy with BAL and molecular detection techniques applied to BAL fluid or induced sputum. Although superior to histochemical staining at detecting *Pneumocystis*, they currently do not reliably discriminate between colonization and disease. The use of adjunctive biomarkers, such as serum 1, 3-beta-D-glucan, needs further evaluation. First-line treatment of PCP, regardless of severity, is TMP-SMX (co-trimoxazole); adjunctive corticosteroids are given if PaO_2 is <9.3 kPa or A–a oxygen gradient is >4.7 kPa. Both US and UK treatment guidelines recommend initiating ART 'early' after the diagnosis of PCP, but the optimal time to start ART in those with severe disease ± on the ICU remains uncertain. In the era of ART, mortality from PCP in the UK and the US is between 10% and 12%.

References

1. Smith DE, McLuckie A, Wyatt J, Gazzard B. Severe exercise hypoxaemia with normal or near normal X-rays: a feature of Pneumocystis carinii infection. *Lancet* 1988;**2**:1049–51.
2. Miller RF, Huang L, Walzer PD. Pneumocystis pneumonia associated with human immunodeficiency virus. *Clin Chest Med* 2013;**34**:229–41.
3. Nelson M, Dockrell D, Edwards S *et al.* British HIV Association and British Infection Association guidelines for the treatment of opportunistic infection in HIV-seropositive individuals 2011. *HIV Med* 2011;**12**(Suppl 2):1–140.
4. Walzer PD, Evans HE, Copas AJ, Edwards SG, Grant AD, Miller RF. Early predictors of mortality from Pneumocystis jirovecii pneumonia in HIV-infected patients: 1985–2006. *Clin Infect Dis* 2008;**46**:625–33.
5. Lyles RH, Chu C, Mellors JW *et al.* Prognostic value of plasma HIV RNA in the natural history of Pneumocystis carinii pneumonia, cytomegalovirus and Mycobacterium avium complex. Multicenter AIDS Cohort Study. *AIDS* 1999;**13**:341–9.
6. Gigliotti F, Wright TW. Pneumocystis: where does it live? *PLoS Pathog* 2012;**8**:e1003025.
7. Bates M, Mudenda V, Mwaba P, Zumla A. Deaths due to respiratory tract infections in Africa: a review of autopsy studies. *Curr Opin Pulm Med* 2013;**19**:229–37.
8. Lowe DM, Rangaka MX, Gordon F, James CD, Miller RF. Pneumocystis jirovecii pneumonia in tropical and low and middle income countries: a systematic review and meta-regression. *PLoS One* 2013;**8**:e69969.
9. Buchacz K, Baker RK, Palella FJ Jr *et al.* AIDS-defining opportunistic illnesses in US patients, 1994–2007: a cohort study. *AIDS* 2010;**24**:1549–59.
10. Blaxhult A, Kirk O, Pedersen C *et al.* Regional differences in presentation of AIDS in Europe. *Epidemiol Infect* 2000;**125**:143–51.
11. Maini R, Henderson KL, Sheridan EA *et al.* Increasing Pneumocystis pneumonia, England, UK, 2000–2010. *Emerg Infect Dis* 2013;**19**:386–92.
12. Tasaka S, Tokuda H, Sakai F *et al.* Comparison of clinical and radiological features of pneumocystis pneumonia between malignancy cases and acquired immunodeficiency syndrome cases: a multicenter study. *Intern Med* 2010;**49**:273–81.
13. Oliveira GM, Cordeiro AM, Marsico GA, Rentería JM, Guimarães CA. Induced sputum in HIV- infected patients: diagnosis of acute pulmonary diseases. *Rev Assoc Med Bras* 2009;**55**:617–20.
14. Stover DE, White DA, Romano PA, Gellene RA. Diagnosis of pulmonary disease in acquired immune deficiency syndrome (AIDS). Role of bronchoscopy and bronchoalveolar lavage. *Am Rev Respir Dis* 1984;**130**:659–62.
15. Huggett JF, Taylor MS, Kocjan G *et al.* Development and evaluation of a real-time PCR assay for detection of Pneumocystis jirovecii DNA in bronchoalveolar lavage fluid of HIV-infected patients. *Thorax* 2008;**63**:154–9.
16. Onishi A, Sugiyama D, Kogata Y *et al.* Diagnostic accuracy of serum 1,3-beta-D-glucan for pneumocystis jirovecii pneumonia, invasive candidiasis, and invasive aspergillosis: systematic review and meta-analysis. *J Clin Microbiol* 2012;**50**:7–15.

17. Sax PE, Komarow L, Finkelman MA *et al.* Blood (1->3)-beta-D-glucan as a diagnostic test for HIV-related Pneumocystis jirovecii pneumonia. *Clin Infect Dis* 2011;**53**:197–202.
18. Green MR. A modicum of caution for blood (1->3)-beta-D-glucan testing for Pneumocystis jurovecii in HIV-infected patients. *Clin Infect Dis* 2011;**53**:1039–40; author reply 1040.
19. Wharton JM, Coleman DL, Wofsy CB *et al.* Trimethoprim-sulfamethoxazole or pentamidine for Pneumocystis carinii pneumonia in the acquired immunodeficiency syndrome. A prospective randomized trial. *Ann Intern Med* 1986;**105**:37–44.
20. Sattler FR, Cowan R, Nielsen DM, Ruskin J. Trimethoprim-sulfamethoxazole compared with pentamidine for treatment of Pneumocystis carinii pneumonia in the acquired immunodeficiency syndrome. A prospective, noncrossover study. *Ann Intern Med* 1988;**109**:280–7.
21. Klein NC, Duncanson FP, Lenox TH *et al.* Trimethoprim-sulfamethoxazole versus pentamidine for Pneumocystis carinii pneumonia in AIDS patients: results of a large prospective randomized treatment trial. *AIDS* 1992;**6**:301–5.
22. Benfield T, Atzori C, Miller RF, Helweg-Larsen J. Second-line salvage treatment of AIDS-associated Pneumocystis jirovecii pneumonia: a case series and systematic review. *J Acquir Immune Defic Syndr* 2008;**48**:63–7.
23. Hughes W, Leoung G, Kramer F *et al.* Comparison of atovaquone (566C80) with trimethoprim-sulfamethoxazole to treat Pneumocystis carinii pneumonia in patients with AIDS. *N Engl J Med* 1993;**328**:1521–7.
24. Schneider MM, Hoepelman AI, Eeftinck Schattenkerk JK *et al.* A controlled trial of aerosolized pentamidine or trimethoprim-sulfamethoxazole as primary prophylaxis against Pneumocystis carinii pneumonia in patients with human immunodeficiency virus infection. The Dutch AIDS Treatment Group. *N Engl J Med* 1992;**327**:1836–41.
25. Hardy WD, Feinberg J, Finkelstein DM *et al.* A controlled trial of trimethoprim-sulfamethoxazole or aerosolized pentamidine for secondary prophylaxis of Pneumocystis carinii pneumonia in patients with the acquired immunodeficiency syndrome. AIDS Clinical Trials Group Protocol 021. *N Engl J Med* 1992;**327**:1842–8.
26. Zolopa A, Andersen J, Powderly W *et al.* Early antiretroviral therapy reduces AIDS progression/death in individuals with acute opportunistic infections: a multicenter randomized strategy trial. *PLoS One* 2009;**4**:e5575.
27. The National Institutes of Health-University of California Expert Panel for Corticosteroids as Adjunctive Therapy for Pneumocystis Pneumonia. Consensus statement on the use of corticosteroids as adjunctive therapy for pneumocystis pneumonia in the acquired immunodeficiency syndrome. *N Engl J Med* 1990;**323**:1500–4.

CASE

Intensive care unit and ventilation

Justin Garner

Expert commentary David Treacher

Case history

A 45-year-old gentleman, previously healthy, was brought to his district general hospital with a 3-day history of rapidly worsening shortness of breath, coughing yellow sputum, and feverishness. He denied upper respiratory symptoms, wheeziness, and recent foreign travel but admitted to a 20 pack-year smoking history. A temperature of 39°C, pulse of 120 beats/minute, blood pressure of 99/85 mmHg, respiratory rate of 40 breaths/minute, oxygen saturations of 78% on room air, marked use of accessory muscles, and crepitations throughout his chest were observed. His jugular venous pressure (JVP) was not elevated, and heart sounds were normal. There was no wheeze. An ABG showed a pH of 7.49, $PaCO_2$ of 3.8 kPa, PaO_2 of 5.6 kPa, base excess of −0.4 mmol/L, and HCO_3 of 22.1 mmol/L. Fifteen litres of oxygen per minute delivered via a non-rebreathe face mask increased saturations to 100%.

Clinical tip Respiratory failure and alveolar-arterial (A–a) gradient

Respiratory failure is traditionally divided into two types [1]:

- type 1 respiratory failure: hypoxia (PaO_2 <8 kPa) with a normal $PaCO_2$;
- type 2 respiratory failure: hypoxia with hypercapnia ($PaCO_2$ >6.7 kPa).

The alveolar-arterial (A–a) gradient is helpful in determining the cause of hypoxaemia in patients breathing room air. For example, a normal gradient is observed at high altitude and in alveolar hypoventilation, when the lung parenchyma is normal. An increased gradient reflects defective gas exchange, which may be due to impaired diffusion, V/Q mismatch (commonest), or a right-to-left shunt, this unresponsive to an increase in FiO_2.

A–a gradient = $PAO_2 - PaO_2$

$$PaO_2 = FiO_2 \times (P_{ATM} - P_{H_2O}) - PaCO_2/R$$
$$= FiO_2 \times 95 - PaCO_2/0.8$$

where:

P_{ATM} (atmospheric pressure) at sea level = 101.3 kPa;

P_{H_2O} (partial pressure of water) at body temperature = 6.3 kPa;

R (respiratory exchange ratio, a constant) = 0.8.

Normal A–a gradient = (0.044 × age) − 0.3 kPa

Assuming an FiO_2 of 21% on room air, this gentleman has a significant defect in gas exchange of 9.6 kPa (expected = 1.68 kPa) due to a structural lung problem.

Learning point Lung compliance

Lung compliance is defined as a change in lung volume per unit change in transmural pressure gradient and is the inverse of elastance [1]. Reduced lung compliance is seen in ARDS where alveolar oedema and surfactant dysfunction make the lungs increasingly 'stiff'.

Clinical tip Management of oxygenation and carbon dioxide removal

Oxygenation is achieved by increasing the FiO_2 or the level of PEEP, which recruits alveoli to take place in gas exchange. Carbon dioxide clearance is dependent on minute ventilation and can be controlled by changes in the respiratory rate and/or tidal volume.

Clinical tip Pneumothorax in the ventilated patient

Pneumothorax has been reported in up to 15% of ventilated ICU patients. Ultrasound is increasingly recognized as the imaging modality of choice for diagnosis and management in these patients [2]. The 2010 BTS guidelines recommend intercostal drainage for any pneumothorax in a ventilated patient, as positive pressure tends to maintain the air leak [3].

A portable CXR revealed patchy infiltrates throughout both lungs. Acute respiratory distress syndrome (ARDS) secondary to pneumonia was diagnosed.

The Casualty Officer established IV access and started fluids and antibiotics, a penicillin and a macrolide. Ventilation with a full face mask using an inspiratory positive airways pressure (IPAP) of 15 cmH_2O and an expiratory positive airways pressure (EPAP) of 5 cmH_2O was attempted but poorly tolerated. Within 20 minutes, his respiratory rate had increased to 44 breaths/minute and his pulse to 135 beats/minute, and his blood pressure had fallen to 88/72 mmHg. The intensive care registrar, on arrival, ordered a 500-mL saline bolus and 2 mg of metaraminol IV. The blood pressure increased to 108/87 mmHg. The patient was intubated using a rapid induction sequence. A decreased compliance on manual ventilation was noted.

He was transferred to the ICU for mechanical ventilation. Volume-targeted assist control ventilation (ACV) was selected with the following settings: fraction of inspired oxygen (FiO_2) of 0.9, rate of 16 breaths/minute, tidal volume of 6 mL/kg ideal body weight, peak inspiratory flow of around 60 L/minute (titrated to achieve a peak airway pressure of not more than 30 cmH_2O), and a positive end-expiratory pressure (PEEP) of 10 cmH_2O. A right internal jugular venous catheter and a radial arterial line were sited. Noradrenaline was infused to maintain a mean arterial blood pressure of >65 mmHg.

After 24 hours of invasive ventilation employing an FiO_2 of 0.9 and a PEEP of 20 cmH_2O, his PaO_2 falls from 10 kPa to 7 kPa. A CT chest with contrast demonstrated bilateral diffuse GGO and consolidation and a 1.8-cm left pneumothorax. There was no evidence of PE. A small-bore intercostal drain was inserted using the Seldinger technique and attached to an underwater seal on free drainage.

Expert comment

It is very difficult to identify an anterior pneumothorax on an anteroposterior (AP) CXR. Comments about relative lucency on one side, compared to the other side, may be made with confidence, but usually only after the diagnosis has been confirmed by CT scan! The other advantage of performing an early CT scan is that it quantifies the extent and degree of progression of the lung injury and also allows identification of other pathologies presenting with bilateral infiltrates and severe respiratory failure.

A switch to high-frequency oscillatory ventilation (HFOV) was made in an attempt to improve oxygenation and reduce the risk of further lung injury. Nasogastric feeding was instituted, and fluid restricted to 1 L/day. The microbiology laboratory reported pneumococcal antigen in the urine. The retroviral screen was negative. No changes were made in the antibiotic regime. Overnight, a continuous infusion of low-dose hydrocortisone was commenced on account of hypotension poorly responsive to repeated fluid challenges and increasing vasopressor support. After a further 48 hours, refractory hypoxaemia prompted referral to a tertiary centre offering extracorporeal membrane oxygenation (ECMO). A mobile team retrieved the patient and established venous–venous support, with systemic anticoagulation. Mechanical ventilation was continued using 'lung rest' settings: FiO_2 of 0.3, rate of 10 breaths/minute, tidal volume of 3 mL/kg ideal body weight, peak airway pressure of not more than 20 cmH_2O, and PEEP of 10 cmH_2O.

On the tenth day a percutaneous tracheostomy was performed. After 1 month on ECMO, a favourable response was heralded by falling oxygen requirement and an improving X-ray appearance. He was weaned onto conventional ventilator settings, and ECMO discontinued. Three days later, nursing staff reported fevers of up to 38.5°C and increased respiratory tract secretions. A CXR showed new consolidation in the right lower and mid zones.

Clinical tip Ventilator-associated pneumonia

Ventilator-associated pneumonia (VAP) is the commonest nosocomial infection on the ICU, with an estimated attributable mortality of 9% [4]. It develops 48 hours or more following tracheal intubation and can be classified as early or late onset; after 4 days, the emergence of multidrug-resistant organisms becomes a problem [5]. The presence of a tracheal tube encourages bacterial colonization and entry to the lower respiratory tract via micro-aspiration of pooled oropharyngeal secretions. Lack of consensus criteria makes diagnosis a challenge. VAP should be suspected when there are new or persistent infiltrates on CXR plus two or more of the following:

- purulent tracheal secretions;
- leucocytosis (>12 × 10^9 white cells/L) OR leucopenia (<4 × 10^9 white cells/L);
- temperature >38.3°C.

Obtaining respiratory tract secretions for microbiological analysis is recommended. Tracheal sampling can be performed non-invasively or invasively (using a bronchoscope), and it is unclear which is superior. Diagnostic biomarkers, including soluble triggering receptor expressed on myeloid type 1 (sTREM-1) cells, procalcitonin, and CRP are yet to be validated in clinical practice [6]. Bacteria account for most cases; the predominant organisms are *Staphylococcus aureus*, *Pseudomonas aeruginosa*, and *Enterobacteriaceae* [7]. Prompt empirical antibiotic therapy should be administered. Antimicrobial choice is guided by the laboratory and is influenced by local resistance rates, the duration of hospital stay, severity of illness, and previous antibiotic exposure. Therapy is subsequently rationalized according to culture sensitivities. Measures to prevent VAP include reducing airway colonization with oral antiseptic, nursing in the semi-recumbent position to protect against aspiration, and minimizing the duration of mechanical ventilation delivered as a 'care bundle' [8].

Broad-spectrum antimicrobial therapy, including Gram-negative cover for nosocomial organisms, was started after discussion with the microbiologist. A non-bronchoscopic lung lavage (NBL) specimen cultured *Klebsiella* sensitive to gentamicin, cefotaxime, and imipenem. The antibiotic regime was rationalized to cefotaxime and continued for 7 days.

Combined spontaneous breathing trials with sedation holds were used to facilitate ventilatory weaning, and oral sedation was substituted for IV. The patient's tracheostomy was gradually downsized before decannulation on day 50. He was transferred to a general medical ward for rehabilitation and discharged home on the seventieth day. Reviewed in clinic at 6 months, he had been offered cognitive behavioural therapy and medication for depression by his GP but had returned to work as a computer engineer.

Discussion

During the Copenhagen polio epidemic of 1952, a Danish anaesthetist Björn Ibsen revolutionized the management of respiratory failure and introduced the concept of intensive care medicine [9]. Polio victims with respiratory and bulbar paralysis had been supported with negative pressure ventilation in a tank-like enclosure known as an 'iron lung'. These were effective ventilators, but their numbers were limited, and they did not protect against aspiration of secretions. Bower and Bennet [10] had utilized intermittent positive pressure ventilation as an adjunct to a tank respirator in patients with polio in 1948, but it was Ibsen who adopted this as a first-line therapy using cuffed tracheostomy tubes, minimizing the risk of aspiration and facilitating bronchial toilet. Ibsen's team enlisted thousands of volunteers, medical, nursing, and dental students, to deliver manual positive pressure ventilation around the clock to his patients. The dramatic improvements in survival encouraged him to extend his methods to all cases of respiratory failure in a centralized area manned by an MDT, creating the first 'intensive care unit' in 1953. The modern mechanical ventilator is a sophisticated microprocessor device that incorporates feedback loops and alarm systems to enable precise and safe regulation of breathing. Negative pressure devices have become obsolete.

The indications for ventilation can be broadly categorized into problems of oxygen transfer, hypoventilation, and increased work of breathing. Mechanical ventilation improves gas exchange, reduces V/Q mismatching, and assists the patient's work of breathing. Ventilation can be delivered non-invasively using a nasal or orofacial interface or invasively via a tracheostomy or an endotracheal tube. The decision-making process is guided by the patient's clinical condition, i.e. the security of the airway, the degree of respiratory distress or exhaustion, and the likelihood of deterioration, and is supported by pulse oximetry, haemodynamic status, and ABG analysis (Box 9.1) [11].

Expert comment

The indication for intubation and ventilation is not solely respiratory pathology. Other organ failure may result in the need for intubation and ventilation: (i) neurological: bulbar dysfunction, loss of respiratory drive, (ii) pharmacological/metabolic: excess sedation/analgesia/overdose, need for general anaesthesia, hepatic encephalopathy, severe metabolic acidosis, (iii) cardiac: severe left ventricular myocardial failure, cardiac arrest, recalcitrant ventricular tachycardia/ventricular fibrillation, and (iv) abdominal: distension, severe pain, post-major abdominal surgery. Few patients require 'weaning' after a relatively brief period of ventilation; when the precipitating cause has resolved sufficiently, they can be extubated without delay.

NIV is an option for patients with a secure airway who have hypercapnic respiratory failure or cardiogenic pulmonary oedema. Invasive ventilation is preferred for most other patients.

Box 9.1 Criteria for intubation and ventilation

Criteria for intubation

Airway protection
Airway obstruction
To assist sedation and neuromuscular paralysis

Criteria for ventilation

Cardiac arrest
Respiratory arrest or profound bradypnoea
Exhaustion
Hypoxia
Hypercapnia
To manipulate alveolar ventilation (e.g. decreased PCO_2 in head injury)
To stabilize the chest wall in traumatic injury
To facilitate investigations and/or treatment of other conditions

Source: Appelboam R. Indications for ventilatory support. Advanced Respiratory Critical Care 2011: 69–72, Oxford University Press.

Learning point The ventilator-assisted breath

Ventilators are classified as pressure, volume, or flow controllers. These parameters, the trigger to inspiration, and the cycling to expiration are programmable and determine the 'shape' of the breath [12]. Volume and flow controllers produce almost identical graphical profiles (Figure 9.1).

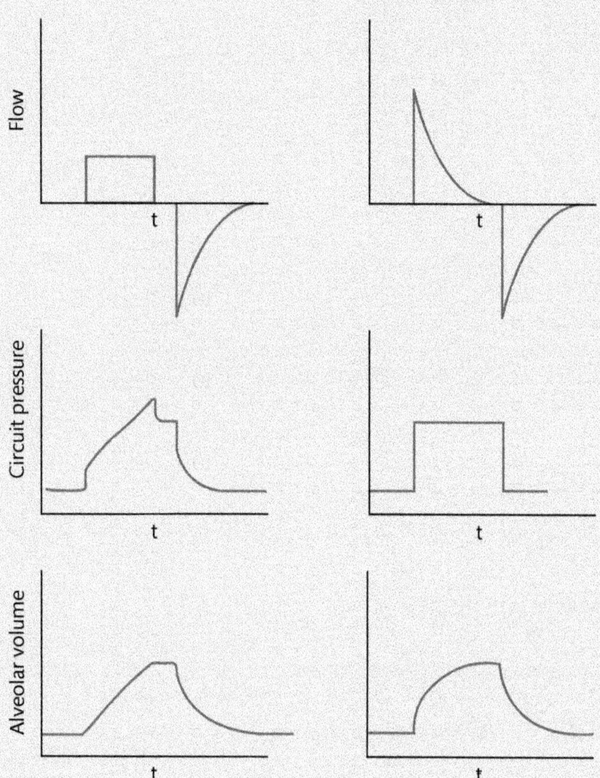

Figure 9.1 Flow, pressure, and volume changes in volume-targeted (left) and pressure-targeted (right) ventilation [12].

During volume-targeted ventilation, the following features are notable:

- **flow-time curve**: a constant flow rate (L/minute), in the shape of a square waveform, delivers a preset tidal volume;
- **volume-time curve**: tidal volume increases linearly;
- **pressure-time curve** (Figure 9.2):
  - peak airway pressure (Pap) is the maximum pressure achieved at end-inspiration (Pap = resistance pressure + compliance pressure + PEEP);
  - plateau pressure (Pplat) is measured at the end of an inspiratory hold manoeuvre and reflects lung elasticity (Pplat = compliance pressure + PEEP)—values >30 cmH2O are associated with lung injury;
  - positive end-expiratory pressure is a baseline pressure set above atmospheric pressure and maintained throughout the respiratory cycle;
  - elevated resistance pressure indicates airways obstruction (e.g. endotracheal blockage, increased intraluminal secretions, or bronchospasm);
  - elevated compliance pressure indicates decreased elasticity (e.g. unilateral lung intubation, ARDS, chest wall deformity, or ascites).

(Continued)

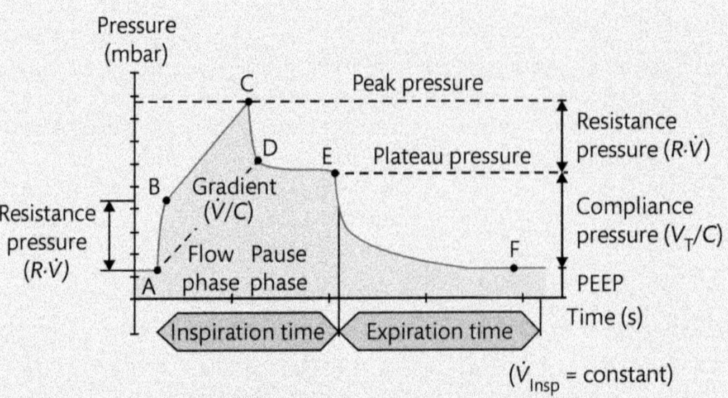

Figure 9.2 Pressure changes during volume-targeted ventilation [12].

During pressure-targeted ventilation, the following features are notable:

- **flow-time curve**: inspiratory flow has a decelerating waveform;
- **volume-time curve**: delivery of tidal volume results in a non-linear waveform;
- **pressure-time curve**: a constant inspiratory pressure delivers a variable tidal volume.

Learning point Invasive ventilator modes

To encourage a principle-based approach, modes have been divided into: volume-targeted, pressure-targeted, flow-targeted, and hybrid/adaptive modes [13].

Volume-targeted mode

Volume-targeted ventilation delivers a preset tidal volume, achieved with a variable pressure. The following parameters can be adjusted: tidal volume (V_t), machine rate, inspiratory:expiratory time ratio (according to peak inspiratory flow rate), and flow-time profile (e.g. decelerating or sinusoidal).

Controlled mechanical ventilation (CMV) is used in unconscious patients and provides full ventilatory support, regardless of respiratory effort. Sedation and neuromuscular blockade are often required, and long-term ventilation leads to disuse atrophy of the respiratory muscles. CMV has evolved into the assist control mode, which facilitates patient-ventilator interaction.

Assist control (AC) ventilation is commonly used in severe respiratory failure. The ventilator 'assists' patient effort with delivery of a set tidal volume. Independent breaths are generated if the respiratory rate falls below a pre-determined rate.

Intermittent mandatory ventilation (IMV) delivers breaths of set tidal volume at a fixed rate, irrespective of patient effort. The patient can trigger additional breaths, but these are unsupported. Asynchrony between patient and ventilator can lead to breath stacking and overinflation.

Synchronized intermittent mandatory ventilation (SIMV) is an improvement on IMV in which a set number of mandatory breaths are synchronized to the patient's inspiratory effort. The patient can trigger additional breaths, which can be unsupported or supported (using pressure support ventilation). SIMV is commonly used post-operatively and in ventilatory weaning, as it encourages the patient to breathe spontaneously.

Pressure-targeted mode

Pressure-targeted ventilation delivers a constant inspiratory pressure with variable tidal volume. The following parameters can be adjusted: target pressure (P_{set}), machine rate, inspiratory:expiratory time ratio, and inspiratory time rise (time to P_{set} or 'ramp'). The same modes are used as for volume-targeted ventilation, in addition to biphasic positive airway pressure ventilation (BIPAP) and airway pressure release ventilation (APRV).

(Continued)

BIPAP delivers alternating high and low continuous positive airways pressure (CPAP), whereas APRV combines high CPAP with very brief timed pressure releases. BIPAP and APRV allow unrestricted spontaneous breathing throughout the mechanical cycle and achieve additional 'passive ventilation'. Of note, CPAP refers to the application of a constant positive pressure and is not strictly a form of ventilation alone, as it does not deliver pressured breaths.

Flow-targeted mode

Pressure support ventilation (PSV) is a patient-triggered, flow-cycled mode that assists spontaneous ventilation. The clinician sets the inspiratory pressure and flow rate at which to cycle (usually 25% of peak inspiratory flow). It is often used as part of a weaning strategy from mechanical ventilation. Proportional assist ventilation (PAV) has developed this mode further by varying pressure support according to patient effort.

Hybrid/adaptive modes

Pressure-regulated volume control (PRVC), adaptive support ventilation (ASV), and neurally adjusted ventilator assist (NAVA) are designed to more closely resemble physiological breath delivery. They are as yet unproven.

Clinical tip Sudden deterioration on a ventilator

Use an 'ABC' approach. Ask for the resuscitation trolley and emergency drugs for intubation and circulatory support to be on standby [14].

Try to answer the following questions.

1. Is a ventilator alarm triggered (oxygen failure, peak airway pressure, minute volume)? What mode and FiO_2 are selected? Are expiratory and inspiratory tidal volumes similar? Is there persistent expiratory flow? Are the tubing connections intact?
2. Is the patient's appearance in keeping with the monitors?
3. Is the tracheal tube displaced? Is there a cuff leak (check using a manometer)?
4. Are both sides of the chest moving?
5. Are there focal chest or cardiac signs?

In the absence of an obvious cause for respiratory distress, the 'feel' on manual ventilation may provide information, e.g. a bouncing or tight character in tube blockage or bronchospasm.

Following the above bedside assessment, perform a full examination, and request urgent baseline investigations (including ABG analysis, ECG, CXR ± echocardiogram).

The vignette illustrates a case of ARDS. ARDS and the less severe acute lung injury (ALI) are characterized by rapid-onset hypoxaemic respiratory failure and non-cardiogenic bilateral pulmonary infiltrates and account for 10–15% of admissions to the ICU [15]. The 1994 American-European Consensus Conference (AECC) definition distinguished ALI from ARDS according to the severity of hypoxaemia, with a PaO_2/FiO_2 ratio of ≤40 kPa (300 mmHg) and ≤27 kPa (200 mmHg), respectively [16]. Patients who fulfil the ARDS criteria have been shown to have higher mortality [17]. However, its validity has been challenged for the following reasons: (i) oxygenation criteria is independent of PEEP and ventilatory mode; (ii) radiological findings are non-specific and subjective; and (iii) pulmonary wedge pressure is not routinely measured. The Murray Lung Injury Score (LIS) expands on the ARDS definition and comprises four components: severity of hypoxaemia (PaO_2/FiO_2 ratio), more specific radiographic findings, level of PEEP, and pulmonary compliance (score 0 = no lung injury; score 1–2.5 = mild to moderate lung injury; score >2.5 = severe lung injury) [18]. However, cardiogenic pulmonary oedema is not excluded. The

Learning point Biomarkers

A number of biomarkers are currently being assessed to establish their role in the diagnosis and prognostication of ARDS, e.g. neutrophil chemotactic factor, IL-8, and surfactant protein D (SP-D), expressed by type 2 alveolar cells [22].

Box 9.2 'Berlin' definition of ARDS

ARDS criteria	
Timing	Acute onset within 1 week of insult
Oxygenation	PaO_2/FiO_2 ratio of ≤40 kPa (300 mmHg) with PEEP ≥5 cmH_2O
Chest radiograph	Bilateral infiltrates
Pulmonary oedema	Not fully explained by cardiac failure or fluid overload
Oxygenation criteria	
Mild	PaO_2/FiO_2 ratio of ≤40 kPa (300 mmHg) with PEEP ≥5 cmH_2O
Moderate	PaO_2/FiO_2 ratio of ≤27 kPa (200 mmHg) with PEEP ≥5 cmH_2O
Severe	PaO_2/FiO_2 ratio of ≤13 kPa (100 mmHg) with PEEP ≥5 cmH_2O

Source: Adapted from ARDS Definition Task Force *et al*. Acute respiratory distress syndrome: the Berlin Definition. JAMA 2012; 307(23):2526–33.

Delphi definition addresses this deficiency using pulmonary artery catheterization or echocardiography. Both the LIS and Delphi definition have greater specificity than the AECC criteria, when correlated to autopsy findings [19]. The Berlin modification of the AECC criteria was proposed in 2011 and is currently in use [20]; ALI is no longer recognized, and ARDS is expanded—ranked as mild, moderate, and severe, according to the PaO_2/FiO_2 ratio with a PEEP of at least 5 cmH_2O. Onset within 1 week of causation is specified. Measurement of pulmonary wedge pressure is not required (Box 9.2).

Expert comment

The 1994 AECC definition has recently been updated. The 'Berlin' definition was presented at the European Society of Intensive Care Medicine (ESICM) meeting held in Berlin in October 2011 and published in 2012 [21]. It defines three categories on the basis of the hypoxaemia index: severe <100 mmHg, moderate >100 and <200 mmHg, and mild >200 and <300 mmHg. It also requires bilateral pulmonary infiltrates, respiratory system compliance of <40 mL/cmH_2O, PEEP ≥10 mmHg, and exp minute volume >10 L/minute. Notably, it does not specify a pulmonary wedge pressure of <18 mmHg.

The incidence of ALI/ARDS has significantly declined over the last decade, but mortality remains high at around 40%. The reasons for this are unclear. ARDS can result from pulmonary or extrapulmonary insults, of which sepsis is the most frequent [23] (Table 9.1).

Table 9.1 Pulmonary and extrapulmonary causes of ALI/ARDS

Pulmonary causes	Extrapulmonary causes
Common	**Common**
Pneumonia	Sepsis
Aspiration of gastric contents	Severe trauma with shock and multiple transfusions
Less common	**Less common**
Pulmonary contusion	Burns
Fat/amniotic fluid embolism	Disseminated intravascular coagulation
High altitude	Cardiopulmonary bypass
Near drowning	Drug overdose (e.g. heroin, barbiturates)
Inhalation injury	Acute pancreatitis
Reperfusion injury	Transfusion of blood products
	Hypoproteinaemia

Laycock H, Rajah A. Acute Lung Injury and Acute Respiratory Distress Syndrome: A Review Article. BJMP 2010; 3(2): 324.

The underlying pathology is diffuse alveolar damage characterized by inflammation, oedema, haemorrhage, and hyaline membrane formation. There is heterogeneous lung involvement, and surfactant function is impaired. This results in impaired gas exchange and reduced lung compliance [25].

Indiscriminate positive pressure ventilation may cause additional injury from overdistension (volutrauma), high plateau pressures (barotrauma), and repeated alveolar opening and collapse that generate injurious shearing forces on adjacent alveoli (atelectrauma). This, in turn, induces a secondary inflammatory response, adding to the traumatic process (biotrauma). Limiting ventilator-induced lung injury (VILI), which is clinically indistinguishable from ALI/ARDS, is now the focus of protective strategies that employ low tidal volumes of 4–6 mL/kg, permissive hypercapnia, and adequate PEEP to minimize cyclical atelectasis [26].

Low tidal volume

A 2009 meta-analysis of four RCTs (n = 1149), comparing low and high tidal volume ventilation at similar PEEP, supports a lower tidal volume strategy in reducing hospital mortality (odds ratio 0.75; 95% CI 0.58 to 0.96; p = 0.02) [27].

Evidence base The ARMA trial

The ARDS Network is a US-based multicentre clinical trials programme that was set up in 1994 to test emerging treatments and management protocols for patients with ARDS. The ARMA trial, conducted between March 1996 and July 1999, randomized 861 patients to either a low tidal volume (6 mL/kg ideal body weight) or conventional tidal volume (12 mL/kg ideal body weight) ventilation strategy [28]. Plateau pressure was limited to ≤30 cmH_2O and ≤50 cmH_2O, respectively. The lower tidal volume group had significantly reduced mortality at 180 days (31% versus 39.8%; p = 0.007) and more ventilator-free days (mean [± standard deviation, SD] 12 ± 11 versus 10 ± 11; p = 0.007). This was associated with reduced IL-6 levels.

A recently published multicentre prospective cohort study compared the 2-year mortality of patients with ALI whose ventilator settings, recorded twice a day, satisfied the criteria for lung protection throughout their stay with those whose settings were satisfactory only half the time and with those whose settings were never satisfactory. The improvement in survival for the first two groups was 7.8% and 4%, respectively [29].

Expert comment

Following the ARDS Network ARMA trial, there was considerable controversy about whether the higher level of tidal volume used in this study reflected routine clinical practice or indeed was ethical. Did it tell us whether a tidal volume of 8 mL/kg was more harmful than a tidal volume of 6 mL/kg? Subsequent studies have shown that, if indexed, as in the ARMA study, to ideal body weight, many clinicians were using a tidal volume of up to 12 mL/kg, and it is now generally accepted that the lowest tidal volume possible should be used to limit 'volutrauma', provided unacceptable respiratory acidosis (pH <7.15) does not result.

Of interest, despite the evidence and although nearly all clinicians will say that they do adhere to a tidal volume of 6 mL/kg ideal body weight, when audited, the tidal volume used in their units is frequently considerably higher!

Radiological correlation suggests that tidal volumes as low as 6 mL/kg may cause additional harm in those individuals with more significant lung injury, lending support to an ultralow volume strategy [30].

> **Expert comment**
>
> I would consider a respiratory acidosis of <7.10 as being too permissive. Most clinicians would accept a raised $PaCO_2$, provided the pH is not <7.15. At this stage, if no reversible factors can be identified, including reducing carbohydrate intake and cooling to <37.5°C, the patient should be considered for referral for extracorporeal CO_2 removal using the Novolung or a pumped veno-venous circuit or for ECMO if oxygenation is also markedly impaired with an FiO_2 of >0.6 (see CESAR criteria).

Permissive hypercapnia

Low tidal volume ventilation, without a sufficient rise in respiratory rate, may lead to hypercapnia with associated respiratory acidosis. Attempts to normalize gas exchange are relaxed, in order to minimize volume- and pressure-induced trauma to the already injured lung. The benefit of permissive hypercapnia is yet to be demonstrated in an RCT [31]. The physiological effects of this are often opposing and difficult to predict in an individual. Physicians will have varying thresholds before intervention, and, in the absence of any contraindication (e.g. cerebral pathology limiting a rise in intracranial pressure from vasodilation), a $PaCO_2$ of <15 kPa and a pH of 7.05–7.1, without the need for buffering, can be tolerated [32].

Positive end-expiratory pressure

PEEP is applied in an attempt to maximize alveolar recruitment, minimize trauma from alveolar overdistension (more open alveoli share tidal volume) and cyclical atelectasis, and increase oxygenation. Conversely, too much PEEP can cause barotrauma and reduced cardiac output. An 'open lung' strategy employs low tidal volumes combined with sufficient PEEP. The optimal level of PEEP is not known and is likely to vary according to the extent of recruitable lung [26]. In practice, PEEP can be titrated to SpO_2, PaO_2/FiO_2 ratio, lung compliance, or oxygen delivery. An RCT evaluated a decremental PEEP regimen following an alveolar recruitment manoeuvre, compared to table-based PEEP (control) titration from the ARDS Network. Despite an initial improvement in oxygenation in the decremental PEEP group, there was no difference in patient outcomes [33]. Five recent meta-analyses, including data from three large multicentre RCTs (ALEVOLI, LOVS, and EXPRESS), have looked at the role of a high versus low PEEP strategy in patients with ARDS. The evidence suggests a potential mortality benefit of using a higher PEEP strategy in those with severe ARDS [34–38].

Ventilatory mode

The majority of patients with ALI/ARDS require invasive ventilation. There are no trials directly comparing volume- with pressure-targeted ventilation. Assist control is generally favoured (Box 9.3). Alternative ventilatory modes used in ARDS include airway pressure release ventilation (APRV) and biphasic positive airways pressure ventilation (BIPAP), but neither have been shown to be superior to conventional ventilation. Inverse ratio ventilation is a strategy that prolongs inspiration relative to expiration (inspiration:expiration >1:1), designed to increase total PEEP (intrinsic and extrinsic) and mean airway pressure (mPaw) without increasing peak airway pressures. This facilitates alveolar recruitment and improves oxygenation, respectively. Too short an expiratory time can result in breath stacking and cardiovascular instability [26].

Box 9.3 Initial ventilator settings for assist control

Ventilator settings	
FiO_2	1.0
Frequency	14–16/minute
Tidal volume	6 mL/kg
Peak inspiratory flow rate	50–60 L/minute
Flow trigger sensitivity	2 L/minute

Learning point Recruitment manoeuvres and prone ventilation

A recruitment manoeuvre is the brief application of high pressure (e.g. 30–40 cmH_2O for 30–40 seconds) to reinflate collapsed alveoli used before setting PEEP and is used following ventilator circuit disruption or as a salvage technique for severe hypoxaemia. A 2009 Cochrane review of trials comparing recruitment manoeuvres to standard ventilatory care in patients with ALI/ARDS found no significant difference in 28-day mortality or risk of barotrauma and did not recommend their routine use [39].

Prone ventilation has been shown to reduce mortality in those individuals with severe acute hypoxaemic respiratory failure [40]. The mechanism is speculative. Nursing is difficult. Accidental extubation and displacement of lines are amongst the complications discouraging universal use [41].

High-frequency oscillatory ventilation

HFOV employs high respiratory rates of 3–10 Hz (180–600 breaths/minute) and very small tidal volumes (1–4 mL/kg), which may be less than the anatomical dead space. Peak airway pressures are reduced, avoiding overdistension, but an increase in mPaw is permitted, preventing alveolar collapse. The objective of HFOV is to improve oxygenation and minimize volutrauma. It is one of several options available to patients whose conventional ventilator settings within the lung protection range do not achieve adequate oxygenation [42, 43] (Figure 9.3).

The traditional concept of bulk flow cannot explain gas exchange. Novel mechanisms have been proposed, including bulk convection, convective dispersion due to asymmetric velocity profiles, pendelluft (asynchronous filling of adjacent alveoli due to varied emptying times), cardiogenic mixing, and augmented and molecular diffusion [44].

The oscillatory piston, analogous to a vibrating speaker diaphragm, intermittently compresses entrained gas (bias flow) to generate a sinusoidal waveform of inspiratory and expiratory pressures, which attenuates from ventilator to alveoli [45]. The bias flow is humidified and facilitates CO_2 removal. A resistance valve is used to control the mPaw (also termed the continuous distending pressure), which determines alveolar recruitment and lung volume. Oxygenation is regulated by the FiO_2 and mPaw. Ventilation or CO_2 removal is a function of tidal volume, which is directly related to the pressure excursion or amplitude of the piston (ΔP) but inversely related to respiratory frequency. The smaller tidal volumes, active expiratory phase (versus passive elastic lung recoil), and the facility to independently adjust oxygenation and ventilation distinguish it from conventional ventilation.

On initiation of HFOV, haemodynamic instability may occur, higher mPaws increasing the intrathoracic pressure and reducing the venous return. Prior adequate fluid replacement is recommended. Recruitment manoeuvres are recommended on commencing HFOV and after circuit interruption (e.g. for bronchoscopy). A closed suction system should be used to prevent derecruitment. Sedation and neuromuscular blockade are almost always needed.

Haemodynamic status, mPaw and ΔP, ABG analysis, and plain chest film are observed. Symmetrical chest vibration ('chest wiggle') is a useful sign confirming endotracheal tube placement, an airway clear of mucus, and the exclusion of a pneumothorax. Lung overdistension is suggested by worsening gas exchange (particularly rising pCO_2) with hypotension or a reduction in cardiac output. Consider weaning to conventional ventilation when the mPaw is <22 cmH_2O and the FiO_2 is 0.4 for at least 24 hours [46].

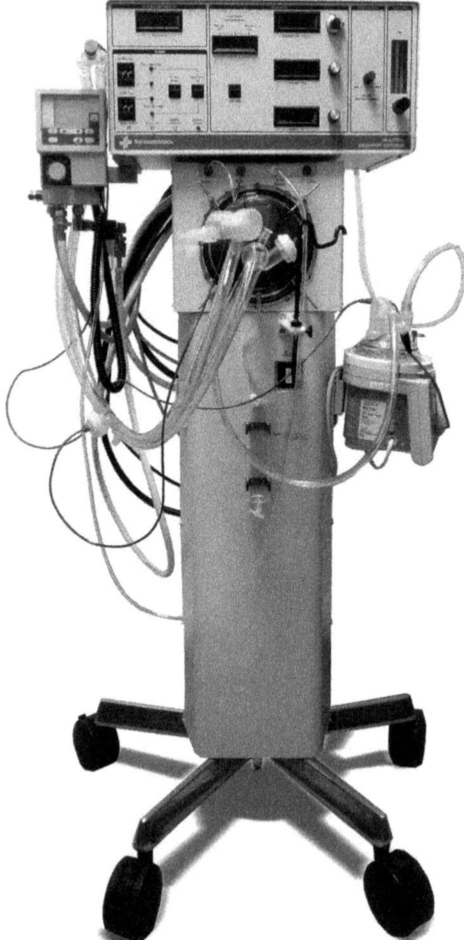

Figure 9.3 SensorMedics 3100B high-frequency oscillatory ventilator.

Source: photography by Evonne Tam.

Evidence base The MOAT trial

The Multicentre Oscillatory Ventilation for Acute Respiratory Distress Syndrome (MOAT) trial was the first randomized controlled study comparing HFOV with conventional ventilation (CV) in adults with ARDS (defined as a $PaO_2/FiO_2 \leq 200$ mmHg on ≥ 10 cmH_2O PEEP) in 2002 and is the largest to date [47]. A total of 148 patients were randomized to HFOV (n = 75) or continued conventional ventilation (n = 73). The primary outcome of survival without the need for ventilation at 30 days was similar at 36% and 31%, respectively (p = 0.686). Although the study was not powered to demonstrate mortality, HFOV was associated with a non-significant trend toward reduced mortality at 30 days (HFOV = 37%, CV = 52%; p = 0.102) and 6 months (HFOV = 47%, CV = 59%; p = 0.143).

A 2010 meta-analysis looking at eight RCTs of HFOV in adults and children (n = 419) was inconclusive. Limited data, heterogeneity in physiological parameters, and the lack of universal lung-protective ventilation strategies in the studies make interpretation challenging [48]. Two recently published large multicentre RCTs were designed to address these deficiencies. The OSCAR trial (Oscillation in ARDS) randomized around 800 patients to HFOV or conventional ventilation (CV). No difference in all-cause 30-day mortality was shown (HFOV = 41.7%, CV = 41.1%; p = 0.85) [49]. The OSCILLATE trial (Oscillation for Acute Respiratory Distress Syndrome Treated Early) was discontinued after enrolment of 548 patients when mortality reached 45%, compared to 35% in the CV group (relative risk of death with HFOV = 1.33, 95% CI 1.09 to 1.64; p = 0.005) [50]. The future for HFOV in ARDS is still uncertain.

Extracorporeal life support

Extracorporeal life support (ECLS) refers to the provision of artificial organ function necessary to maintain life, including oxygenation, CO_2 removal, and haemodynamic assistance. Unlike cardiopulmonary bypass used during cardiac surgery for a number of hours, ECLS can be employed for days, weeks, or even months. ECMO is an emerging technique used as a salvage therapy in patients with ARDS [51].

Extracorporeal membrane oxygenation

Early RCTs using ECMO were disappointing [52,53]. However, they were limited by small numbers of patients. Furthermore, the selection criteria, medical therapies, ventilation strategies, and extracorporeal circuitry employed are not comparable to current practice.

Evidence base The CESAR trial

The Conventional Ventilation or ECMO for Severe Adult Respiratory Failure (CESAR) trial was a recent multicentre RCT that recruited 180 patients aged 18–65 years with severe (Murray score >3.0 or pH <7.20) respiratory failure [54]. Subjects were randomly assigned to receive continued conventional ventilation (n = 90) or referral for consideration of ECMO (n = 90). The primary outcome was death or severe disability at 6 months. Of those patients allocated to the consideration of ECMO arm, 63% survived to 6 months without disability, compared with 47% in the conventional ventilation arm (relative risk 0.69; 95% CI 0.05–0.97; p = 0.03).

The Conventional Ventilation or ECMO for Severe Adult Respiratory Failure (CESAR) trial demonstrated improved survival in carefully selected adult ARDS patients referred for ECMO in a specialist centre. Controls received conventional ventilation in other centres. Not all the patients randomized to ECMO received it. It proved impossible to agree a standardized protocol for the controls. The trial demonstrated the benefit of a dedicated unit, rather than of ECMO itself. The length of hospital stay and costs were doubled [55]. A recent cohort study of influenza A H1N1-related ARDS also showed that transfer to a specialist ECMO centre was associated with lower hospital mortality [56]. A multicentre RCT—Extracorporeal Membrane Oxygenation to Rescue Lung Injury in Severe ARDS (EOLIA)—evaluating early intervention and specifying a standardized ventilator protocol is in progress [57].

The ECMO circuit comprises tubing taking deoxygenated blood from the patient, a pump, a semi-permeable membrane, a heat exchanger, and tubing returning oxygenated blood to the patient [59] (Figure 9.4). The two commonest configurations are: venous–venous (VV) used for patients with respiratory failure who are haemodynamically stable, and venous–arterial (VA) for patients requiring cardiovascular support. Wide-bore cannulae (21–23 French in adults) are inserted using ultrasound or fluoroscopic guidance by the retrieval team at the referring hospital or on arrival to the ECMO centre.

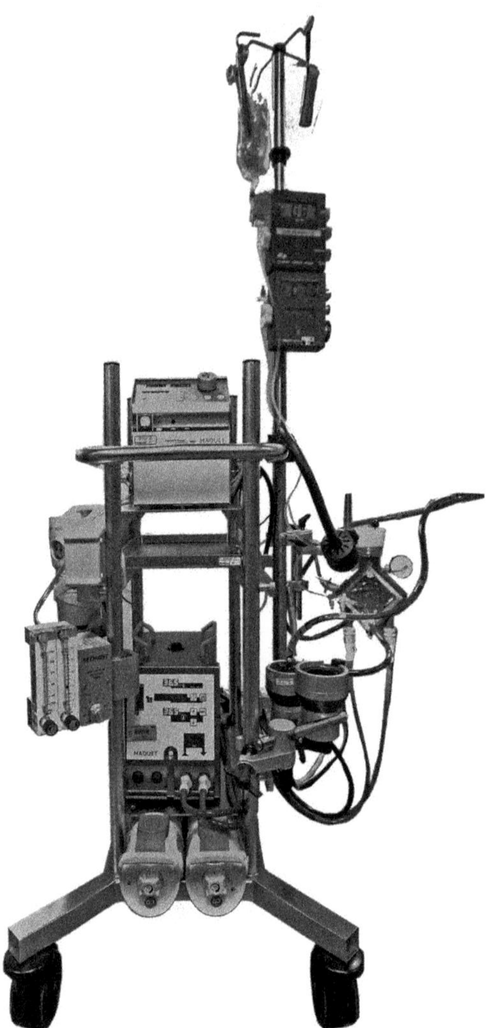

Figure 9.4 Maquet extracorporeal membrane oxygenation apparatus.

Source: photography by Evonne Tam.

In VV ECMO, a mechanical pump withdraws blood from a central vein (internal jugular or femoral vein) into an oxygenator. A semi-permeable membrane facilitates exchange of oxygen and CO_2 between extracorporeal blood and sweep gas (a mixture of air and oxygen adjusted by the blender). Oxygen carriage is saturation-dependent and determined by the haemoglobin concentration and the rate of extracorporeal blood flow (usually 3.5–5 L/minute). The objective is an arterial oxygen saturation of 88% or more. CO_2 removal is partial pressure-dependent and governed by the flow rate of sweep gas, titrated to the desired pH level. Thermostatic regulation of blood occurs before reinfusion into a central vein. A single (bicaval dual-lumen) or dual (single-lumen) site approach may be employed.

Patients on ECMO continue to be ventilated using a 'lung rest' strategy, although the optimal settings have not been established. Many centres advocate aggressive diuresis and blood transfusion to optimize oxygen delivery. Systemic anticoagulation with unfractionated heparin is required to prevent thromboembolism within the circuit, which also presents pharmacological challenges in terms of drug adsorption, increased volume of distribution, and flow dynamics. Monitoring of drug levels is therefore recommended for medications that have a narrow therapeutic window such as vancomycin and gentamicin.

By far, the commonest complication is bleeding (around 50%), which is managed by reducing or temporarily stopping anticoagulation and supplementing with blood products. Others include infection and problems relating to the ECMO circuit, e.g. oxygenator failure and clots within the circuit [60].

Patients are weaned onto lung-protective ventilator settings when clinical and/or radiological parameters improve. Experience has been described of ambulatory ECMO in patients awaiting lung transplantation—use of this technique in patients with ARDS is awaited [61, 62].

ECMO is complex, expensive, and labour-intensive, requiring 24 hours' supervision by a dedicated team of trained personnel, and has not been widely implemented in ICU units. The long-term functional outcome of patients undergoing ECMO is still not clear.

Expert comment

Following publication of the CESAR study and the recent outbreak of H1N1 influenza producing severe viral pneumonitis which was successfully treated using ECMO, the Department of Health established five regional ECMO centres for England and Wales. Over the past 18 months, these centres have produced remarkable results, with survival from severe respiratory failure of approximately 80%. This can be attributed to the regionalization of care, so that patients are referred early to a specialist centre, to better technology in terms of heparin-bonded access lines and extracorporeal circuitry, to the development of centrifugal pumps to replace the old roller pumps, and to the use of polymethylpentene (PMP) membranes in the oxygenator. This results in less inflammatory response, less haemolysis and destruction of platelets, and a lower incidence of bleeding, with unfractionated heparin only required at a dose to achieve an activated partial thromboplastin time (APTT) of 1.5–2.

With the recent publication of the two major HFOV studies showing no benefit (Oscar) and possible harm (Oscillate) from this mode of ventilation, it now seems that, despite no studies yet showing benefit, it looks probable that ECMO is the future for patients with severe ARDS.

Learning point Pharmacotherapies

Steroid therapy

The rationale for steroids is to modulate the inflammatory response. Their use is controversial and is limited to those individuals with early severe ARDS or septic shock, as in this gentleman's case [63].

Surfactant therapy

Adult ARDS is associated with surfactant dysfunction due to reduced surface activity and large aggregate depletion in the context of a complex heterogeneous inflammatory process. RCTs of exogenous surfactant therapy have shown no benefit [64].

Inhaled nitric oxide and prostacyclin therapies

Nitric oxide is a potent vasodilator that has been administered via inhalation to improve V/Q mismatch in ARDS. A 2010 meta-analysis including 11 RCTs in adults showed transient improvement in oxygenation, but no benefit in the duration of ventilation, ventilator-free days, length of hospital stay, and survival [65].

Furthermore, it was associated with an increased risk of renal impairment. Prostacyclin has been used for its vasodilatory and antiplatelet effects in ARDS. No RCTs have been published to demonstrate its efficacy. Both nitric oxide and prostacyclin have been used as salvage therapies in patients with refractory hypoxaemia [66].

Expert comment

A recent systematic review of the use of steroids in ARDS did demonstrate reduced morbidity and mortality with the use of low-dose (0.5–2.5 mg/kg/day) corticosteroid therapy. The mortality reduction was relevant, with a number needed to treat (NNT) of 4 [67].

Supportive care

Patients with ALI/ARDS often require higher levels of analgesia (e.g. fentanyl or morphine) and sedation (e.g. propofol, midazolam, lorazepam) to reduce stress, promote tolerance of the endotracheal tube, and optimize ventilator–patient synchrony. Neuromuscular blockade is associated with residual weakness and is avoided, if at all possible. Judicious use of sedation and analgesia titrated to a light sedation score (e.g. Richmond Agitation Sedation Scale) is suggested. In addition, conservative fluid management to reduce pulmonary oedema, nutritional support with gastric protection, prevention and early treatment of nosocomial infection (mouth care, regular subglottic aspiration, early ventilator weaning to minimize VAP), and thromboprophylaxis are recommended. All of the above measures have yet to be conclusively shown to improve clinical outcomes [68].

Learning point Nutritional therapy

ARDS is characterized by an inflammatory response and catabolic state. Nutritional support is generally instituted early in the form of nasogastric or nasojejunal feeding to meet increased energy expenditure and maintain respiratory muscle strength. However, the evidence base is limited in terms of timing, formulation, and amount of enteral nutrition. Calorific provision is often estimated, according to premorbid nutritional reserve and severity of illness. The use of an immune-modulatory diet (omega-3 fatty acids and antioxidants) remains controversial [69].

Ventilatory weaning

A standardized weaning protocol is recommended [70]. An integrated algorithm for sedation and ventilatory weaning, as part of an 'awake and breathing' strategy, has been shown to reduce the length of hospital stay and improve 1-year survival [71].

A weaning protocol comprises: (i) 'readiness to wean' criteria; (ii) guidelines for reducing ventilatory support; and (iii) 'readiness to extubate or decannulate' criteria [72].

'Readiness to wean'

The potential or 'readiness' for reducing ventilatory support can be assessed using the following screening criteria:

- the underlying cause of respiratory failure is resolving;
- adequate oxygenation, e.g. PaO_2/FiO_2 ≥20–27 kPa (150–200 mmHg) or SpO_2 ≥90% on FiO_2 ≤0.4–0.5 and PEEP ≤5–8 cmH_2O, and pH ≥7.25;
- haemodynamic stability with minimal vasopressor support;
- spontaneous respiratory effort.

Some patients may not meet the criteria, e.g. those with chronic hypoxaemia who are otherwise stable, and therefore their application must be individualized. The Rapid Shallow Breathing Index (respiratory rate to tidal volume ratio in breaths per minute/L) is a commonly used weaning predictor but has not been shown to improve clinical outcomes, including reintubation rate and hospital mortality rate [73].

Box 9.4 Complications of ventilation

Respiratory complications

Ventilator-induced lung injury—clinically indistinguishable from ALI/ARDS
Pneumothorax and air leaks—pneumomediastinum, pneumoperitoneum, surgical emphysema
VAP

Systemic complications

Reduced cardiac output
Gastrointestinal bleeding
Renal failure
Raised intracranial pressure
Neuromuscular weakness
Inflammation

Source: McLellan S, Nimmo G. Complications of ventilation. Advanced Respiratory Critical Care 2011: 244–256, Oxford University Press.

Guidelines for reducing ventilator support

Spontaneous breathing trials (SBTs) are the preferred weaning strategy [74]. They can be unsupported (using a T-piece adaptor) or supported (low-level pressure support, CPAP, or automatic tube compensation—used to overcome endotracheal tube resistance) and initially last 30 minutes. Weaning ventilatory modes include pressure support ventilation and synchronized intermittent mandatory ventilation (SIMV). Newer computerized weaning programmes include adaptive support ventilation and proportional assist ventilation. Tracheostomy should be performed for patients who require prolonged mechanical ventilation (>7–10 days), reducing the need for sedation, etc. The optimal timing remains unclear.

Extubation and decannulation criteria

Extubation or decannulation (removal of tracheostomy) are considered when a patient can safely protect their airway (as assessed by an adequate level of consciousness typically Glasgow Coma Scale (GCS) >8, sufficient cough strength, and minimal airway secretions) and maintain adequate gas exchange. This should be performed by a physician prepared to immediately reintubate, if necessary.

Ventilatory complications

Mechanical ventilation is associated with a number of problems involving the lungs and other systems of the body (Box 9.4) [75].

Outcomes

The long-term outcome of survivors of ARDS is influenced more by neuromuscular, cognitive, and psychological impairments than by pulmonary dysfunction, and this persists at 5 years following the critical illness [76]. Patients with pre-existing health problems and functional disability have poorer outcomes and higher health-care utilization and incur greater financial burden. There is also emerging evidence of psychological morbidity in family members supporting them and is prompting moves to early rehabilitation before discharge from the ICU. However, it should be noted that the majority of data predate the widespread use of lung-protective strategies. Research is needed to improve prediction, prevention, and treatment of these sequelae and to observe the effects of lung-protective strategies on long-term outcomes (Table 9.2) [77].

Table 9.2 Long-term outcomes in ARDS survivors and caregivers

Major morbidity in patient	Minor morbidity in patient	Caregiver morbidity
Neuromuscular:	Tracheostomy site complications	Depression
Critical illness polyneuropathy	Pulmonary dysfunction	Post-traumatic stress disorder
Critical illness myopathy	Entrapment neuropathy	
Neurocognitive:	Heterotopic ossification	
Memory	Frozen joints	
Attention	Striae	
Concentration		
Executive function		
Neuropsychological:		
Depression		
Anxiety		
Post-traumatic stress disorder		

Rubenfeld GD, Herridge MS. Epidemiology and Outcomes of Acute Lung Injury. Chest 2007; 131; 554–562.

Conclusions

Intensive care is now an integral component of the curriculum for respiratory trainees. A general knowledge of ventilation and its modes and applications will hopefully prove worthwhile and beneficial. For those wishing to pursue joint accreditation in intensive care medicine, referral to specialist anaesthetic texts is recommended.

A final word from the expert

For most of the last two decades of the last century, ICU clinicians made little progress in the treatment of ALI/ARDS. In fact, we harmed our patients by overly aggressive ventilation with high tidal volumes and excessive PEEP levels, by fluid overloading them in pursuit of inappropriately high levels of oxygen delivery, and by the indiscriminate use of steroids and other pharmacological interventions. We have now learnt that 'less is more'.

One of the reasons for the failure of certain interventions, however, has been the heterogeneity of the patients studied in terms of the true underlying pathological diagnosis. As intensivists, we seem to be wedded to diagnosing **syndromes**, and, whether defined by the 1994 or the Berlin criteria, we must always remember that identifying the underlying pathological diagnosis causing the ARDS will direct the appropriate treatment and determine the prognosis.

References

1. Church C, Roditi G, Banham S (2011). Diagnosis of respiratory failure. In: Hughes M, Black R (eds.) *Advanced Respiratory Critical Care*. Oxford: Oxford University Press, pp. 22–48.
2. Yarmus L, Feller-Kopman D. Pneumothorax in the critically ill patient. *Chest* 2012;**141**:1098–105.
3. Havelock T, Teoh R, Laws D, Gleeson F; BTS Pleural Disease Guideline Group. Pleural procedures and thoracic ultrasound: British Thoracic Society Pleural Disease Guideline 2010. *Thorax* 2010;**65**(Suppl 2):ii61–76.

4. Melsen WG, Rovers MM, Koeman M, Bonten MJ. Estimating the attributable mortality of ventilator-associated pneumonia from randomized prevention studies. *Crit Care Med* 2011;**39**:1–7.
5. Hunter JD. Ventilator associated pneumonia. *BMJ* 2012;**344**:e3325.
6. Palazzo SJ, Simpson T, Schnapp L. Biomarkers for ventilator-associated pneumonia: review of the literature. *Heart Lung* 2011;**40**:293–8.
7. Chastre J, Fagon JY. Ventilator-associated pneumonia. *Am J Respir Crit Care Med* 2002;**165**:867–903.
8. Morris AC, Hay AW, Swann DG *et al.* Reducing ventilator-associated pneumonia in intensive care: impact of implementing a care bundle. *Crit Care Med* 2011;**39**:2218–24.
9. Ibsen B. The anaesthetist's viewpoint on the treatment of respiratory complications in poliomyelitis during the epidemic in Copenhagen, 1952. *Proc R Soc Med* 1954;**47**:72–4.
10. Bower AG, Bennett VR, Dillon JB, Axelrod B. Investigation on the care and treatment of poliomyelitis patients. *Ann West Med Surg* 1950;**4**:561–82.
11. Appelboam R. Indications for ventilatory support. In: Hughes M, Black R (eds.) *Advanced Respiratory Critical Care*. Oxford: Oxford University Press, pp. 69–72.
12. Cranshaw J. Pressure vs volume delivery. In: Hughes M, Black R (eds.) *Advanced Respiratory Critical Care*. Oxford: Oxford University Press, pp. 111–18.
13. Hall JB, McShane PJ (2013). *Overview of mechanical ventilation*. Available at: <http://www.merckmanuals.com/professional/critical_care_medicine.html>.
14. Black R, Hughes M. Sudden deterioration on a ventilator. In: Hughes M, Black R (eds.) *Advanced Respiratory Critical Care*. Oxford: Oxford University Press, pp. 301–4.
15. Siegel MD (2016). *Acute respiratory distress syndrome: epidemiology; pathophysiology; pathology; and etiology*. Available at: <http://www.uptodate.com/contents/acute-respiratory-distress-syndrome-epidemiology-pathophysiology-pathology-and-etiology-in-adults>.
16. Bernard GR, Artigas A, Brigham KL *et al.* The American-European Consensus Conference on ARDS. Definitions, mechanisms, relevant outcomes, and clinical trial coordination. *Am J Respir Crit Care Med* 1994;**149**:818–24.
17. Roupie E, Lepage E, Wysocki M *et al.* Prevalence, etiologies and outcome of the acute respiratory distress syndrome among hypoxemic ventilated patients. SRLF Collaborative Group on Mechanical Ventilation. Société de Réanimation de Langue Française. *Intensive Care Med* 1999;**25**:920–9.
18. Murray JF, Matthay MA, Luce JM *et al.* An expanded definition of the adult respiratory distress syndrome. *Am Rev Respir Dis* 1988;**138**:720–3.
19. Ferguson ND, Frutos-Vivar F, Esteban A *et al.* Acute respiratory distress syndrome: underrecognition by clinicians and diagnostic accuracy of three clinical definitions. *Crit Care Med* 2005;**33**:2228–34.
20. ARDS Definition Task Force, Ranieri VM, Rubenfeld GD *et al.* Acute respiratory distress syndrome: the Berlin Definition. *JAMA* 2012;**307**:2526–33.
21. Ranieri VM, Rubenfeld GD, Thompson BT *et al.* Acute respiratory distress syndrome: the Berlin Definition. *JAMA* 2012;**307**:2526–33.
22. Barnett N, Ware LB. Biomarkers in acute lung injury—making forward progress. *Crit Care Clin* 2011;**27**:661–83.
23. Blank R, Napolitano LM. Epidemiology of ARDS and ALI. *Crit Care Clin* 2011;**27**:439–58.
24. Laycock H, Rajah A. Acute lung injury and acute respiratory distress syndrome: a review article. *BJMP* 2010;**3**:324
25. Tomashefski JF Jr. Pulmonary pathology of acute respiratory distress syndrome. *Clin Chest Med* 2000;**21**:435–66.
26. Haas C. Mechanical ventilation with lung protective strategies: what works? *Crit Care Clin* 2011;**27**:469–86.
27. Putensen C, Theuerkauf N, Zinserling J, Wrigge H, Pelosi P. Meta-analysis: ventilation strategies and outcomes of the acute respiratory distress syndrome and acute lung injury. *Ann Intern Med* 2009;**151**:566–76.

28. ARDS Clinical Trials Network. The Acute Respiratory Distress Syndrome Network. Ventilation with lower tidal volumes as compared with traditional tidal volumes for acute lung injury and the acute respiratory distress syndrome. *N Engl J Med* 2000;**342**:1301–8.
29. Needham DM, Colantuoni E, Mendez-Tellez PA *et al.* Lung protective mechanical ventilation and two year survival in patients with acute lung injury: prospective cohort study. *BMJ* 2012;**344**:e2124.
30. Terragni PP, Rosboch G, Tealdi A *et al.* Tidal hyperinflation during low tidal volume ventilation in acute respiratory distress syndrome. *Am J Respir Crit Care Med* 2006;**175**:160–6.
31. Broccard AF. Respiratory acidosis and acute respiratory distress syndrome: time to trade in a bull market? *Crit Care Med* 2006;**34**:229–31.
32. Hughes M, Black R. Hypercapnia while on a ventilator. In: Hughes M, Black R (eds.) *Advanced Respiratory Critical Care*. Oxford: Oxford University Press, pp. 296–304.
33. Huh JW, Jung H, Choi HS, Hong SB, Lim CM, Koh Y. Efficacy of positive end-expiratory pressure titration after the alveolar recruitment manoeuver in patients with acute respiratory distress syndrome. *Crit Care* 2009;**13**:R22.
34. Putensen C, Theuerkauf N, Zinderling J *et al.* Meta-analysis: ventilation strategies and outcomes of the acute respiratory distress syndrome and acute lung injury. *Ann Intern Med* 2009;**151**:566–76.
35. Briel M, Meade M, Mercat A *et al.* Higher vs lower positive end-expiratory pressure in patients with acute lung injury and acute respiratory distress syndrome. *JAMA* 2010;**303**:865–73.
36. Phoenix SI, Paravastu S, Columb M *et al.* Does a higher positive end expiratory pressure decrease mortality in acute respiratory distress syndrome? A systematic review and meta-analysis. *Anesthesiology* 2009;**110**:1098–105.
37. Oba Y, Thameen D, Zaza T. High levels of PEEP may improve survival in acute respiratory distress syndrome: a meta-analysis. *Respir Med* 2009;**103**:1174–81.
38. Dasenbrook EC, Needham DM, Brower RG *et al.* Higher positive end-expiratory pressure in patients with acute lung injury: a systematic review and meta-analysis. *Respir Care* 2011;**56**:568–75.
39. Fan E, Wilcox ME, Brower RG *et al.* Recruitment maneuvers for acute lung injury. *Am J Respir Crit Care Med* 2008;**178**:1156–63.
40. Cesana BM, Antonelli P, Chiumello D, Gattinoni L. Positive end-expiratory pressure, prone positioning, and activated protein C: a critical review of meta-analyses. *Minerva Anestesiol* 2010;**76**:929–36.
41. Dickinson S, Park PK, Napolitano LM. Prone-positioning therapy in ARDS. *Crit Care Clin* 2011;**27**:511–23.
42. Chan KP, Stewart TE, Mehta S. High-frequency oscillatory ventilation for adult patients with ARDS. *Chest* 2007;**131**:1907–16.
43. Ali S, Ferguson ND. High-frequency oscillatory ventilation in ALI/ARDS. *Crit Care Clin* 2011;**27**:487–99.
44. Slutsky AS, Drazen JM. Ventilation with small tidal volumes. *N Engl J Med* 2002;**29;347**:630–1.
45. Krishnan JA, Brower RG. High-frequency ventilation for acute lung injury and ARDS. *Chest* 2000;**118**:795–807.
46. Camporota L. High-frequency oscillatory ventilation. In: Hughes M, Black R (eds.) *Advanced Respiratory Critical Care*. Oxford: Oxford University Press, pp. 158–64.
47. Derdak S, Mehta S, Stewart TE *et al.*; the Multicenter Oscillatory Ventilation for Acute Respiratory Distress Syndrome Trial (MOAT) Study Investigators. High-frequency oscillatory ventilation for acute respiratory distress syndrome in adults: a randomized controlled trial. *Am J Respir Crit Care Med* 2002;**166**:801–8.

48. Sud S, Sud M, Friedrich JO *et al.* High frequency oscillation in patients with acute lung injury and acute respiratory distress syndrome (ARDS): systematic review and meta-analysis. *BMJ* 2010;**340**:c2327.
49. Young D, Lamb SE, Shah S *et al.* High-frequency oscillation for acute respiratory distress syndrome. *N Engl J Med* 2013;**368**:806–13. Available at: <http://www.oscar-trial.org/index.php>.
50. Ferguson ND, Cook DJ, Guyatt GH *et al.* High-frequency oscillation in early acute respiratory distress syndrome. *N Engl J Med* 2013;**368**:795–805. Available at: <http://www.oscillatetrial.com/>.
51. Gaffney AM, Wildhirt SM, Griffin MJ, Annich GM, Radomski MW. Extracorporeal life support. *BMJ* 2010;**341**:c5317.
52. Zapol WM, Snider MT, Hill JD *et al.* Extracorporeal membrane oxygenation in severe acute respiratory failure. A randomized prospective study. *JAMA* 1979;**242**:2193–6.
53. Morris AH, Wallace CJ, Menlove RL *et al.* Randomized clinical trial of pressure-controlled inverse ratio ventilation and extracorporeal CO_2 removal for adult respiratory distress syndrome. *Am J Respir Crit Care Med* 1994;**149**:295–305.
54. Peek GJ, Mugford M, Tiruvoipati R *et al.* Efficacy and economic assessment of conventional ventilatory support versus extracorporeal membrane oxygenation for severe adult respiratory failure (CESAR): a multicentre randomised controlled trial. *Lancet* 2009;**374**:1351–63.
55. Zwischenberger JB, Lynch JE. Will CESAR answer the adult ECMO debate? *Lancet* 2009;**374**:1307–8.
56. Noah MA, Peek GJ, Finney SJ *et al.* Referral to an extracorporeal membrane oxygenation center and mortality among patients with severe 2009 influenza A(H1N1). *JAMA* 2011;**306**:1659–68.
57. ClinicalTrials. gov (2016). *Extracorporeal Membrane Oxygenation for Severe Acute Respiratory Distress Syndrome (EOLIA)*. Available at: <https://clinicaltrials.gov/ct2/show/NCT01470703>.
58. Brodie D, Bacchetta M. Extracorporeal membrane oxygenation for ARDS in adults. *N Engl J Med* 2011;**365**:1905–14.
59. Park PK, Napolitano LM, Bartlett RH. Extracorporeal membrane oxygenation in adult acute respiratory distress syndrome. *Crit Care Clin* 2011;**27**:627–46.
60. Paden ML, Conrad SA, Rycus PT, Thiagarajan RR; ELSO Registry. Extracorporeal Life Support Organization Registry Report 2012. *ASAIO J* 2013;**59**:202–10.
61. Garcia JF, Iacono A, Kon ZN *et al.* Ambulatory extracorporeal membrane oxygenation: a new approach for bridge-to-lung transplantation. *J Thorac Cardiovasc Surg* 2010;**139**:e137–8.
62. Mangi AA, Mason DP, Yun JJ *et al.* Bridge to lung transplantation using short-term ambulatory extracorporeal membrane oxygenation. *J Thorac Cardiovasc Surg* 2010;**140**:713–15.
63. Marik PE, Umberto Meduri G, Rocco PRM, Annane Djillali. Glucocorticoid treatment in acute lung injury and acute respiratory distress syndrome. *Crit Care Clin* 2011;**27**:589–607.
64. Raghavendran K, Wilson D, Notter RH. Surfactant therapy for acute lung injury and acute respiratory distress syndrome. *Care Clin* 2011;**27**:525–59.
65. Afshari A, Brok J, Møller AM, Wetterslev J. Inhaled nitric oxide for acute respiratory distress syndrome (ARDS) and acute lung injury in children and adults. *Cochrane Database Syst Rev* 2010;**112**:1411–21.
66. Puri N, Dellinger RP. Inhaled nitric oxide and inhaled prostacyclin in acute respiratory distress syndrome: what is the evidence? *Care Clin* 2011;**27**:561–87.
67. Tang BM, Craig JC, Eslick GD, Seppelt I, McLean AS. Use of corticosteroids in acute lung injury and acute respiratory distress syndrome: a systematic review and meta-analysis. *Crit Care Med* 2009;**37**:1594–603.

68. Siegel MD (2016). *Acute respiratory distress syndrome: supportive care and oxygenation in adults*. Available at: <http://www.uptodate.com/contents/acute-respiratory-distress-syndrome-supportive-care-and-oxygenation-in-adults>.
69. Krzak A, Pleva M, Napolitano LM. Nutrition therapy for ALI and ARDS. *Care Clin* 2011;**27**:647–59.
70. Blackwood B, Alderdice F, Burns K, Cardwell C, Lavery G, O'Halloran P. Use of weaning protocols for reducing duration of mechanical ventilation in critically ill adult patients: Cochrane systematic review and meta-analysis. *BMJ* 2011;**342**:c7237.
71. Girard TD, Kress JP, Fuchs BD *et al.* Efficacy and safety of a paired sedation and ventilator weaning protocol for mechanically ventilated patients in intensive care (Awakening and Breathing Controlled trial): a randomised controlled trial. *Lancet* 2008;**371**:126–34.
72. MacIntyre NR, Cook DJ, Ely EW Jr *et al.*; American College of Chest Physicians; American Association for Respiratory Care; American College of Critical Care Medicine. Evidence-based guidelines for weaning and discontinuing ventilatory support: a collective task force facilitated by the American College of Chest Physicians; the American Association for Respiratory Care; and the American College of Critical Care Medicine. *Chest* 2001;**120**(6 Suppl):375S–95S.
73. Tanios MA, Nevins ML, Hendra KP *et al.* A randomized, controlled trial of the role of weaning predictors in clinical decision making. *Crit Care Med* 2006;**34**:2530–5.
74. Esteban A, Frutos F, Tobin MJ *et al.* A comparison of four methods of weaning patients from mechanical ventilation. Spanish Lung Failure Collaborative Group. *N Engl J Med* 1995;**332**:345–50.
75. McLellan S, Nimmo G. Complications of ventilation. In: Hughes M, Black R (eds.) *Advanced Respiratory Critical Care*. Oxford: Oxford University Press, pp. 244–56.
76. Herridge MS, Tansey CM, Matté A *et al.*; Canadian Critical Care Trials Group. Functional disability 5 years after acute respiratory distress syndrome. *N Engl J Med* 2011;**364**:1293–304.
77. Rubenfeld GD, Herridge MS. Epidemiology and outcomes of acute lung injury. *Chest* 2007;**131**;554–62.

CASE

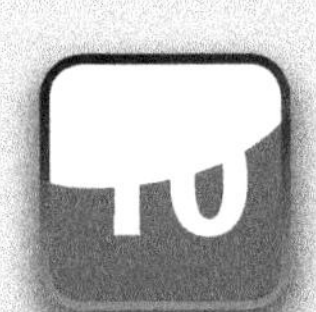

Idiopathic pulmonary fibrosis

Clare Ross

Expert commentary Athol Wells

Case history

A 55-year-old gentleman was referred to the interstitial lung diseases (ILD) unit by his GP, with a 4-month history of shortness of breath and intermittent chest tightness on exertion. He had quit smoking 3 months prior to presentation but had a 30-pack year history. He had a cough, recently productive of thick green sputum, with associated fevers and a weight loss of 2.5 kg. Initial examination by the GP revealed bibasal crepitations, and he was started on amoxicillin and azithromycin, with a salbutamol inhaler to use as needed. The patient returned to the GP a few weeks later with persisting breathlessness and lethargy. He was prescribed a further course of antibiotics and referred to the respiratory department of the local hospital as a 2-week wait, in view of his smoking history and lack of response to antibiotics.

At his outpatient appointment, his history and symptoms were unchanged, and his exercise capacity was several kilometres on the flat, although he stopped regularly to catch his breath. His oxygen saturation was 94% on air at rest, and a CXR was consistent with a fibrotic process. He was given a provisional diagnosis of 'accelerating cryptogenic fibrosing alveolitis (CFA)' and was booked for an outpatient CT scan. He was started on oral prednisolone 50 mg od for 1 month, to be tapered thereafter, with a plan to be seen again 4 months later. 'Steroid trials', such as this, are commonly used in suspected ILD but are not advisable in likely idiopathic pulmonary fibrosis (IPF) and should certainly be avoided before imaging is available.

Learning point Classification of the idiopathic interstitial pneumonias

In 2002, the ATS and European Respiratory Society (ERS) published an international consensus defining the clinical manifestations, pathology, and radiological features of idiopathic interstitial pneumonias (IIPs), i.e. a subset of acute and chronic lung disorders collectively referred to as interstitial lung diseases (ILDs) or diffuse parenchymal lung disorders (DPLDs) of unknown aetiology [1]. The previous lack of an international standard had resulted in confusing diagnostic criteria and made interpretation of clinical trials difficult. The term 'cryptogenic fibrosing alveolitis', traditionally used in the UK, was used interchangeably with the term idiopathic pulmonary fibrosis (IPF) but was often broadly applied to a range of disease entities with varying histological patterns. These different patterns carry with them different prognoses, and recent advances in HRCT has revolutionized the classification of ILDs. The new classification includes seven clinico-radiologic-pathologic entities, listed in order of relative frequency:

- **idiopathic pulmonary fibrosis (IPF);**
- non-specific interstitial pneumonia (NSIP);
- cryptogenic organizing pneumonia (COP);
- acute interstitial pneumonia (AIP);
- respiratory bronchiolitis-associated interstitial lung disease (RB-ILD);
- desquamative interstitial pneumonia (DIP);
- lymphoid interstitial pneumonia (LIP).

Expert comment

The 2002 IIP classification was of immediate practical value. Historically, when the IIPs were lumped as 'cryptogenic fibrosing alveolitis' (CFA), subgroups with a 5-year survival of 15% (IPF), a 5-year survival of 50–80% (NSIP), and a 5-year survival of over 90% (the remaining disorders) were amalgamated. As the major purposes of making a diagnosis are to reach conclusions on the likely natural history and treated outcome, it is difficult to justify ignoring these survival differences and viewing all the IIP entities as the same diagnostic entity. It has been argued that 'CFA' is a clinical presentation which is required for the purposes of epidemiological studies. However, the outcome differences detailed above make it very clear that the clinical presentation of 'CFA' should be viewed as a diagnostic starting point, but not as a final diagnosis. The IIP classification also ensured that, for the first time, terminology was unified and there was certainty that clinicians in different countries were, in truth, describing the same entities. This, in turn, facilitated large multinational treatment trials which have become a core part of the IPF landscape.

Learning point Pathophysiology of IPF

IPF is defined as a specific form of chronic progressive fibrosing interstitial pneumonia of unknown cause, occurring primarily in older adults, limited to the lungs, and associated with the histopathological and/or radiological pattern of usual interstitial pneumonia (UIP) (defined in Learning point, p. 113) [2]. It is the most prevalent IIP. The incidence in the UK is 7.4/100,000 person years and is increasing every year [3]. It is a devastating condition that carries a mean survival of 2.9–5.0 years [4]. As the name implies, the aetiology of IPF is unknown, and research has therefore focussed on identifying the natural history and pathogenesis of the disease in order to develop targeted therapies. Historical hypotheses attributed the fibrosis to a series of inflammatory responses to cellular injury; however, more recent research suggests that inflammation is neither necessary nor sufficient for the progression of fibrosis [5] and that IPF is a disease perpetuated by aberrant wound healing, rather than primarily by chronic inflammation [6]. Fibrosis results from excessive fibroblastic proliferation and accumulation of extracellular matrix in response to alveolar epithelial cell injury [7]. Additional pathways involving coagulation, apoptosis, and oxidative stress have also been implicated in the pathogenesis of IPF.

Expert comment

The revision of the IIP classification did also have disadvantages. There has been a tendency to view the pathways and mediators identified in IPF as specific to IPF and to see IPF pathogenesis as entirely different from the pathogenesis of other fibrosing lung diseases. Certainly, the role of inflammation does differ broadly between IPF and almost all the other pulmonary fibrosing disorders, in which progression from inflammation to fibrosis can still be viewed as the best disease model. However, even in IPF, recent data suggest that immunological dysregulation may be pathogenetically important in a subset of patients. By contrast, adverse outcomes with warfarin therapy in IPF indicate that the pro-thrombotic milieu in IPF may represent a protective mechanism (although, it should be acknowledged, not a very effective one!). More importantly, the same biomarker/mediator signal in IPF is also present in other fibrosing disorders. It is likely that many of the pathways studied in IPF are relevant to the phenotype of progressive fibrosis in general and are not, in reality, specific to IPF.

The patient deteriorated rapidly over the next few weeks and was subsequently referred to a tertiary centre for a second opinion.

At the time of assessment by the ILD unit (almost 3 months after his initial presentation to his GP), his exercise tolerance had reduced, and he had an MRC dyspnoea score of 3. History taking revealed that the patient had experienced discoloration of his fingers in the cold for the last 18 months. He remembered having difficulty climbing steep or multiple staircases over a similar duration. He had been referred to the local rheumatology department with possible Raynaud's phenomenon but had been lost to follow-up, with no reported diagnosis or treatment. The patient's grandmother and daughter had been diagnosed with systemic lupus erythematosus (SLE), but, other than possible Raynaud's, the patient did not describe or display any other features of connective tissue disease (CTD). He had no particular occupational or environmental exposures and had worked for nearly all his life in information technology. The patient was a keen hill walker and was used to hill walking carrying significant weights. The patient had no symptoms of gastro-oesophageal reflux disease (GORD).

Learning point History taking in ILD

Diagnosis of IPF relies on a combination of thorough history taking and objective data. The mean age of presentation is 70 years of age, and the disease is unlikely to present below the age of 50. It is commoner in men than women and classically presents with an insidious onset of breathlessness, often in association with a troubling dry cough. As with this patient, presentation often follows an acute infective episode, but the history of breathlessness predates this, usually by several months. Although, traditionally, the clinical course has been viewed as one of relentless progression, there is now growing evidence that some patients experience prolonged periods of stability.

History taking should include specific questions relating to occupational exposure (including metal dust, wood dust, farming, hairdressing, and stone cutting), environmental exposure (e.g. to vegetable or animal dust), and features suggestive of CTD (including Raynaud's phenomenon, arthritis, rashes, myopathies, or sicca symptoms). Previous medical history and medication history should identify any potential related conditions that could have resulted in pulmonary fibrosis. Triggers of other ILDs should be sought such as antigen exposure relevant to hypersensitivity pneumonitis (HP), occupational exposures, and the use of therapies known to be complicated by pulmonary fibrosis (such as nitrofurantoin and amiodarone).

Particular attention has been paid to the aetiological role of micro-aspiration and GORD in IPF in recent years. GORD tends to be clinically silent in IPF patients, but one prospective study demonstrated abnormal gastro-oesophageal reflux (on manometry and pH studies) in 87% of patients [8].

Smoking is relevant, and the majority of patients with IPF have a history of cigarette smoking. It has been postulated that smokers with IPF have a better prognosis than those who do not smoke; however, this is more likely to be due to an earlier presentation due to coexisting COPD. IPF is an independent risk factor for lung cancer, and, compared to a patient without IPF, the risk of developing lung cancer in IPF increases around 200-fold in a 20/day smoker.

Unlike other IIPs, some cases of IPF may be hereditary, although these cases account for only 0.5–2.2% of all cases [9].

Learning point CTD-associated ILD

Our patient's history included a few features suggestive of a CTD, and he was relatively young to be diagnosed with IPF. The relevance of this should not be underestimated, as, on average, CTD-associated interstitial pneumonias have a better prognosis than their idiopathic counterparts [10].

The suspicion of CTD-related disease should be high in younger patients like this, and they may well go on to develop clinical or serological features of a CTD after their presentation with ILD [11].

The latest guidelines recommend serological testing in the majority of patients with IPF and should include antinuclear antibody (ANA), rheumatoid factor (RF), and anti-cyclic citrullinated peptide (CCP). Other additional tests may be indicated in individual patients, and the 2008 BTS guidance recommends extractable nuclear antigen testing, in addition [2, 12]. Our patient's auto-antibody screen was negative.

Clinical tip Clinical signs in IPF

Clubbing is noted in about 50% of patients with IPF, whilst the characteristic bibasal end-inspiratory Velcro-like crepitations are heard in >90% of cases [11].

Expert comment

It should be stressed that neither sign is specific to IPF. Bilateral basal crackles are present in a great many fibrosing diseases, and their diagnostic value is confined to their absence, as is the rule in sarcoidosis. Clubbing also occurs in NSIP, asbestosis, fibrotic HP, and rheumatoid lung, although commoner in IPF.

Expert comment

The presence of Raynaud's and the family history of CTD both raise the possibility that a CTD might eventually emerge. The development of rheumatoid arthritis, systemic sclerosis, and inflammatory myopathy after the onset of ILD are all well recognized scenarios. The prognostic significance of these observations varies between patients as, in general, CTD-related ILD has a worse outcome, closer to that of IPF, when lung involvement is the first disease manifestation. However, the subsequent identification of a CTD does change the approach to treatment, with greater emphasis on anti-inflammatory therapies than in IPF.

On examination, the patient was clubbed, with bibasal end-inspiratory Velcro-like crepitations heard on auscultation. He had no features consistent with pulmonary hypertension (PH) or right ventricular failure and no signs suggestive of an underlying cause for his fibrosis.

Following the initial clinic assessment, the patient was electively admitted for a full ILD work-up. This consisted of pulmonary function tests (PFTs), 6-minute walk test (6MWT), overnight oximetry, HRCT, bronchoscopy with BAL and cell differential, blood tests (including an auto-antibody screen, avian and *Aspergillus* precipitins, and brain natriuretic peptide (BNP) level), echocardiogram, and bone density scan.

The results of serial PFTs are shown in Table 10.1. Typically, all fibrotic diseases show a restrictive defect, with a reduced TLCO. The patient's forced expiratory ratio was 86%, and his TLCO was markedly reduced at 30.4% of predicted. His flow–volume loop revealed a degree of scalloping towards the end of expiration, implying an additional mild obstructive component (Figure 10.1). This is not surprising, given his smoking history, but is worth noting, as concurrent emphysema will contribute to a reduction in the TLCO. The patient's saturations at rest were 95% on air. He had a 6MWT in which he walked 532 m and desaturated to 84%. As such, he was eligible for ambulatory oxygen, but the patient declined this. Overnight oximetry was reassuring, with saturations maintained at 95% throughout the night.

Table 10.1 The patient's serial pulmonary function tests

	Pred LL	Pred UL	Presentation		3 months		9 months		12 months	
			Actual	% pred	Actual	% pred	Actual	% pred	Actual	% pred
TLC	5.99	8.29	3.77	52.8	3.00	42.0	3.75	52.5	3.77	52.8
RV	1.66	3.01	1.23	52.6	0.93	39.7	1.02	43.6	1.17	50.0
FEV_1	2.70	4.38	2.21	61.8	1.71	47.9	2.13	60.1	2.09	58.9
FVC	3.46	5.46	2.57	57.6	2.03	45.2	2.61	58.7	2.64	59.2
TLCOc	7.73	12.37	3.07	30.4	1.76	17.4	2.42	24.0	2.87	28.5
KCOc	1.03	1.91	0.91	61.9	0.66	44.9	0.78	52.9	0.84	57.0

Clinical tip Interpretation of PFTs in IPF

Patients with IPF can sometimes present with a normal FVC. This implies coexisting emphysema, and the TLCO should be interpreted with caution, as both conditions will have contributed to impaired gas exchange.

(Continued)

It is useful to note the gap between the % predicted FVC and the % predicted TLCO. If the % predicted TLCO seems disproportionately reduced, in the absence of coexisting emphysema, pulmonary vascular involvement should be considered. Similarly, if, on serial PFTs, the lung volumes remain stable but the TLCO falls, a pulmonary vascular component may be present.

PFTs are used to predict prognosis in IPF. A gas transfer of <35–40% predicted, combined with HRCT scores, has an 80% sensitivity and specificity for predicting death within 2 years [13].

Change in the FVC is the serial lung function measurement most consistently predictive of mortality, possibly reflecting the good reproducibility of the test. A fall from baseline of ≥10% in FVC or ≥15% in TLCO in the first 6–12 months identifies patients with a much higher mortality. In general, follow-up is recommended every 3–6 months to assess disease progression and potential complications (either due to the disease itself or due to therapeutic interventions).

Learning point Exercise testing in IPF

The 2008 BTS guideline states that desaturation during the 6MWT at presentation is a stronger prognostic determinant in IPF than resting lung function [12]. A study of 197 patients with IPF reported that desaturation to ≤88% was associated with a median survival of 3.21 years, compared to 6.63 years in those who did not desaturate to this extent [14]. Subsequent follow-up revealed that different lung function variables served as better prognostic indicators, depending on which 6MWT category the patients fell into. These findings have not informed current guidance (mostly due to issues with reproducibility of the 6MWT); however, our unit advocates repetition of the 6MWT as the disease advances, in order to identify patients who may benefit from ambulatory oxygen.

The patient's CXR (Figure 10.2) shows coarse reticulation, greatest in a subpleural, mid- and lower-zone distribution. The lung volumes are reduced.

The patient's HRCT is shown in Figure 10.3.

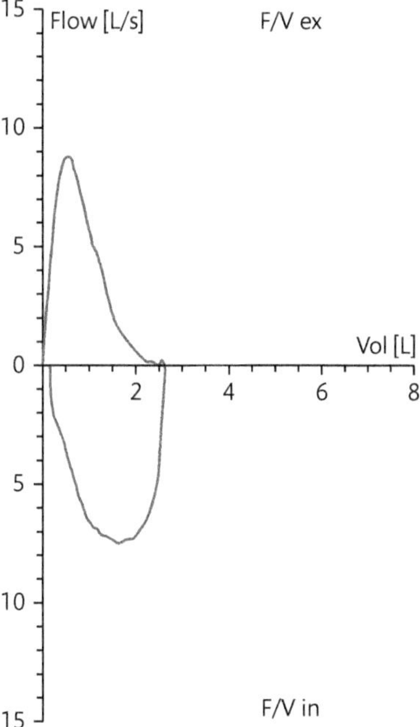

Figure 10.1 The patient's flow–volume loop.

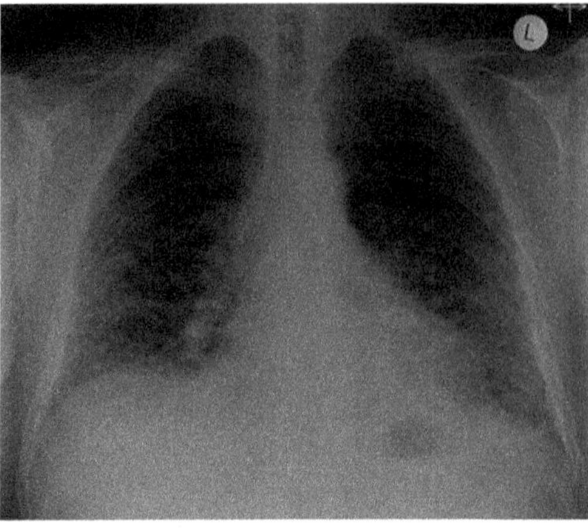

Figure 10.2 CXR showing coarse reticulation, greatest in the subpleural areas with a mid- and lower-zone distribution. The lung volumes are reduced.

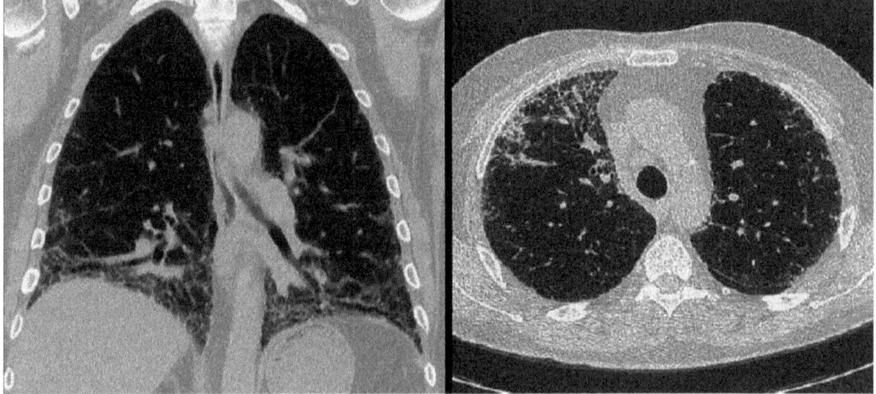

Figure 10.3 The patient's HRCT scan showing a UIP pattern with reticular shadowing in a predominantly subpleural distribution, with evidence of traction bronchiectasis and honeycombing.

Clinical tip Radiology in IPF

A baseline CXR can be useful to allow disease progression to be identified by a subsequent CXR, without the considerable radiation of repeated HRCTs. However, CXRs are unable to distinguish reliably between different forms of ILD and may be more useful in detecting complications relating to IPF such as lung cancer, pneumonia, or pneumothoraces. It should be remembered that false positives can occur, especially in obese patients, and that a normal CXR does not rule out ILD.

UIP on HRCT is characterized by reticular abnormalities with subpleural and basal distribution, honeycombing with or without traction bronchiectasis, and the absence of features inconsistent with UIP such as extensive GGOs, diffuse mosaic attenuation, profuse micronodules, and consolidation. It has been demonstrated by several groups that the extent of fibrosis and honeycombing on HRCT are predictive of survival in IPF [15,16].

A UIP pattern on HRCT is highly accurate for the presence of UIP on biopsy, and, when the CT appearances are consistent with UIP, the diagnosis is correct in >90% of cases [17]. However, the classical CT findings of UIP are present in, at most, two-thirds of patients with IPF. The main differential diagnoses are NSIP, which typically has more extensive ground glass shadowing, and fibrotic HP. In the absence of honeycombing, the diagnosis is less certain, and a surgical biopsy is necessary to make a definite diagnosis, although contraindicated in many patients by age, disease severity, major co-morbidity, or patient disinclination to undergo the procedure. The overall complication rate from open lung biopsy is <6% [18], with a mortality rate of 1–2%. VATS approaches are now commonplace and facilitate

(Continued)

multi-lobe biopsies, whilst being associated with less post-operative pain. Transbronchial biopsies are not sufficient for the diagnosis of IPF.

Honeycombing is critical for making a definitive diagnosis. The appearance is one of clustered cystic airspaces, typically similar in diameter to each other, usually between 3 and 10 mm, but occasionally as large as 2.5 cm. It can be hard to differentiate between honeycombing and paraseptal emphysema, but emphysematous cystic spaces will have less well-defined walls [19]. Honeycombing can also occur in NSIP in around 5% of cases but is typically microcystic (as opposed to macrocystic in IPF).

Learning point Diagnosis of IPF

Evidence-based international guidance for the diagnosis of IPF has recently been issued in a joint statement from the ATS, ERS, Japanese Respiratory Society (JRS), and the Latin American Thoracic Association (ALAT) [2]. The diagnosis of IPF requires:

1. exclusion of other known causes of ILD (e.g. domestic and occupational environmental exposures, CTD, and drug toxicity);
2. the presence of a UIP pattern on HRCT in patients not subjected to surgical lung biopsy;
3. specific combinations of HRCT and surgical lung biopsy pattern in patients subjected to surgical lung biopsy.

Learning point UIP histopathology features

The hallmark feature of UIP on histology at low magnification is a heterogeneous appearance, in which areas of fibrosis with scarring and honeycombing alternate with areas of less affected or normal parenchyma. It must be stressed that a UIP pattern on biopsy does not, in itself, differentiate between diseases in which this pattern may occur, including CTDs (especially rheumatoid arthritis), chronic HP, and asbestosis—once again stressing how important the history-taking process and other investigations are.

The accuracy of diagnosis of IPF increases in the context of a multidisciplinary approach, utilizing clinicians, radiologists, and pathologists who are experienced in the diagnosis of ILD [20]. All patients with ILD should have access to an MDT based in a regional centre of expertise.

It is also important to note that discordant histological patterns can be seen at surgical biopsy, whereby fibrotic NSIP is identified in one area, but UIP in another. Patients with so-called 'discordant UIP' seem to behave similarly to those with concordant UIP [21]. This highlights how important it is to choose biopsy sites carefully (as part of the MDT discussion) and to ensure that samples are taken from several areas. It is recommended that areas of intermediate abnormality, or comparatively normal lung adjacent to areas of honeycombing, are sampled [12].

Our patient had a fibreoptic bronchoscopy with BAL during his work-up. This was predominantly performed to rule out potentially reversible conditions. His cell differential revealed mild neutrophilia and eosinophilia. His lymphocyte count was normal, and no bacteria were isolated.

Clinical tip The role of BAL in IPF

Cell differentials of BAL fluid can be useful in the diagnosis of ILD. In the context of IPF, the main purpose is to differentiate IPF from chronic HP. A prominent lymphocytosis (>40%) favours the latter. If this is high on the list of differential diagnoses, a BAL is recommended. A finding of raised neutrophils (>4%) and raised eosinophils (>2%) is more characteristic of IPF, but this is also a feature of fibrotic NSIP. BAL may be most useful if targeted to the most affected segment [22].

BAL is also indicated to identify complications, once the diagnosis of IPF is established. This may include infection (especially in an immunocompromised host) and malignancy.

Expert comment

It should be stressed that the diagnostic value of BAL in IPF is critically dependent on the clinical context. In patients with clinical and HRCT features typical of IPF, it has been argued that the added diagnostic value of BAL is doubtful, although this view can be questioned. In some patients with chronic HP, the presence of an environmental antigen is not immediately evident, and the HRCT appearances mimic those of IPF. A BAL lymphocytosis may prompt the clinician to identify an antigen with a more detailed history or may indicate that an identified exposure, previously weighted as of doubtful significance, does indeed have major diagnostic significance. Separately, BAL does often add major value in patients in whom HRCT appearances are not definitive for IPF or an alternative disorder, a frequent scenario, and continues to play a major diagnostic role in our unit, especially with regard to decisions on whether to proceed to a diagnostic surgical biopsy.

By and large, diagnostic BAL tends to be performed in regional centres. The acquisition and laboratory evaluation of BAL samples undoubtedly increases in quality with the frequent performance of BAL, and thus the introduction of diagnostic BAL in peripheral centres may be difficult to justify on cost/ benefit grounds.

Our patient underwent non-invasive cardiac investigations to look for potential right heart failure secondary to his lung disease. His BNP was normal at 8 pmol/L, and an echocardiogram revealed normal ventricular function and right-sided pressures. The patient did not warrant further cardiac investigations in view of these results.

Learning point Pulmonary hypertension in IPF

Pulmonary hypertension (PH) is known to occur in IPF and is a poor prognostic indicator. It should be considered in all patients whose breathlessness, lung function, or oxygenation seems disproportionate to the degree of fibrosis. A right heart catheter is required to accurately confirm the presence of PH, but, given the invasiveness of this procedure, simple alternatives are often used. Transthoracic Doppler echocardiography is used to estimate the right ventricular systolic pressure (RSVP) and, when combined with BNP testing, can be used to identify patients who may warrant further investigation. These two tests in combination have also been shown to predict mortality in IPF [23]. If PH is identified, long-term oxygen should be prescribed for chronic hypoxia, and referral to a specialist PH unit should be considered.

Expert comment

Currently, there is no evidence that targeted therapies for PH are beneficial in IPF patients with PH, and there are concerns that, in occasional patients, PH therapy may cause worsening of V/Q mismatch (although, based on limited clinical information, this problem appears to be relatively infrequent). Referral to a PH unit should therefore be confined to IPF patients in whom PH is severe, impairs the quality of life, and is likely to have major prognostic significance. Regardless of whether such patients are entered into trials of PH treatment or receive empirical targeted therapy on compassionate grounds, a prior right heart study is essential, with measurement of the pulmonary capillary wedge pressure. Occult left ventricular diastolic dysfunction is sometimes present in IPF and may lead to fatal pulmonary oedema with the use of vasodilator therapies.

There is ongoing debate about whether a minority subset of IPF patients with 'disproportionate PH', which is out of keeping with the severity of ILD [24], might have a greater benefit from targeted treatment, but this decision is best taken on a case-by-case basis by a PH specialist.

Given the patient's family history of SLE and his own history of Raynaud's, the patient's initial working diagnosis was that of 'CTD-related ILD', and he had a single dose of IV cyclophosphamide in September 2010. He was due to receive his second dose 1 month later, but, at the time he presented, he was very unwell with an exacerbation of his ILD and was admitted instead. At this point, his lung function had deteriorated, and his TLCO was only 17.4%. He required 1 L of oxygen at rest. Inflammatory markers were normal, and his sputum was unremarkable. He was treated with three doses of IV methylprednisolone (750 mg on day 1, and 1 g on days 2 and 3), with antibiotic cover. However, the patient failed to respond, and, on further review of his imaging and results to date, his diagnosis was changed to that of 'rapidly progressive IPF' in the context of an acute exacerbation.

Learning point Diagnosis and management of exacerbations in IPF

Acute exacerbations are not uncommon in IPF and carry a mortality of over 70%, as well as being a predictor of poor survival after the event [24]. Acute exacerbations must be distinguished from other causes of rapid clinical deterioration, and all of the following should be considered:

- infection;
- PE;
- heart failure;
- pneumothorax;
- respiratory failure;
- bronchogenic carcinoma;
- PH.

If a cause for the acute respiratory decline cannot be identified, the term 'acute exacerbation of IPF' is used. These exacerbations can occur at any point in the disease course. High-dose steroids are commonly prescribed for the treatment of acute IPF exacerbations. However, no controlled trials have been performed to assess the efficacy of this. Nevertheless, the international consensus states that the majority of patients with an acute exacerbation should be treated with corticosteroids (based on the fact that a prominent organizing pneumonia component, present in 10–15% of cases, cannot be excluded based on HRCT appearances), but specific recommendations regarding the dose, route, and duration have not been given [2].

Expert comment

The 2011 consensus statement is an important advance because it has been difficult to draw confident conclusions on many aspects of acute exacerbations, due to the highly variable inclusion criteria in small historical series. The definition of an acute exacerbation requires worsening dyspnoea for up to 4 weeks and evidence of diffuse alveolar damage on imaging, superimposed on abnormalities ascribable to IPF. It is not yet clear whether the prevalence of acute exacerbations (average annual incidence of 5–10%) is linked to chronic disease severity. Acute exacerbations may be the presenting feature in IPF, and, in some cases, underlying abnormalities due to IPF cannot be seen, even with careful HRCT evaluation.

In the 2011 consensus statement, it is argued that infection should be excluded by means of BAL or culture of tracheal aspirate samples and that, by definition, the presence of a clinically significant infection rules out a diagnosis of an acute exacerbation. This view is a little contentious. If it is argued that acute exacerbations are triggered by a number of extraneous factors, a supposition that is supported by the fact that acute exacerbations may be caused by a diagnostic surgical biopsy, it appears counterintuitive to exclude patients in whom an infective trigger can be clearly identified. Diffuse alveolar damage due to infection is a relatively rare event in ILDs other than IPF, and the outcome in IPF in this context is identical to that of acute exacerbations. Management differs little, as it is common practice, as in our unit, to use broad-spectrum antibiotic therapy in acute exacerbations to cover the possibility of an occult infective trigger (although, in many cases, a viral trigger may be responsible).

The patient was discharged from our unit on a weaning regimen of oral steroids.

Learning point Pharmacological therapy in IPF

The 2000 ATS/ERS consensus statement for IPF diagnosis and treatment stated that therapy was not indicated for all patients and that, given the limited success of available treatments, the potential benefits of any treatment protocol for an individual patient with IPF may be outweighed by an increased risk for treatment-related complications [25]. Nevertheless, the consensus also stated that, until further studies were conducted, combination therapy (corticosteroid and either azathioprine or cyclophosphamide) was advised for those patients who had been given adequate information regarding the merits and pitfalls of treatment.

With advanced understanding of IPF, the contribution of inflammation to the pathogenesis has been marginalized. As a result, the role of corticosteroids and azathioprine as first-line therapy was drawn into question.

NICE issued a clinical guideline in June 2013 [26] in light of recent trials which updated recommendations for treatment, compared to the 2000 ATS/ERS consensus statement and the 2011 guidelines. The recommendation is not to use any of the drugs listed, either alone or in combination, to attempt to modify disease progression in IPF: ambrisentan, azathioprine, bosentan, co-trimoxazole, mycophenolate mofetil, prednisolone, sildenafil, or warfarin.

Of course, exceptions to this rule exist, but often such decisions come down to the individual clinician and patient. As such, routine therapy with combination corticosteroid and immunomodulators, therapy with combination corticosteroid, azathioprine, and N-acetylcysteine (NAC), and NAC monotherapy are now not recommended.

Other therapeutic targets which have been assessed in clinical trials include interferon-γ 1b (an agent with antifibrotic and immunomodulatory properties, recently studied in the 'INSPIRE' trial [27]), colchicine (which has been shown to inhibit fibroblast proliferation and collagen synthesis *in vitro*), ciclosporin A, and etanercept (a recombinant soluble human tumour necrosis factor (TNF) receptor which binds to TNF—also implicated in IPF pathogenesis—and neutralizes its activity *in vitro*). None of these have been shown to reliably improve survival in IPF. Cyclophosphamide has also not been shown to have any long-term benefits in IPF but has been shown to be of benefit in CTD-associated ILDs.

Endothelin-1 (ET-1) has also been postulated as a potential therapeutic target. ET-1 is a powerful vasoconstrictor, which may be implicated in the pathogenesis of IPF, as well as PH. Bosentan (a dual endothelin receptor A and B antagonist) was tested in a phase 2 RCT in IPF ('BUILD-1'), looking for a change in the modified 6MWT [28]. This primary end point was not reached, but post hoc analysis suggested that patients who had undergone surgical lung biopsy did benefit from the drug. As a result, a larger study ('BUILD-3') [29] was undertaken. Over 600 patients were recruited (407 in the bosentan arm and 297 in the placebo arm), and there was no significant difference found between the two treatment groups over the 1-year trial. There is no current recommendation for IPF patients to be treated with bosentan routinely.

Anticoagulation in IPF has also received recent interest in IPF, since a link between activation of the coagulation cascade and fibrogenesis has been suggested. A Japanese trial compared corticosteroids alone to corticosteroids plus anticoagulation, and a survival benefit was seen in the anticoagulation arm [30]. In-hospital mortality during acute exacerbations was far lower in the anticoagulated group. Although this has led some clinicians to adopt this practice during acute exacerbations, flaws in the study design have meant that anticoagulation is not currently recommended in IPF (be it routinely or during exacerbations) in international or British guidance. This view has recently been endorsed by a high-quality placebo-controlled trial of oral anticoagulant therapy, in which mortality was actually seen to **increase** with active treatment, although this was not ascribable to the expected side effects of anticoagulant therapy. There is also no current indication for anticoagulation in PH in IPF, unless there is coexisting evidence of thromboembolic disease.

Given the limited, and often conflicting, data, it remains vital to consider all patients for recruitment to high-quality clinical trials of therapy and/or for lung transplantation, if appropriate.

(Continued)

The role of best supportive care should not be underestimated and is relevant to all patients with IPF, irrespective of potential concurrent disease-modifying therapy; this may well include withdrawal of treatment that is proving to be ineffective.

Patients with evidence of GORD (including asymptomatic GORD) should be treated with a PPI.

Oral opiates may be effective in relieving distressing breathlessness or cough. Many clinicians use small doses of benzodiazepines to relieve breathlessness, although there is no evidence to support this practice [31].

Evidence base The IFIGENIA trial and subsequent findings

Several studies have suggested that an antioxidant imbalance may contribute to the disease process in IPF, evidenced by depleted pulmonary glutathione levels in IPF [32]. Restoration of glutathione levels can be achieved with the administration of NAC, at a daily dose of 1800 mg [33], and has been shown to result in a statistically significant improvement in lung function in patients classified as having 'fibrosing alveolitis' after 12 weeks of therapy [34].

The IFIGENIA trial was the first study in IPF to reach its primary end point, namely a change between baseline and 12-month vital capacity and single-breath TLCO, and was the evidence behind the previous BTS guideline's weak recommendation for triple therapy. This multicentre RCT enrolled 155 patients and randomized them to receive standard therapy alone (prednisolone and azathioprine) or standard therapy plus NAC, 600 mg tds. The addition of NAC was shown to preserve the vital capacity and TLCO better than standard therapy alone, but more recent additional analyses have shown that these effects were confined to patients with earlier disease, with a composite physiologic index (CPI, a composite scoring system that uses values from FEV_1, FVC, and TLCO to predict the extent of disease on HRCT and that is able to predict mortality better than any individual lung function measure) threshold of 50 units, providing the most discriminatory cut-off [35].

The effect of NAC as a stand-alone treatment (versus placebo and versus triple therapy) was assessed in patients with mild to moderate IPF (the 'PANTHER-IPF' trial). However, in October 2011, analysis of interim data revealed an increase in mortality, serious adverse events, and drug discontinuation in the triple therapy arm [36].

Interestingly, the mortality rates for the triple therapy and standard therapy arms in the IFIGENIA study interim analysis were similar to those found in the triple therapy arm of the PANTHER-IPF interim analysis, highlighting the need for more placebo-controlled clinical trials. If a placebo arm had been included in the IFIGENIA trial, the final recommendations from the trial may well have been very different. The BTS ILD Specialist Advisory Group recommends that new patients with definite IPF should not be initiated on a regimen containing prednisolone plus azathioprine; for patients with definite IPF already receiving triple therapy, it is recommended that azathioprine therapy, in particular, should be withdrawn if there is evidence of disease progression (declining lung function). In patients established on triple therapy with 'stable' disease, the decision to withdraw should be on a case-by-case basis, but the threshold for withdrawing azathioprine from elderly patients should be low.

The other two arms of the study (placebo versus NAC) were reported in 2014. The trial did not find any significant benefit with the use of NAC alone in preserving the FVC in patients with IPF and a mild to moderate impairment in lung function. Therefore, the use of NAC alone is not recommended, based on this evidence [37].

Expert comment

The recent PANTHER data have thrown current treatment recommendations into disarray, and an update of the ATS/ERS treatment guidelines is definitely needed. Strikingly, the adverse outcomes in the PANTHER study co-segregated with high-dose corticosteroid therapy in the first 16 weeks of the study, and it is entirely unclear, from this prematurely terminated trial, whether

(Continued)

the pulmonary function benefits seen in the IFIGENIA study at 1 year would also have become evident with time in the PANTHER cohort with lower-dose, longer-term treatment. Recent data have suggested that immune dysregulation is present in at least 30% of IPF patients. The possibility that a separate IPF patient subset exists, in which immune modulation might provide major benefits but will not be trialled because of short-term toxicity in the PANTHER study, is deeply disturbing. It should therefore be stressed that the PANTHER data should emphatically not be extrapolated to disorders other than IPF, in which an inflammatory/fibrotic disease model remains appropriate.

Evidence base The CAPACITY trial and subsequent findings

Pirfenidone is a novel antifibrotic and anti-inflammatory agent, which inhibits the progression of fibrosis in animal models. A Japanese RCT in 107 IPF patients was terminated prematurely when an interim analysis revealed significantly more exacerbations in the placebo group, compared to the pirfenidone group [38]. However, due to the early termination of the trial, the overall results were inconclusive, and two further trials (the 'CAPACITY' trials) were developed, with the aim of confirming the findings [39]. Only one of these trials met its primary end point of absolute change from baseline in % predicted FVC, and, although some secondary end points were supportive of pirfenidone, there were inconsistencies between the two trials. Pirfenidone is associated with significant gastrointestinal adverse events, derangement of LFTs, photosensitivity, and rashes.

NICE issued a guideline on pirfenidone for treating IPF in April 2013, with the following guidance [40]

Pirfenidone is recommended for treating patients with IPF only if:

- FVC between 50% and 80% predicted;
- treatment with pirfenidone is discounted if there is evidence of disease progression (FVC decline of 10% or more over a 12-month period).

The potential benefits of pirfenidone have been replicated in a phase 3 trial (ASCEND) published in 2014 [41]. A total of 555 patients were randomized to pirfenidone or placebo. There was a relative reduction of 47.9% in the proportion of patients who had an absolute decline of 10 percentage points or more in the % predicted FVC. The pirfenidone group also had a reduced decline in 6MWT ($p = 0.04$) and improved progression-free survival ($p < 0.001$) at 52 weeks. Side effects included gastrointestinal and skin symptoms, but the majority of patients were able to continue with the treatment.

The NHS Commissioning Board in the UK has limited the initiation of pirfenidone to a number of highly specialist respiratory centres. This will lead to increased expertise and research within these centres but risks delays in treatment initiation.

Our patient was considered for pirfenidone, but unfortunately his lung function had declined, with an FEV_1 of 45% predicted, and therefore he was not eligible for this treatment.

This demonstrates that, whilst recent trials provide a major breakthrough for patients with IPF, questions remain regarding their efficacy in patients whose lung function falls outside the recruitment criteria for these trials. Of note, the INPULSIS trials did not exclude patients with a normal FVC, resulting in a cohort of patients with less severe disease than we encounter in our clinical practice, and even than the average patient in the ASCEND trial. To date, these trials provide little data about their use in patients with more severe disease (FVC <50% predicted) and also provide little data about their effects beyond 52 weeks.

Our patient was also referred for consideration of lung transplantation due to the progression of his IPF, his age, and the severe reduction in FVC and TLCO. There were no contraindications to transplantation, given his age, normal echocardiogram and subsequent normal CT coronary angiogram, and normal bone density. He was discharged home from our unit, with long-term oxygen, ambulatory oxygen, and community palliative care support.

Learning point Non-pharmacological therapy in IPF

Oxygen

Although no studies directly address the benefits of oxygen in patients with IPF, extrapolation of data from trials in other respiratory conditions suggests that IPF patients with clinically significant resting hypoxaemia should receive long-term oxygen. Similarly, patients who desaturate on exercise should be considered for ambulatory oxygen, after formal ambulatory assessment. Nocturnal hypoxaemia has been demonstrated in IPF patients and may have an impact on HRQoL [42]; however, there has been minimal research into this area, and there is currently no evidence to suggest that supplemental oxygen is beneficial in this setting.

Lung transplantation

This is the only treatment shown to offer a survival benefit in IPF. IPF is now the commonest indication for transplantation. The international 2009 1-, 5-, and 10-year survival rates were 74%, 45%, and 22%, respectively, somewhat lower than other indications [43]. Criteria for transplant referral include advanced (TLCO <40% predicted) or progressive (≥10% decline in FVC or ≥15% decline in TLCO during 6 months of follow-up) disease in patients usually ≤65 years of age with no significant co-morbidities. Previous pleurodesis (e.g. following a pneumothorax, a recognized complication of IPF) is not a contraindication to transplantation. Discussions about transplantation should be encouraged in suitable candidates soon after diagnosis, and further assessment for transplant should begin at the first sign of an objective deterioration. Mechanical ventilation should not be used as a bridge to transplantation, due to a high risk of post-operative complications and increased mortality. Similarly, the majority of IPF patients with respiratory failure should not receive mechanical ventilation, given the very high mortality rate in ventilated patients [44].

Smoking cessation

All patients with IPF who smoke should be referred for smoking cessation.

Pulmonary rehabilitation

Pulmonary rehabilitation has been shown to improve exercise tolerance, symptoms, and quality of life in IPF. It should be offered to all patients in whom it is not contraindicated. However, as with the use of ambulatory oxygen, the decision of the patient should not be questioned. In quality of life matters and related treatment decisions, the patient is the 'world expert' on their personal morbidity and its impact on their day-to-day life [44].

Palliative care

As stated earlier, the role of best supportive care should not be underestimated, and palliative care is central to this, paying careful attention to symptom relief and comfort. Health-care professionals should be honest with patients regarding their prognosis and current uncertainties regarding disease-modifying therapy. Advanced directives and end-of-life care issues should be addressed in the ambulatory setting, and palliative care specialists should be involved when and where appropriate.

Since his referral for lung transplantation, the patient has now completed a course of pulmonary rehabilitation and remains on the transplant waiting list.

Discussion

As our patient demonstrates, the onset of IPF tends to be insidious, with patients presenting following an additional acute insult. On presentation, it is important to look carefully for underlying causes or associated features that may point to an alternative diagnosis. As with our patient, the diagnosis is not always clear-cut, and it is fair to say that considerable overlap can exist between the IIPs. This simply re-enforces the need for a thorough multidisciplinary approach in all patients with suspected ILD, and more regional centres are emerging. There is now growing evidence that patients can experience prolonged periods of stability, and clinicians must be careful not to over-treat patients. There is clearly a need for more placebo-controlled trials into the treatment of IPF, including further combination therapy trials (including the possible combination of pirfenidone with nintedanib) to address the complex pathogenesis of this devastating disease.

A final word from the expert

In addition to these important points, early discussion of advanced care and of the efficacy of palliative measures in end-stage disease should be considered. It is increasingly clear that many IPF patients have major loss of quality of life throughout their disease because of anxieties about what may happen late in disease, including a fear of slow 'suffocation'. In a recent IPF 'patients' day' at our institution, this issue was polled, and it was considered by 68 or 69 patients that discussion of end-stage care was highly desirable at, or shortly after, diagnosis.

References

1. American Thoracic Society, European Respiratory Society. American Thoracic Society/ European Respiratory Society International Multidisciplinary Consensus Classification of the Idiopathic Interstitial Pneumonias. This joint statement of the American Thoracic Society (ATS), and the European Respiratory Society (ERS) was adopted by the ATS board of directors, June 2001 and by the ERS Executive Committee, June 2001. *Am J Respir Crit Care Med* 2002;**165**:277–304.
2. Raghu G, Collard HR, Egan JJ *et al.* ATS/ERS/JRS/ALAT Committee on Idiopathic Pulmonary Fibrosis. An official ATS/ERS/JRS/ALAT statement: idiopathic pulmonary fibrosis: evidence-based guidelines for diagnosis and management. *Am J Respir Crit Care Med* 2011; **183**: 788–824.
3. Navaratnam V, Fleming KM, West J *et al.* The rising incidence of idiopathic pulmonary fibrosis in the U.K. *Thorax* 2011;**66**:462–7.
4. Nicholson AG, Colby TV, du Bois RM, Hansell DM, Wells AU. The prognostic significance of the histologic pattern of interstitial pneumonia in patients presenting with the clinical entity of cryptogenic fibrosing alveolitis. *Am J Respir Crit Care Med* 2000;**162**:2213–17.
5. Strieter RM. Pathogenesis and natural history of usual interstitial pneumonia: the whole story or the last chapter of a long novel. *Chest* 2005;**128**:526S–32S.
6. Gross TJ, Hunninghake GW. Idiopathic pulmonary fibrosis. *N Engl J Med* 2001;**345**:517–25.
7. Selman M, King TE, Pardo A; American Thoracic Society; European Respiratory Society; American College of Chest Physicians. Idiopathic pulmonary fibrosis: prevailing and evolving hypotheses about its pathogenesis and implications for therapy. *Ann Intern Med* 2001;**134**:136–51.
8. Raghu G, Freudenberger TD, Yang S *et al.* High prevalence of abnormal acid gastro-oesophageal reflux in idiopathic pulmonary fibrosis. *Eur Respir J* 2006;**27**:136–42.
9. Marshall RP, Puddicombe A, Cookson WO, Laurent GJ. Adult familial cryptogenic fibrosing alveolitis in the United Kingdom. *Thorax* 2000;**55**:143–6.

10. Antoniou KM, Margaritopoulos G, Economidou F, Siafakas NM. Pivotal clinical dilemmas in collagen vascular diseases associated with interstitial lung involvement. *Eur Respir J* 2009;**33**:882–96.
11. Nadrous HF, Myers JL, Decker PA, Ryu JH. Idiopathic pulmonary fibrosis in patients younger than 50 years. *Mayo Clin Proc* 2005;**80**:37–40.
12. Bradley B, Branley HM, Egan JJ *et al.* British Thoracic Society Interstitial Lung Disease Guideline Group, British Thoracic Society Standards of Care Committee; Thoracic Society of Australia; New Zealand Thoracic Society; Irish Thoracic Society. Interstitial lung disease guideline: the British Thoracic Society in collaboration with the Thoracic Society of Australia and New Zealand and the Irish Thoracic Society. *Thorax* 2008;**63**(Suppl 5):v1–58.
13. Mogulkoc N, Brutsche MH, Bishop PW, Greaves SM, Horrocks AW, Egan JJ; Greater Manchester Pulmonary Fibrosis Consortium. Pulmonary function in idiopathic pulmonary fibrosis and referral for lung transplantation. *Am J Respir Crit Care Med* 2001;**164**:103–8.
14. Flaherty KR, Andrei AC, Murray S *et al.* Idiopathic pulmonary fibrosis: prognostic value of changes in physiology and six-minute-walk test. *Am J Respir Crit Care Med* 2006;**174**:803–9.
15. Best AC, Meng J, Lynch AM *et al.* Idiopathic pulmonary fibrosis: physiologic tests, quantitative CT indexes, and CT visual scores as predictors of mortality. *Radiology* 2008;**246**:935–40.
16. Sumikawa H, Johkoh T, Colby TV *et al.* Computed tomography findings in pathological usual interstitial pneumonia: relationship to survival. *Am J Respir Crit Care Med* 2008;**177**:433–9.
17. Flaherty KR, Thwaite EL, Kazerooni EA *et al.* Radiological versus histological diagnosis in UIP and NSIP: survival implications. *Thorax* 2003;**58**:143–8.
18. Shah SS, Tsang V, Goldstraw P. Open lung biopsy: a safe, reliable and accurate method for diagnosis in diffuse lung disease. *Respiration* 1992;**59**:243–6.
19. Wells AU, King AD, Rubens MB, Cramer D, du Bois RM, Hansell DM. Lone cryptogenic fibrosing alveolitis: a functional-morphologic correlation based on extent of disease on thin-section computed tomography. *Am J Respir Crit Care Med* 1997;**155**:1367–75.
20. Flaherty KR, King TE Jr, Raghu G *et al.* Idiopathic interstitial pneumonia: what is the effect of a multidisciplinary approach to diagnosis? *Am J Respir Crit Care Med* 2004;**170**:904–10.
21. Monaghan H, Wells AU, Colby TV, du Bois RM, Hansell DM, Nicholson AG. Prognostic implications of histologic patterns in multiple surgical lung biopsies from patients with idiopathic interstitial pneumonias. *Chest* 2004;**125**:522–6.
22. Agusti C, Xaubet A, Luburich P, Ayuso MC, Roca J, Rodriguez-Roisin R. Computed tomography-guided bronchoalveolar lavage in idiopathic pulmonary fibrosis. *Thorax* 1996;**51**:841–5.
23. Corte TJ, Gatzoulis MA, Parfitt L, Harries C, Wells AU, Wort SJ. The use of sildenafil to treat pulmonary hypertension associated with interstitial lung disease. *Respirology* 2010;**15**:1226–32.
24. Song JW, Hong SB, Lim CM, Koh Y, Kim DS. Acute exacerbation of idiopathic pulmonary fibrosis: incidence, risk factors and outcome. *Eur Respir J* 2011;**37**:356–63.
25. American Thoracic Society. Idiopathic pulmonary fibrosis: diagnosis and treatment. International consensus statement. American Thoracic Society (ATS), and the European Respiratory Society (ERS). *Am J Respir Crit Care Med* 2000;**161**:646–64.
26. National Institute for Health and Care Excellence (2013). *Idiopathic pulmonary fibrosis in adults: diagnosis and management.* NICE guidelines CG163. Available at: <https://www.nice.org.uk/guidance/cg163>.
27. King TE Jr, Albera C, Bradford WZ *et al.* INSPIRE Study Group. Effect of interferon gamma-1b on survival in patients with idiopathic pulmonary fibrosis (INSPIRE): a multicentre, randomised, placebo-controlled trial. *Lancet* 2009;**374**:222–8.

28. King TE Jr, Behr J, Brown KK *et al.* BUILD-1: a randomized placebo-controlled trial of bosentan in idiopathic pulmonary fibrosis. *Am J Respir Crit Care Med* 2008;**177**:75–81.
29. King TE Jr, Brown KK, Raghu G *et al.* BUILD-3: a randomized, controlled trial of bosentan in idiopathic pulmonary fibrosis. *Am J Respir Crit Care Med* 2011;**184**:92–9.
30. Kubo H, Nakayama K, Yanai M *et al.* Anticoagulant therapy for idiopathic pulmonary fibrosis. *Chest* 2005;**128**:1475–82.
31. Simon ST, Higginson IJ, Booth S, Harding R, Bausewein C. Benzodiazepines for the relief of breathlessness in advanced malignant and non-malignant diseases in adults. *Cochrane Database Syst Rev* 2010;**1**:CD007354.
32. Cantin AM, Hubbard RC, Crystal RG. Glutathione deficiency in the epithelial lining fluid of the lower respiratory tract in idiopathic pulmonary fibrosis. *Am Rev Respir Dis* 1989;**139**:370–2.
33. Meyer A, Buhl R, Magnussen H. The effect of oral N-acetylcysteine on lung glutathione levels in idiopathic pulmonary fibrosis. *Eur Respir J* 1994;**7**:431–6.
34. Behr J, Maier K, Degenkolb B, Krombach F, Vogelmeier C. Antioxidative and clinical effects of high-dose N-acetylcysteine in fibrosing alveolitis. Adjunctive therapy to maintenance immunosuppression. *Am J Respir Crit Care Med* 1997;**156**:1897–901.
35. Behr J, Demedts M, Buhl R *et al.* IFIGENIA study group. Lung function in idiopathic pulmonary fibrosis-extended analyses of the IFIGENIA trial. *Respir Res* 2009;**10**:101.
36. Idiopathic Pulmonary Fibrosis Clinical Research Network Raghu G, AnstromKJ, King TE Jr, Lasky JA, Martinez FJ. Prednisone, azathioprine, and N-acetylcysteine for pulmonary fibrosis. *N Engl J Med* 2012;**366**:1968–77.
37. Idiopathic Pulmonary Fibrosis Clinical Research Network, Martinez FJ, de Andrade JA, Anstrom KJ, King TE Jr, Raghu G. Randomized trial of acetylcysteine in idiopathic pulmonary fibrosis. *N Engl J Med* 2014;**370**:2093–101.
38. Azuma A, Nukiwa T, Tsuboi E *et al.* Double-blind, placebo-controlled trial of pirfenidone in patients with idiopathic pulmonary fibrosis. *Am J Respir Crit Care Med* 2005;**171**:1040–7.
39. Noble PW, Albera C, Bradford WZ *et al.* CAPACITY Study Group. Pirfenidone in patients with idiopathic pulmonary fibrosis (CAPACITY): two randomised trials. *Lancet* 2011;**377**:1760–9.
40. National Institute for Health and Care Excellence (2013). *Pirfenidone for treating idiopathic pulmonary fibrosis.* NICE technology appraisal guidance TA282. Available at: <https://www.nice.org.uk/guidance/TA282?UNLID=248563829201426101 62>.
41. King TE Jr, Bradford WZ, Castro-Bernardini S *et al.* ASCEND Study Group. A phase 3 trial of pirfenidone in patients with idiopathic pulmonary fibrosis. *N Engl J Med* 2014;**370**:2083–92.
42. Clark M, Cooper B, Singh S, Cooper M, Carr A, Hubbard R. A survey of nocturnal hypoxaemia and health related quality of life in patients with cryptogenic fibrosing alveolitis. *Thorax* 2001;**56**:482–6.
43. Christie JD, Edwards LB, Aurora P *et al.* The Registry of the International Society for Heart and Lung Transplantation: Twenty-sixth Official Adult Lung and Heart-Lung Transplantation Report-2009. *J Heart Lung Transplant* 2009;**28**:1031–49.
44. Mallick S. Outcome of patients with idiopathic pulmonary fibrosis (IPF) ventilated in intensive care unit. *Respir Med* 2008;**102**:1355–9.

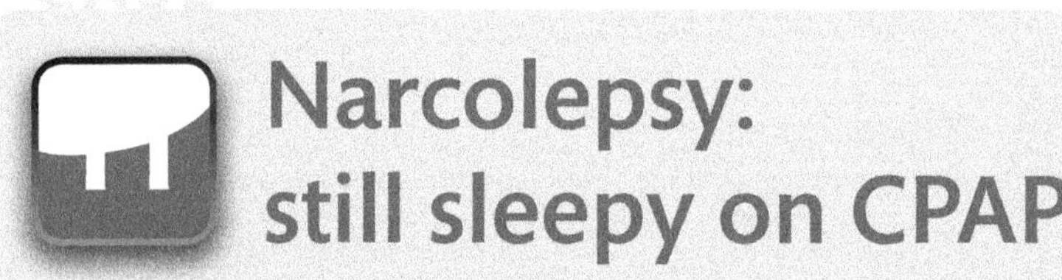

Narcolepsy: still sleepy on CPAP

Dave Walder

Expert commentary Paul Reading

Case history

A 35-year-old man initially presented to his GP complaining of heavy snoring and feeling sleepy throughout the day. His partner had noticed him having episodes at night where he appeared to 'stop breathing'. He had no past medical history and was taking no regular medications. Systemic enquiry was unremarkable. He was unemployed and a non-smoker, and his average alcohol intake was 10 units/week. He drank approximately two caffeine-containing drinks per day.

Examination revealed him to be obese with a thick set neck (height 1.93 m, weight 177.8 kg, BMI 47.7). Cardiovascular, respiratory, abdominal, and neurological examinations were normal. His GP was concerned he may have obstructive sleep apnoea (OSA) and arranged an overnight sleep study and referral to his local sleep clinic (Figure 11.1).

Based on his overnight pulse oximetry, he was found to have moderate to severe OSA and was started on nocturnal CPAP at a pressure of 15 cmH_2O.

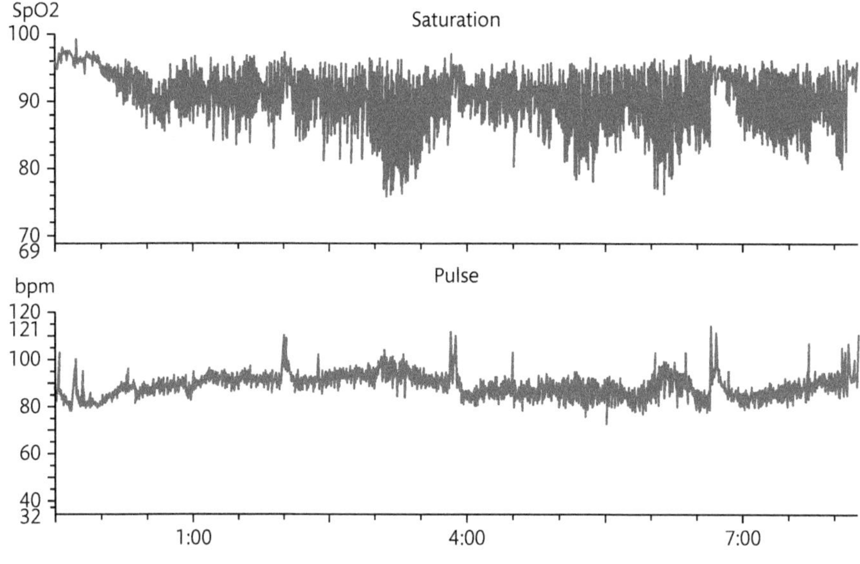

Figure 11.1 Results of overnight oximetry.

Expert comment

One of the clues that excessive daytime sleepiness may be due to a primary (neurological) sleep disorder is the longevity of symptoms. It is important to establish exactly when symptoms were first noticed by the subject, and not necessarily when first discussed with doctors. Most cases of narcolepsy start at around, or even before, puberty, and falling asleep in the classroom is a symptom that needs to be actively explored, even if not mentioned spontaneously in routine history taking.

Clinical tip

When reviewing a patient on CPAP who remains excessively sleepy, it is essential to check compliance. At least 4, and preferably >6, hours are required to relieve excessive daytime sleepiness [1].

Learning point Obstructive sleep apnoea

Diagnosis of OSA is made by combination of a focussed sleep history, physical examination, and sleep testing. Specific features to illicit include witnessed apnoeas, gasping episodes, snoring, and excessive daytime sleepiness. The severity of sleepiness should be quantified with the ESS.

Accepted objective measurements for OSA are by PSG or portable pulse oximetry. An AHI of >5 in the presence of suggestive symptoms is diagnostic. When using pulse oximetry, an apnoeic/hypopnoeic episode is scored if there is a >4% oxygen desaturation.

- Mild: AHI 5–15.
- Moderate: AHI 15–30.
- Severe: AHI >30.

The gentleman was distressed that his symptoms had not improved despite CPAP and asked for a referral to a tertiary centre for a second opinion. The data were downloaded from his CPAP machine, and compliance was found to be good with an average daily use of 6.4 hours. The respiratory registrar agreed the history was in keeping with OSA. His ESS score was 13/24. His weight had now increased to 184 kg, and there was concern that his CPAP pressures were now insufficient.

The repeat oximetry on CPAP showed that his sleep apnoea was well controlled, with a 4% oxygen desaturation index (ODI) of 1/hour. However, he was noted to have a dense heart rate variability, suggesting arousals. The decision was made to perform a more detailed PSG (Table 11.1).

Table 11.1 **Full polysomnography results**

Sleep summary				
Total recording time:	525.0 minutes	Apnoea + hypopnoea (A+H):	2	0.3/h
Sleep period:	514.5 minutes	Obstructive apnoea:	0	0.0/h
Wake after sleep onset:	110.0 minutes	Central apnoea:	2	0.3/h
Total sleep time:	404.5 minutes	Mixed apnoea:	0	0.0/h
Sleep onset:	10.5 minutes	Hypopnoea (all):	0	0.0/h
Sleep efficiency:	78.6%	Obstructive hypopnoea:	–	–/h
Number of awakenings:	35	Central hypopnoea:	–	–/h
Sleep latency to N1:	96.0 minutes	Mixed hypopnoea:	–	–/h
Sleep latency to N2:	10.5 minutes	Oxygen desaturation events (OD)	14	2.1/h
Sleep latency to N3 (SWS):	31.0 minutes			
Stage R latency from sleep onset:	67.0 minutes	Snore time:	169.1 minutes	41.8

Arousal statistics	Number	Index		Number	Index
Arousals	–	–	Spontaneous arousals	40	5.9
Apnoea arousals	–	–	Hypopnoea arousals	–	–
Desaturation arousals	–	–	Snore arousals	–	–
Respiratory arousals	0	0.0	RERA	49	7.3
User-defined arousals	1	0.1	Total arousals	93	13.8

Learning point Polysomnography

PSG is a multi-parametric test used in the diagnosis of sleep disorders that measures the biophysical changes occurring during sleep. The range of inputs available will vary from centre to centre but typically include electroencephalography (EEG), electro-oculography (EOG), electromyography (EMG), ECG, pulse oximetry, respiratory effort (via chest wall and upper abdominal pressure belts), and nasal and oral airflow. Additionally, most centres video the patient and record any snoring.

The data are analysed by a scorer who divides each channel into 30-second epochs, from which the following data are given (normal values):

1. **sleep latency**: time taken to fall asleep from time lights turned off (<20 minute);
2. **sleep efficiency**: time asleep divided by time in bed, as a percentage (85–95%);
3. **sleep stages**: scored based on information from EEG, EOG, and chin EMG. Each 30-second epoch is divided between awake and each of the four stages of sleep. Stage 4 is rapid eye movement (REM) sleep. Stages 1–3 are classified as non-REM sleep. (REM sleep 25%);
4. **apnoea/hypopnoea index (AHI)**: information from airflow meters, chest wall pressure transducers, and oxygen saturation calculate the number of apnoeic episodes and hypopnoeic episodes. These are divided by the total time asleep to give the AHI (normal <5/hour, mild 5–15/hour, moderate 15–30/hour, severe >30/hour);
5. **respiratory-related arousal index**: combination of apnoeic, hypopnoeic, and respiratory effort-related arousals (RERAs) divided by total sleep time. RERAs are episodes of 10 seconds or more of increased respiratory effort leading to arousal (same range as AHI).

The results of the full PSG were reviewed by the registrar who noticed a sleep latency of 10.5 minutes, a sleep efficiency of 78.6%, an AHI of 0.3/hour, and a respiratory-related arousal index of 7.3/hour. In light of these findings, the continued snoring, and reduced airflow, the decision was made to increase the CPAP to 17.6 cmH_2O.

The patient was reviewed in clinic 5 months later. He was still complaining of excessive sleepiness. His repeat ESS score was 18/24. On questioning, he revealed that he was having very vivid dreams which were often quite disturbing. He had also noticed episodes where, when he laughed, his head, legs, and arms felt weak. He described the sensation that he had no strength in his legs and felt as if he was going to fall down. Observers had noticed that his head fell forward at these times. He went on to have a repeat overnight sleep study, with subsequent multiple sleep latency testing (MSLT) (Table 11.2).

Expert comment

One would normally expect a sleep efficiency of well over 80% in a gentleman of this age. In narcolepsy, sleep continuity is often 'destructured' with general fragmentation and an abnormal distribution of slow-wave sleep overnight. REM sleep may occur earlier than average and be associated with body movement, in contrast to the normal complete muscle atonia during REM periods.

Learning point Multiple sleep latency testing

MSLT is the accepted standard objective test for excessive daytime sleepiness. It is usually performed on the day following overnight PSG, as a minimum of 6 hours of recorded sleep is recommended on the night before MSLT.

The MSLT consists of four or five scheduled sleeps of 20-minute duration, separated by periods of 2 hours. The patient is required to stay awake between naps. The patient is connected to the polysomnogram during these naps to allow the time taken to fall asleep to be calculated and the presence or absence of REM sleep. When REM sleep occurs within 15 minutes of sleep onset, it is termed sleep-onset REM sleep (SOREM).

Expert comment

This appears to be a good description of cataplexy which is virtually diagnostic for narcolepsy, given that it is never seen in other disorders. Some cases can cause diagnostic doubt if the cataplexy attacks are partial or subtle. A stuttering dysarthria when telling jokes or slight 'bobbing' of the head may be the only manifestation in mild cases.

The repeat PSG showed a sleep latency of 9 minutes, with a REM sleep latency of 1.5 minutes. The AHI was again controlled on his CPAP at 0.5/hour. Sleep fragmentation was again noticed. The MSLT over four naps showed a mean sleep latency of 1.6 minutes, and three out of the four naps included SOREM. He went

Table 11.2 Multiple sleep latency testing result

	Nap 1	Nap 2	Nap 3	Nap 4
Lights off clock time	08:43	10:31	12:34	14:37
Lights on clock time	09:01	10:49	12:51	14:55
Total record time	17.5	17.5	16.5	17.5
Total sleep time	15.5	15.5	15.0	15.0
Sleep efficiency	88.6	88.6	90.9	85.7
Latency to sleep	1.5	2.0	1.5	1.5
Latency to N1	1.5	2.0	1.5	1.5
Latency to N2	–	–	3.0	5.5
Latency to N3	–	–	–	–
Latency to R (from lights out)	4.0	7.5	–	4.5
Latency to R (from sleep onset)	2.5	5.5	–	4.5
Minutes of REM	13.0	10.0	–	11.5

Sleep efficiency	88.4%
Mean sleep latency of the first four naps	1.6 min
Mean sleep latency of the first three naps	1.7 min
Mean sleep latency of the first two naps	1.8 min
Number of naps with stage R Sleep	3
Average latency to R (from lights out)	5.8
Average latency to R (from sleep onset)	4.2

on to have human leucocyte antigen (HLA) testing which was positive for HLA DQB1*0602 allele, the common haplotype seen in narcolepsy. Diagnosis of narcolepsy is based on a combination of clinical history, objective measures of excessive daytime sleepiness, and laboratory testing. The lack of specificity of each of these tests means that reliance on any one alone may lead to misdiagnosis. Based on a combination of the history and these findings, a diagnosis of narcolepsy with cataplexy was made.

Learning point The International Classification of Sleep Disorders for narcolepsy

Narcolepsy with cataplexy

- Excessive daytime sleepiness almost daily for at least 3 months.
- Definite history of cataplexy.
- Diagnosis should be confirmed, whenever possible, by one of the following:

1. PSG and MSLT; mean sleep latency should be ≤8 minutes and at least 2 SOREMs;
2. Cerebrospinal fluid (CSF) hypocretin level ≤110 pg/mL or one-third of mean normal controls;
3. hypersomnia is not better explained by another disorder or medication.

Narcolepsy without cataplexy

- Excessive daytime sleepiness almost daily for at least 3 months.
- Definite cataplexy is not present.
- Diagnosis must be confirmed by PSG or MSLT; mean sleep latency should be ≤8 minutes and ≥2 SOREMs.
- Hypersomnia is not better explained by another disorder or medication.

Secondary narcolepsy (narcolepsy due to medical condition)

- Excessive daytime sleepiness almost daily for at least 3 months.
- One of the following is present:

(Continued)

1. definite history of cataplexy; if cataplexy is not present, diagnosis must be confirmed by PSG and MSLT; mean sleep latency should be ≤8 minutes and at least 2 SOREMs;
2. CSF hypocretin level ≥110 pg/mL;
3. underlying medical or neurological condition accounts for the sleepiness;
4. hypersomnia is not better explained by another disorder or medication [2].

Clinical tip HLA haplotype

The aetiology of narcolepsy is unclear, but family clustering supports a genetic component. Of those patients that have narcolepsy with cataplexy, >85% are positive for the HLA allele HLA DQB1*0602. This is often seen in combination with HLA DRB1*1501 [3]. The correlation is much less in patients with narcolepsy without cataplexy, and hence it is not routinely tested in this group. Importantly, the allele is found in between 12% and 38% of the general population and therefore lacks both the sensitivity and specificity to be used as a routine diagnostic test [4].

Learning point Hypocretins

Hypocretins 1 and 2 are dorsolateral hypothalamic neuropeptides. A mutated hypocretin receptor 2 gene in dogs causes narcolepsy that is inherited in an autosomal recessive pattern [5]. A study by Nishino *et al.* showed seven patients with narcolepsy and cataplexy had undetectable CSF hypocretin levels which were detectable in their matched controls [6]. In humans, rather than a defective gene, post-mortem examination of narcoleptic patients reveals a loss of hypocretin neurons and associated gliosis [7]. Hypocretin measurement requires lumbar puncture and is not recommended as part of routine testing. It should be considered in patients who are unable to perform MSLT or who cannot stop medications that may affect the result of MSLT and in those patients who have an excellent history of narcolepsy with cataplexy but have a normal MSLT. Hypocretin-1 level below 110 pg/mL is highly suggestive of narcolepsy [2].

The patient was noticed to have a gallop rhythm on examination. He had an ECG which showed sinus rhythm, and a subsequent echocardiogram was normal. He was started on treatment with modafinil 200 mg mane and 200 mg at midday. He was also started on venlafaxine XR 75 mg mane.

Evidence base Randomized trial of modafinil as treatment for excessive daytime somnolence of narcolepsy: US Modafinil in Narcolepsy Multicenter Study Group

- 21 US centres, double-blind RCT comparing modafinil 200 mg od (n = 89), modafinil 400 mg od (n = 89), and placebo (n = 93) [8].
- Maintenance of wakefulness test (MWT), MSLT, Epworth Sleepiness Scale (ESS), and Clinical Global Impression of change (CGI-S) measured before and after 9 weeks of treatment.
- All parameters significantly improved with both treatment groups, compared to placebo (p <0.001).
- **Conclusion**: no significant difference between the two treatment groups.

Evidence base Dose effects of modafinil in sustaining wakefulness in narcolepsy patients with residual evening sleepiness

- Four-centre, randomized, double-blind study [10].
- A total of 56 patients randomized to modafinil 200 mg od (n = 11), 400 mg od (n = 23), 200 mg bd (n = 10), or 400 mg mane and 200 mg noon (n = 12).
- A randomized, single-blind, 1- or 2-week placebo washout period was given prior to the study period.
- An extended MWT was used, allowing testing into the early evening, CGI-S, and ESS.
- All treatment groups improved MWT from baseline (p <0.01).
- **Conclusion**: late-afternoon/evening MWT was significantly improved in the split-dose regimes, compared to 200 mg od (p <0.05).

Evidence base Randomized, double-blind, placebo-controlled cross-over trial of modafinil in the treatment of excessive daytime sleepiness in narcolepsy

- Cross-over trial in nine Canadian centres [9].
- Each of 75 patients assigned in order to placebo for 2 weeks, modafinil 200 mg od for 2 weeks, and modafinil 200 mg bd for 2 weeks.
- MWT, ESS, and patient sleep diary recorded at each stage.
- **Conclusion**: MWT and ESS significantly improved with modafinil, but no significant difference between doses.

On next review in clinic, he was much improved but still troubled by both excessive daytime sleepiness and episodes of cataplexy. Sodium oxybate was added to his regimen, titrated to a dose of 4.5 g bd (bedtime and 4 hours later). This led to complete resolution of his cataplexy and marked improvement in his daytime symptoms.

Evidence base US Xyrem Multicenter Study Group 2002

- Randomized, double-blind, placebo-controlled trial (n = 136) [11].
- Following gradual withdrawal and washout of previous medication, allocated to placebo or sodium oxybate at 3 g, 6 g, or 9 g/night in two equally divided doses at bedtime and 2.5–4 hours later for 4 weeks.
- Patient diary recording of number of cataplexy attacks (primary outcome), nocturnal awakenings, total time asleep, hypnagogic hallucinations, and adverse events.
- **Conclusion**: weekly cataplexy attacks reduced at 6 g ($p = 0.0529$) and significantly at 9 g ($p = 0.0001$).

Evidence base Sodium oxybate improves excessive daytime sleepiness in narcolepsy

- International multicentre, randomized, placebo-controlled, double-blind study [12].
- A total of 270 patients already receiving modafinil for excessive daytime sleepiness (dose range 200–600 mg daily).
- Following baseline PSG and MWT, assigned to:

1. modafinil placebo and sodium oxybate placebo; or
2. sodium oxybate (6 g/night for 4 weeks, increased to 9 g/night for 4 weeks) plus modafinil placebo; or
3. modafinil (established dose) plus sodium oxybate placebo; or
4. sodium oxybate and modafinil.

- Primary outcome measure MWT: sleep latency decreased in placebo group from 9.84 minutes to 6.87 minutes at 8 weeks ($p < 0.001$).
- No change in sodium oxybate group; suggests sodium oxybate as effective as modafinil in reducing excessive daytime sleepiness.
- Sodium oxybate and modafinil combination: sleep latency increased from 10.43 minutes to 13.15 minutes ($p < 0.001$).

Discussion

This case highlights the difficulty of a patient presenting with similar symptoms from dual pathologies. Thorough history taking was the key to making the correct diagnosis of narcolepsy with cataplexy. In the majority of OSA cases where CPAP treatment has failed, the reason will be either insufficient pressures, equipment failure such as a large air leak, or poor compliance. It is imperative, when reviewing a patient who remains sleepy on CPAP, to check that these issues have been addressed.

Narcolepsy is a rare disabling lifelong REM sleep disorder of unknown cause. It is characterized by excessive daytime sleepiness, with irresistible sleep attacks, cataplexy, and other REM sleep manifestations such as sleep paralysis and hypnagogic hallucinations. Patients also complain of disturbed nocturnal sleep and parasomnias. Cataplexy is a feature unique to narcolepsy and is characterized by sudden bilateral loss of muscle tone. Such events are often triggered by a strong emotion such as laughter, elation, anger, or surprise. Cataplexy may be localized to regional muscle groups such as the neck, upper or lower limbs, waist, or eyelids. In some cases, all skeletal muscle groups will be affected. Respiratory muscles remain intact, and consciousness remains clear [13].

The diagnosis in the absence of cataplexy is particularly fraught. The differential diagnosis should include idiopathic hypersomnia, recurrent hypersomnia, restless legs syndrome, OSA, periodic limb movement disorder, and insufficient sleep syndrome. Chronic medical conditions associated with sleepiness, such as COPD, congestive cardiac failure, chronic renal or hepatic failure, should be considered. Degenerative neurological conditions, such as Parkinson's disease, Alzheimer's disease, and multiple sclerosis, may be associated with sleepiness and REM sleep behavioural disorder [13]. The characteristic finding in narcolepsy is that of two or more SOREMs on MSLT which can be particularly helpful in differentiating the cause, as SOREMs are not seen in idiopathic hypersomnia.

Expert comment

Although MSLT is widely used as a diagnostic tool, the results can be misleading. It is a test particularly vulnerable to protocol violations, especially in units not experienced in managing sleep disorders. False-negative results are probably common and may be due, for example, to treatment with antidepressant drugs which almost invariably suppress REM sleep. Adequate monitoring of overnight sleep prior to MSLT is highly recommended, but not always undertaken in many units.

Treatments in narcolepsy are aimed at symptom control by pharmacological methods. Rogers *et al.* showed there is some benefit to scheduled naps and routine bed timing to combat sleepiness, but there is insufficient improvement to act as a primary therapy [14].

Excessive daytime sleepiness has historically been treated with stimulants. Originally, this was with caffeine and then, since the 1930s, with amphetamines and their derivatives. These drugs act to release dopamine and noradrenaline via monoaminergic transporters. At low doses, there is an established history from clinical practice that they are effective, but they are associated with a significant side effect profile, including irritability, headache, nervousness, palpitations, insomnia, anorexia, nausea, excessive sweating, and psychosis [15]. There is a lack of RCTs with this group of drugs which may be partly explained by limited research funding for medications already available in generic form. The only controlled trial comparing amphetamines with placebo was performed by Mitler *et al.* in 1990 [16] (see Evidence base, p. 135). The AASM recommends the use of amphetamine, methamphetamine, dextroamphetamine, and methylphenidate as effective treatment for daytime sleepiness due to narcolepsy with a moderate degree of clinical certainty [24].

Evidence base Multicentre, single-blind, controlled trial comparing methylphenidate, pemoline, dexamfetamine, and protriptyline with placebo

- A total of 42 patients with narcolepsy, nine control patients with no sleep disorder [16].
- Subject performance (Wilkinson Addition Test (WAT) and Digit-Symbol Substitution Test (DSST)), ability to stay awake (MWT), and clinical status (questionnaire) were assessed at baseline and after 1 week of treatment at each dose.
- Profound deficit between narcolepsy patients and controls at baseline in all parameters.
- **Conclusions**: methylphenidate, dexamfetamine (all doses), and pemoline >112.5 mg improved the ability to stay awake, performance, and sleep-related symptoms. Protriptyline and pemoline <112.5 mg were not effective.

Learning point Maintenance of wakefulness test

The MWT is a variation on MSLT. It is more accurately a measure of alertness than sleepiness, and hence it is primarily used in clinical trials to establish benefit of therapies and to assess the safety of individuals whose jobs require a high level of alertness. It consists of four or five trials, each separated by 2 hours, of trying to stay awake whilst lying down in a dark room. If no sleep occurs within 40 minutes, the trial is terminated. Sleep latency and REM sleep latency are calculated for each trial.

The monoamine oxidase type B inhibitor selegiline has randomized controlled evidence supporting its efficacy for treating excessive daytime sleepiness and cataplexy [17]. The Standards of Practice Committee (SPC) of the AASM in 2005 cited significant reservations to the use of this agent as the initial choice for sleepiness in narcolepsy. This is due to a combination of limited clinical experience of its use in narcolepsy and significant drug and diet interactions associated with this class of drug [18].

Modafinil is currently the established first-choice treatment for treatment of excessive daytime sleepiness and is recommended by the ASSM. Its method of action is unclear. Side effects include headache, dry mouth, insomnia, nausea and vomiting, anxiety, tachycardia, palpitation, chest pain, and dermatological reactions, including Stevens–Johnson syndrome [19]. A split-dosing strategy is more effective at controlling sleepiness in the evening [10].

The treatment of REM sleep manifestations, including cataplexy, has primarily been with tricyclic antidepressants. This is based on case reports dating back to the 1960s. Their mode of action is by inhibiting the reuptake of catecholamines. There are significant side effects associated with their anticholinergic action, including nausea, anorexia, dry mouth, urinary retention, constipation, and sexual dysfunction [20].

In more recent times, there have been case reports and open-label studies of the efficacy of serotonin-selective reuptake inhibitors (SSRIs) [21], the noradrenergic reuptake inhibitor reboxetine [22], and the noradrenaline and serotonin reuptake inhibitor venlafaxine [23] in the treatment of cataplexy. Despite the lack of strong evidence, based on the case reports and clinical experience, tricyclic antidepressants, SSRIs, venlafaxine, and reboxetine are recommended by the AASM for effective treatment of cataplexy. There is only anecdotal evidence for their efficacy in the treatment of sleep paralysis and hypnagogic hallucinations [18].

Gamma hydroxybutyrate is a natural metabolite of gamma aminobutyrate (GABA). It was initially noted to be effective in the treatment of both cataplexy and excessive daytime sleepiness in the 1970s. Due to concerns over its misuse as a date rape drug, owing to its rapid sedative effects, its use was largely restricted. In recent years, in the form of its sodium salt (sodium oxybate), it has been subject to multiple randomized, double-blind, placebo-controlled trials in the treatment of cataplexy. Three large multicentres from the US have shown a dose-dependent reduction in the number of cataplexy attacks (3 or 4.5–9 g nightly) which becomes significant at a dose of 6 or 9 g/night [11, 24, 25]. The Xyrem International Study Group have also shown sodium oxybate to be effective in the treatment of excessive daytime sleepiness [26]. A subsequent study by Black *et al.* compared combination therapy of active or placebo preparations of modafinil and sodium oxybate [12]. Interestingly, patients receiving the combination therapy of modafinil and sodium oxybate showed the most improvement in objective and subjective measures of sleepiness. This study suggests there is an additive effect of the combination treatment.

Conclusions

The diagnosis of narcolepsy is based on a combination of good history taking, including collateral history from witnesses, and subjective and objective testing of excessive daytime sleepiness. Laboratory tests, such as HLA typing and hypocretin level measurement, can add further supportive evidence when there is diagnostic uncertainty. There is level I evidence to support the use of modafinil, at a split dose of between 100 mg and 400 mg/day, in the treatment of excessive daytime sleepiness in narcolepsy. This can be augmented with sodium oxybate at a starting dose of 4.5 g/night. First-line treatment for cataplexy is with venlafaxine, reboxetine, or sodium oxybate.

A final word from the expert

This case highlights the absolute need for accurate and full history taking in diagnosing sleep disorders, as opposed to relying simply on data from sleep investigations. Narcolepsy is far commoner than is realized (prevalence at least one in 3000), and a spectrum of severity exists. The syndrome often has metabolic consequences, and most narcoleptics are overweight, potentially fuelling additional sleep problems such as OSA. The dual presence of narcolepsy and OSA can be a particular management problem. Most narcoleptic subjects tolerate respiratory masks extremely badly because of dream-like phenomena, hallucinations, and sleep fragmentation in general. The combination of sodium oxybate with CPAP therapy can be very useful in practice, despite any theoretical concerns regarding breathing control when taking the drug.

References

1. Antic NA, Catcheside P, Buchan C *et al*. The effect of CPAP in normalizing daytime sleepiness, quality of life, and neurocognitive function in patients with moderate to severe OSA. *Sleep* 2011;**34**:111–19.
2. American Academy of Sleep Medicine (2005). *International Classification of Sleep Disorders. Diagnostic and Coding Manual*, second edition. Westchester, IL: American Academy of Sleep Medicine.
3. Tafti M. Genetic aspects of normal and disturbed sleep. *Sleep Med* 2009;**10**(Suppl 1):S17–21.
4. Mignot E. Genetic and familial aspects of narcolepsy. *Neurology* 1998;**50**(2 Suppl 1):S16–22.
5. Lin L, Faraco J, Li R *et al*. The sleep disorder canine narcolepsy is caused by a mutation in the hypocretin (oxretin) receptor 2 gene. *Cell* 1998;**98**:365–76.
6. Nishino S, Ripley B, Overeem S, Lammers GJ, Mignot E. Hypocretin (orexin) deficiency in human narcolepsy. *Lancet* 2000;**355**:39–40.
7. Thannickal TC, Moore RY, Nienhuis R *et al*. Reduced number of hypocretin neurons in human narcolepsy. *Neuron* 2000;**27**:469–74.
8. [No authors listed]. Randomized trial of modafinil as treatment for the excessive daytime somnolence of narcolepsy: US Modafinil in Narcolepsy Multicenter Study Group. *Neurology* 2000;**54**:1166–75.
9. Broughton RJ, Fleming JA, George CF *et al*. Randomized double-blind, placebo controlled crossover trial of modafinil in the treatment of excessive daytime sleepiness in narcolepsy. *Neurology* 1997;**49**:444–51.
10. Schwarz JR, Feldman NT, Bogan RK. Dose effects of modafinil in sustaining wakefulness in narcolepsy patients with residual evening sleepiness. *J Neuropsychiatry Clin Neurosci* 2005;**17**:405–12.
11. [No authors listed]. A randomized, double blind, placebo-controlled multicenter trial comparing the effects of three doses of orally administered sodium oxybate with placebo for the treatment of narcolepsy. *Sleep* 2002;**25**:42–9.
12. Black J, Houghton WC. Sodium oxybate improves excessive daytime sleepiness in narcolepsy. *Sleep* 2006;**29**:939–46.
13. Akintomide GS, Rickards H. Narcolepsy: a review. *Neuropsychiatr Dis Treat* 2011;**7**:507–18.
14. Rogers AE, Aldrich MS, Lin X. A comparison of three different sleep schedules for reducing daytime sleepiness in narcolepsy. *Sleep* 2001;**24**:385–91.

15. Ohayon MM, Priest RG, Zulley J, Smirne S, Paiva T. Prevalence of narcolepsy symptomatology and diagnosis in the European general population. *Neurology* 2002;**58**:1826–33.
16. Mitler MM, Hajdukovic R, Erman MK, Koziol JA. Narcolepsy. *J Clin Neurophysiol* 1990;**7**:93–118.
17. Mayer G, Ewert Meier K, Hephata K. Selegiline hydrochloride treatment in narcolepsy. A double-blind, placebo-controlled study. *Clin Neuropharmacol* 1995;**18**:306–19.
18. Morgenthaler TI, Kapur VK, Brown T *et al.*; Standards of Practice Committee of the AASM. Practice parameters for the treatment of narcolepsy and other hypersomnias of central origin. *Sleep* 2007;**30**:1705–11.
19. Peacock J, Benca RM. Narcolepsy: clinical features, co-morbidities and treatment. *Indian J Med Res* 2010;**131**:338–49.
20. Thorpy M. Therapeutic advances in narcolepsy. *Sleep Med* 2007;**8**:427–40.
21. Langdon N, Shindler J, Parkes JD, Bandak S. Fluoxetine in the treatment of cataplexy. *Sleep* 1986;**9**:371–3.
22. Larrosa O, de la Llave Y, Bario S, Granizo JJ, Garcia-Borreguero D. Stimulant and anticataplectic effects of reboxetine in patients with narcolepsy: a pilot study. *Sleep* 2001;**24**:282–5.
23. Smith M, Parkes JD, Dahlitz M. Venlafaxine in the treatment of the narcoleptic syndrome. *J Sleep Res* 1996;**5**:217.
24. U.S. Xyrem Multicenter Study Group. Sodium oxybate demonstrates long-term efficacy for the treatment of cataplexy in patients with narcolepsy. *Sleep Med* 2004;**5**:119–23.
25. Xyrem International Study Group. Further evidence supporting the use of sodium oxybate for the treatment of cataplexy: a double-blind, placebo-controlled study in 228 patients. *Sleep Med* 2005;**6**:415–21.
26. Xyrem International Study Group. A double-blind, placebo-controlled study demonstrates sodium oxybate is effective for the treatment of excessive daytime sleepiness in narcolepsy. *J Clin Sleep Med* 2005;**1**:391–7.

Non-invasive ventilation and chronic obstructive pulmonary disease

Michelle Ramsay

Expert commentary Mike Polkey

Case history

A 72-year-old male smoker presented to the A&E department with a 12-hour history of progressive shortness of breath and productive cough. He had not responded to his usual inhaled therapy and had taken one dose of antibiotics, as he thought he was developing a chest infection. He called for help through his 'careline' who contacted the London ambulance team. Before arrival in hospital, he was given three 5-mg doses of nebulized salbutamol, 500 micrograms of nebulized ipratropium bromide and placed on 4 L of oxygen.

On arrival in the A&E department, he was short of breath, with an audible wheeze; he was tachypnoeic, with a respiratory rate of 34 breaths/minute and using accessory muscles for respiration. He was able to speak in short sentences but unable to perform spirometry.

On examination, his trachea was central, and his chest was hyperinflated. He had bilateral air entry, with an expiratory wheeze and bronchial breathing described at the left base. Cardiovascular and neurological examinations were normal. His abdomen was distended, but soft and not tender, and an indwelling urethral catheter was empty.

He was placed on 24% oxygen via a 'Venturi' mask and given continuous salbutamol nebulizers, IV antibiotics, and hydrocortisone.

An ABG identifying type 2 respiratory failure was taken 15 minutes later on 24% oxygen (Table 12.1). An ECG was unremarkable. His CXR identified emphysematous lungs with reticular change; there was no focal consolidation or pneumothorax (Figure 12.1).

Table 12.1 An ABG taken on 24% oxygen identifying acidotic type 2 respiratory failure with an elevated $PaCO_2$

Parameter (normal values)	Patient values
pH (7.35–7.45)	7.27
PaO_2 (10.67–13.33)	9.1 kPa
$PaCO_2$ (4.67–6.00)	7.1 kPa
$cHCO_3$ (22–26)	24.2 mmol/L
Base excess (−2 to +2)	−3.5 mEq/L

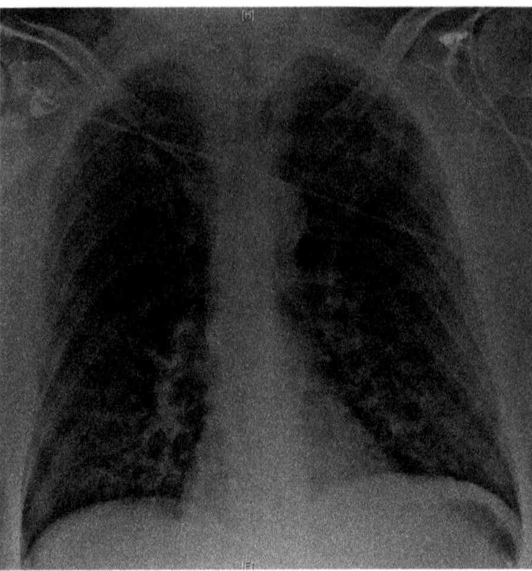

Figure 12.1 A mobile anterior-posterior chest X-ray from the patient on arrival in A&E. It is suggestive of upper lobe emphysema with hyperinflation and crowding of basal lung markings. Large lung volumes are seen extending below the sixth rib anteriorly, with flattening of the hemidiaphragm bilaterally and a narrow heart diameter.

Discussion with the patient's family revealed one previous admission to the ICU a year ago with an exacerbation of COPD, for which he was invasively ventilated, but he has had no further admissions since. He had no previous NIV use. He was diagnosed with limited-stage prostate cancer 3 years previously and had a small bowel obstruction secondary to adhesions operated on 9 months earlier. He lived alone. He is a smoker with a 40- to 50-pack year history. He does not drink alcohol and has an exercise tolerance of 10–20 yards. His most recent spirometry 3 months ago demonstrated an FEV_1 of 0.4 L (15% predicted) with an FVC of 1.2 L (35% predicted).

Learning point Combined assessment of COPD, described by Global Initiative for Chronic Obstructive Lung Disease (GOLD), 2011

In view of the earlier limitations of stratifying the severity of COPD based solely on the airflow obstruction new guidelines have been developed to better incorporate all aspects of the disease. The goals of this approach have been to better determine the severity of disease, the impact on the patient's quality of life and the risk of future deterioration to guide therapy [1].

The assessment includes four components: symptoms, spirometry, risk of exacerbation, and co-morbidity.

Assessment of symptoms

Validated questionnaires—either the COPD assessment test (CAT) or the modified Medical Research Council (mMRC) breathlessness scale—should be used to assess symptoms.

Assessment of the severity of airflow obstruction

$FEV_1/FVC < 0.70$ plus:

	Characteristics
1. Mild COPD	$FEV_1 \geq 80\%$ predicted*
2. Moderate COPD	$50\% \leq FEV_1 < 80\%$ predicted*
3. Severe COPD	$30\% \leq FEV_1 < 50\%$ predicted*
4. Very severe COPD	$FEV_1 < 30\%$ predicted* or<50% with chronic respiratory failure

* Based on post-bronchodilator FEV_1.

The limitations of spirometry include; that patients are frequently unable to perform spirometry or the results are unreliable during an acute exacerbation of COPD which can make a diagnosis at first presentation challenging. Currently alternative physiological biomarkers are under investigation [2].

Learning point Combined Assessment of COPD, described by Global Initiative for Chronic Obstructive Lung Disease (GOLD), 2011

Assessment of the risk of exacerbations: the best predictor of having frequent exacerbations (defined as >2 per year) is having a history of previous treated exacerbations. The risk also increases as airflow obstruction increases.

Assessment of co-morbidities: to identify and treat other diseases commonly occurring in patients with COPD such as cardiovascular disease, osteoporosis, depression, skeletal muscle dysfunction, metabolic syndrome, and lung cancer.

COPD patients are then graded A–D, depending on the results of the four assessments above. These grades provide the physician with a profile of symptom burden and risk of exacerbation. The risk component is determined by the spirometry or exacerbation history, and the patient should be allocated to the grade with the higher score.

For example, a COPD patient with a CAT score of <10, with one exacerbation in the previous year, but an FEV1/FVC of <70% and an FEV1 of 40% predicted, would be **grade C** (spirometry scoring higher than the exacerbation risk).

Grade	*Characteristics*	*Spirometric classification*	*Exacerbations per year*	*mMRC*	*CAT*
A	Low risk, few symptoms	GOLD 1–2	≤1	0–1	≤10
B	Low risk, many symptoms	GOLD 1–2	≤1	≥2	≥10
C	High risk, few symptoms	GOLD 3–4	≥2	0–1	≤10
D	High risk, many symptoms	GOLD 3–4	≥2	≥2	≥10

As the patient remained in type 2 respiratory failure on controlled oxygen therapy of 24%, he was commenced on NIV with an IPAP of 15 cmH_2O, EPAP of 5 cmH_2O, and 1 L of entrained oxygen in the circuit (Table 12.2).

Learning point RCP and BTS national guidelines on the use of NIV in COPD for the management of type 2 respiratory failure [3]

NIV has been shown to reduce intubation rates and mortality in COPD patients with decompensated respiratory acidosis following appropriate medical therapy [4]. It is recommended that NIV be considered within the first 60 minutes for all patients with persistent respiratory acidosis despite treatment with controlled oxygen, to maintain saturations at 88–92%, nebulized salbutamol 5 mg, nebulized ipratropium bromide 500 micrograms, oral prednisolone 30 mg, and antibiotic therapy (where appropriate). A plan stating the appropriate escalation of therapy must be documented when prescribing NIV.

Initiating NIV therapy

This should be performed by a doctor with previous experience of NIV (Specialist Trainee 2 level of training or above). It is recommended that a full face mask be used for the first 24 hours and then changed if NIV is still required, depending on patient comfort.

BTS/RCP guidelines suggest starting an IPAP of 15 cm H_2O and EPAP of 3 cmH_2O and titrating up the IPAP gradually as tolerated by 2–5 cm H_2O every 2–5 mins (until effective tidal volume is achieved and leak minimized) [3]. A target IPAP of 20 cmH_2O is advised or until the therapeutic target or patient tolerability is reached.

Expert comment

The admitting team has tried to get a feeling for the patient's premorbid functional capacity, presumably in order to decide whether the patient would be for invasive mechanical ventilation and/or cardiopulmonary resuscitation in the event that they fail to respond to NIV, in line with BTS/RCP guidelines. The GOLD stages provide an unreliable guide to prognosis once the FEV_1 is <50% predicted, whereas physical activity and muscle weakness may be more reliable [5, 6].

Learning point Mechanism of action of NIV

NIV assists alveolar ventilation, reducing arterial CO_2 levels and oxygen levels. Improved gas exchange may be achieved through many different mechanisms; altering pulmonary mechanics, reducing the threshold effect of PEEP on the instigation of inspiratory flow, and pushing the lung volume along the linear part of the pressure–volume curve. Over time, NIV has also been shown to facilitate lung emptying during expiration and reduce hyperinflation [7]. Mechanical ventilation with EPAP also assists recruitment of areas of atelectasis to improve V/Q ratios and oppose fluid extravasation from the capillary bed [8]. Importantly, NIV facilitates the administration of higher inspired oxygen concentrations to correct hypoxia without an increase in arterial CO_2.

NIV improves respiratory muscle unloading and the work of breathing, reducing the transdiaphragmatic pressure, the pressure–time product of the diaphragm, and the diaphragm electrical activity measured by EMG [9]. This helps to reduce the respiratory rate, normalize the breathing pattern, and improve minute ventilation [10].

Improvements in central chemoreceptor sensitivity to arterial CO_2 have also been demonstrated with longer use of NIV, reflected by an improved hypercapnic ventilatory response [7].

Table 12.2 Inclusion and exclusion criteria for starting NIV

Inclusion criteria	Exclusion criteria
Primary diagnosis of COPD exacerbation (known diagnosis or history and examination consistent with the diagnosis)	Predominantly hypoxaemic respiratory failure or absence of hypercapnia
Able to protect airway*	Severe co-morbidity
Conscious and cooperative*	Confusion/agitation/severe cognitive impairment
Potential for recovery for an acceptable quality of life	Facial burns/trauma/recent facial or upper airway surgery
Patient's wishes considered	Vomiting
	Fixed upper airway obstruction
	Untreated pneumothorax
	Recent upper abdominal surgery
	Inability to protect the airway
	Copious respiratory secretions
	Haemodynamically unstable requiring inotropes/vasopressors (unless in critical care environment)
	Patient moribund
	Bowel obstruction
	NIV should not be the modality of choice for patients with pneumonia or heart failure but may be used in COPD patients with these complications that are not for further escalation

* NIV can be used in unconscious patients if endotracheal intubation is not deemed appropriate or NIV is to be provided in a critical care setting. There is evidence for the use of NIV in comatosed patients secondary to COPD-induced hypercapnia.

Clinical tip Starting non-invasive ventilation

An explanation to the patient of what NIV therapy involves helps to alleviate anxiety. Holding the mask first to the arm and then to the face, without straps attached, helps the patient to gain control and synchronize their pattern of breathing with the ventilator and may aid adherence. Patients that are struggling to tolerate NIV may benefit from low-dose opiates or benzodiazepines, with suitable monitoring for changes in respiratory rate and conscious levels. It is important to take time to improve a patient's first experience of NIV, as this may assist compliance to future therapy.

Table 12.3 An ABG taken on NIV at 1 hour and 4 hours, identifying improving acidotic type 2 respiratory failure with an elevated $PaCO_2$

Parameter (normal values)	Patient values at 1 hour	Patient values at 4 hours
pH (7.35–7.45)	7.31	7.34
PaO_2 (10.67–13.33)	8.7 kPa	9.0 kPa
$PaCO_2$ (4.67–6.00)	6.6 kPa	6.2 kPa
$cHCO_3$ (22–26)	24.4 mmol/L	25 mmol/L
Base excess (−2 to +2)	−2.4 mEq/L	−1.3 mEq/L

One hour later, a blood gas taken on NIV showed some improvement (Table 12.3). The pressures on the NIV were titrated to an IPAP of 18 cmH_2O and an EPAP of 4 cmH_2O, and 2 L of oxygen were entrained in the circuit.

The patient was transferred to an HDU, and a further ABG was repeated 4 hours later on the above settings (Table 12.3). Transcutaneous CO_2 and oxygen were monitored overnight.

Learning point RCP and BTS national guidelines on the use of NIV in COPD for the management of type 2 respiratory failure [3]

Monitoring of NIV

This should be performed in an appropriate environment where both physiological and clinical parameters can be adequately monitored. Assessments carried out over the first 4 hours should guide the physician on the need to escalate treatment to endotracheal intubation.

Observation guidelines

Observations should include heart rate, respiratory rate, patient conscious level (GCS), patient comfort, patient–ventilator synchrony, chest wall expansion, and accessory muscle use.

It is recommended that these are performed every 15 minutes in the first hour, every 30 minutes for the first 1–4 hours, and every hour from 4 hours to 12 hours.

Blood gas guidelines

ABGs should be monitored at 30 minutes to 1 hour after initiating therapy and then in 2 to 3 hours, and earlier if there is any clinical deterioration.

ABGs should be performed 30 minutes to an hour after any change in settings.

In the early hours of the morning, he became very agitated and refused to continue NIV therapy. His respiratory rate was 24. With perspiration and agitation, the transcutaneous oximetry and capnography (TOSCA) was difficult to keep in place. Transcutaneous readings were inaccurate, but his saturations were 92%. He was given 1 mg haloperidol for agitation, and an ABG was obtained on air with local anaesthetic (Table 12.4).

Despite improving ABGs, the patient's agitation continued to increase, and he was reviewed by the intensive care outreach team. He was given lorazepam 0.5 mg orally, to good effect, and he was prescribed subcutaneous morphine 2.5 mg for further episodes of agitation. NIV was removed overnight, and his oxygen levels were maintained at 92% with oxygen.

Expert comment

Clinicians should not be unduly worried if CO_2 levels do not fall rapidly in COPD, if other indicators are favourable. In the pivotal study by Plant *et al.*, $PaCO_2$ fell only by 0.4 kPa more in the intervention group than in the controls at 1 hour [11].

Table 12.4 An ABG taken on air at 9 hours post-admission, identifying improved acidotic type 2 respiratory failure with adequate oxygen levels and near normal $PaCO_2$

Parameter (normal values)	Patient values at 9 hours
pH (7.35–7.45)	7.34
PaO_2 (10.67–13.33)	8.5 kPa
$PaCO_2$ (4.67–6.00)	6.1 kPa
$cHCO_3$ (22–26)	22.9 mmol/L
Base excess (–2 to +2)	–2.1 mEq/L

Table 12.5 An ABG taken on NIV with an IPAP of 34 cmH_2O, an EPAP of 5 cmH_2O, and 4 L of oxygen at 22 hours post-admission, identifying worsening acidotic type 2 respiratory failure with oxygen levels above expected for this COPD patient and elevated $PaCO_2$ levels

Parameter (normal values)	Patient values at 22 hours
pH (7.35–7.45)	7.26
PaO_2 (10.67–13.33)	9.8 kPa
$PaCO_2$ (4.67–6.00)	8.6 kPa
$cHCO_3$ (22–26)	28 mmol/L
Base excess (–2 to +2)	–1.6 mEq/L

The next day, he remained wheezy, and his respiratory rate had increased to 28 breaths/minute. He was prescribed an aminophylline infusion and restarted on NIV with an IPAP of 36 cmH_2O, an EPAP of 5 cmH_2O, with 4 L of oxygen entrained in the circuit.

The patient was reviewed 5 hours later; the settings had been reduced by the HDU staff, because the patient was not tolerating them well, to an IPAP of 34 cmH_2O and an EPAP of 5 cmH_2O. His saturations were now 95%, and a repeat ABG was obtained (Table 12.5).

The plan was to reduce the oxygen and increase the IPAP to 36 cmH_2O and, if the oxygenation drops further, to increase the EPAP to 6 cmH_2O, then to 8 cmH_2O.

Overnight, the ventilator was manipulated, and the patient maintained oxygen saturations of 82% on 5 L of oxygen, with an IPAP of 36 cmH_2O and an EPAP of 8 cmH_2O. Poor synchronization with the ventilator was noted overnight, and regular morphine boluses were given which improved this. A CXR was performed to exclude a pneumothorax with the high pressure ventilation used. Target saturations were set for 88–92%, with a view that a further deterioration would be palliated.

Clinical tip

During NIV, the leak at the mask increases in direct proportion to the pressure support supplied [12]. Ventilators differ in their ability to compensate for mask leak, and most face masks are only tested to inspiratory pressures of 25–30 cmH_2O [13]. Increasing the IPAP above these pressures may increase the leak, rather than produce any beneficial increase in tidal volume delivered to the patient. Substantial mask leak can lead to patient discomfort and sleep disruption that may reduce adherence to therapy [14].

In patients that are very sensitive to oxygen and develop hypercapnia when hypoxia is normalized, it is vitally important to maintain target saturations of 88–92% [15]. This may limit the need for such high pressure support levels because of oxygen-induced hypercapnia.

Learning point Pulmonary mechanics: 'the interaction between the COPD patient and the ventilator'

Due to the underlying pathophysiology of COPD patients, they commonly have difficulties in synchronizing with the non-invasive ventilator. COPD patients have significant expiratory flow limitation which leads to lung hyperinflation and the development of intrinsic PEEP [16]. This PEEP acts as a threshold load and requires the patient to make significantly more inspiratory effort to generate inspiratory flow [16]. Most non-invasive ventilators are now flow-triggered devices, following a study that suggested these were more sensitive than pressure-triggered ventilators [17]. Difficulties in generating inspiratory flow in COPD patients can prevent them from triggering the ventilator, an asynchronous episode referred to as an 'ineffective effort' (Figure 12.2). This leads to a wasted inspiratory effort by the patient and counterproductively increases the work of breathing.

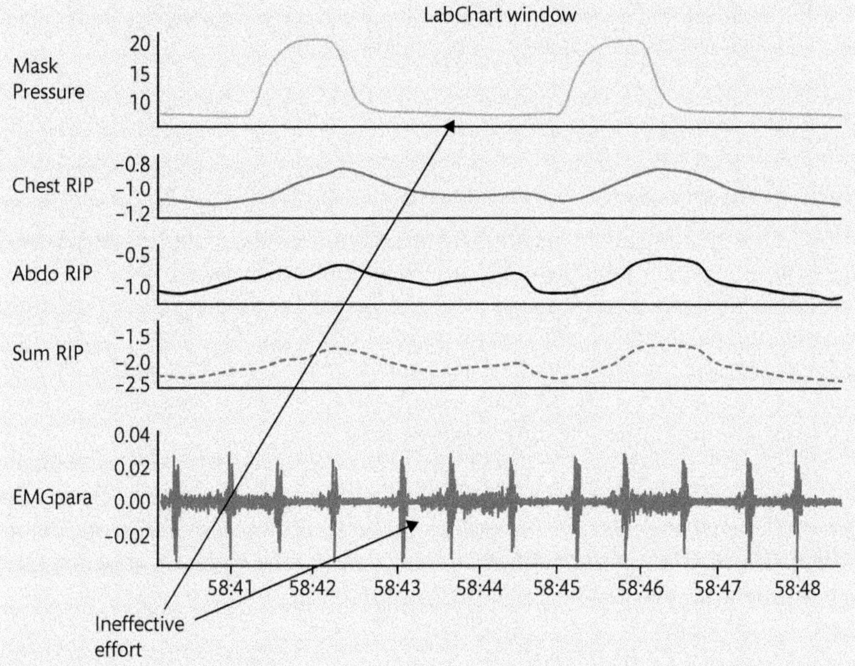

Figure 12.2 An 'ineffective effort' asynchronous event. Patient inspiratory effort is identified by chest wall muscle (EMGpara) activity and chest wall excursion (respiratory inductance plethysmography (chest RIP)), without a corresponding triggered pressure delivery from the ventilator (mask pressure), arrowed [18].

Ineffective efforts are also affected by the pressure support provided by the ventilator and the cycling of the ventilator from inspiration to expiration. High levels of pressure support reduce the neural drive to the respiratory muscles, increase the tidal volume delivered to the patient, and can delay cycling of the ventilator into expiration [7, 16, 19] (Figure 12.3). These all adversely affect the triggering of the ventilator but may be offset by reducing the pressure support applied and adequate titration of extrinsic positive airways pressure (EPAP) [19].

The patient's condition improved with improving synchronization, and the pressures were titrated down to 18/5. A nasogastric tube was placed to deflate abdominal distension, due to the high pressure support, and to give high-calorie feeds. His steroid therapy was changed to an oral preparation for 5 more days, and he continued a

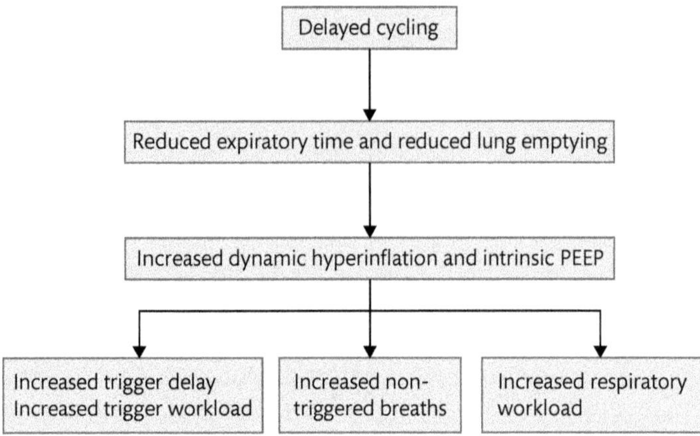

Figure 12.3 Potential consequences of a 'delayed cycling' asynchronous event in a COPD patient.

Source: Adapted from a review by Jolliet *et al.* [16].

7-day course of antibiotic therapy. His aminophylline and nebulizers were weaned and stopped, and he then returned to his usual inhaler therapy.

Whilst an inpatient, he was seen by physiotherapists and occupational therapists to assist his rehabilitation and plan an assisted discharge. Overnight oximetry and capnography were performed when his condition was stable, and he did not meet criteria for home oxygen. Domiciliary non-invasive mechanical ventilation was considered but not felt to be indicated in this patient.

The COPD outreach team assessed the patient and arranged community follow-up. He was referred for smoking cessation and pulmonary rehabilitation. He was discharged home with a package of care. An oxygen form was written for the London Ambulance Service, informing them that the patient is at high risk of hypercapnia and requires controlled oxygen therapy.

Learning point Criteria for home oxygen

The current guidelines recommend long-term oxygen therapy to be used if the COPD patient is chronically hypoxic (PaO_2 <7.3 kPa) when breathing air for 30 minutes [21, 22]. It may also be used if the PaO_2 is between 7.3 kPa and 8 kPa if the patient has signs of polycythaemia or PH [21]. Oxygen should be provided for at least 30 minutes, with the objective of raising the patient's arterial blood oxygen to at least 8 kPa, without a significant rise in $PaCO_2$ [21] A doubling in survival benefit has been shown if oxygen is administered for >15 hours a day, although longer daily use has been shown to improve survival further [23, 24].

Expert comment

The position of NIV for patients with chronic hypercapnia remains uncertain. Several ongoing trials are attempting to resolve the issue, but existing trials have failed to show a benefit, perhaps because participants have had only marginally elevated CO_2 levels or because applied airway pressures have been low [20].

Evidence base Evidence for domiciliary mechanical ventilation

Increasing numbers of patients with chronic hypercapnic respiratory failure secondary to COPD are starting domiciliary mechanical ventilation [25]. Currently, there remains little evidence to suggest that NIV has a significant survival benefit or reduction in exacerbation rate over long-term oxygen therapy alone [8–10]. These studies have been criticized for using small numbers of patients that have had insufficient acclimatization to NIV before starting the study and for using insufficient pressure support to control hypercapnia [22, 26]. However, these studies have suggested that NIV may be poorly

(Continued)

tolerated in the long term in COPD and result in increased sleep disruption [27]. A study by Windisch *et al.* suggested that using higher pressure support (mean IPAP of 28 cmH_2O, mean EPAP of 4 cmH_2O) improved daytime hypercapnia, lung function, and haematocrit, with a possible reduction in exacerbation rate and mortality, compared to previous data [26]. The tolerability of such an approach and sleep efficiency have not yet been assessed.

Currently, a pragmatic approach is often advised. Patients that experience symptoms of nocturnal hypoventilation, such as early morning headaches and daytime somnolence, despite maximal therapy are most likely to benefit [28]. Those that are unable to tolerate long-term oxygen therapy without becoming significantly hypercapnic may also find some improvement [28]. COPD patients with frequent admissions to hospital in hypercapnic respiratory failure may be another subgroup of patients in whom nocturnal ventilation could be considered [28]. Domiciliary nocturnal ventilation is not recommended for patients without daytime hypercapnia.

Clinical tip

All patients should be referred for smoking cessation [29]. Along with long-term oxygen therapy, this is one of the only interventions to improve survival in patients with COPD [30]. Smoking cessation has been shown to reduce the decline in FEV_1, especially in moderate COPD patients, reduce cough and sputum production, improve quality of life, and reduce COPD exacerbations [5, 6]. Current guidelines suggest that nicotine replacement therapy, along with counselling, have the greatest effect of improving abstinence rates in COPD patients who smoke [31]. The average 12-month cessation rate for this approach is estimated at 12.3%, but this has been shown to be cost-effective [32].

All patients should be referred for pulmonary rehabilitation [29]. Numerous RCTs have shown significant benefit in patient-reported outcomes following pulmonary rehabilitation in COPD patients [33, 34]. A Cochrane meta-analysis assessed the efficacy of pulmonary rehabilitation in COPD patients [35]. It identified significant benefits in dyspnoea levels and HRQoL (mastery and fatigue levels) [35, 36]. There was also a significant increase in exercise capacity assessed by the 6MWT (an average increase in walking distance of 49 m) [36, 37]. The largest benefit was observed in severe COPD patients, and this benefit was maintained at 6 months following the rehabilitation programme [36]. Although the Cochrane meta-analysis did not identify any reduction in hospital admissions, some studies have suggested this may occur, resulting in added cost benefits [38].

Clinical tip End-of-life care

The 5-year mortality rates for patients with hypercapnic respiratory failure and COPD have been quoted as 11% [39, 40]. Mortality rates for COPD patients with reversible hypercapnic respiratory failure and normocapnia are slightly better at 28% and 33%, respectively [39, 40]. COPD is a progressively debilitating, and ultimately terminal, disease. It is important that end-of-life decisions are addressed in a sensitive, appropriate manner. As patients are approaching the latter stages of the disease, it is recommended that their wishes regarding ventilation and resuscitation are discussed thoughtfully in an outpatient clinical setting. This prevents inappropriate decisions from being made by teams unfamiliar with the patient during emergency admissions and ensures that palliative care services are involved in a timely fashion to support the patient's care outside the hospital environment.

Discussion

The use of non-invasive positive pressure ventilation to treat acute respiratory failure has increased dramatically over the last two decades, with increasing evidence for its use as first-line treatment for hypercapnic exacerbations of COPD. Many guidelines exist on the use of NIV, but widespread varieties in clinical practice remain, and concerns are voiced over the safety of NIV outside the critical care setting.

The art of NIV settings can often be challenging, and importantly it takes time to optimize in an acutely distressed patient. Correctly assessing the patient, making note of their size and estimated 'ideal' tidal volume, can help with the common pitfalls of using too high or too low pressure support levels. Most non-invasive ventilators also have both an inspiratory and an expiratory trigger that can be manipulated to improve the coordination between the patient and ventilator breathing cycles. Ensuring that bronchodilator medications are given to improve airflow limitation and to act as an adjunct to NIV is important.

The physician must take time to assess the patient's comfort and re-review their response post-changes in ventilator settings. Monitoring is a key component to early recognition of patients that are struggling on NIV. When appropriate, these patients should be moved to a critical care environment where strategies, such as using sedatives or invasive ventilation, can be performed quickly and efficiently.

Hypercapnic exacerbations of COPD represent those with severe underlying disease, and mortality rates in this group of patients are high. Provisions should be made to support patients on discharge and to optimize quality of life. The role of domiciliary ventilation in this group remains unclear, with further RCTs due to be published.

Current research is also focussing on improving ventilator technologies using autotitration mechanisms, such as the forced oscillation technique, to better identify 'individualized' ventilator settings.

A final word from the expert

Planning for an acute exacerbation is key, and the team looking after this patient should have done so after the episode of intubation 1 year previously; at least at the point of admission, the family and team were unaware of the patient's wishes in that regard. Acute exacerbation of COPD has, in some ways, been treated rather nihilistically in the UK where intubation rates are significantly lower than elsewhere in the developed world. Key learning points are that careful high dependency care with NIV may avert endotracheal intubation, but, where this therapy is required, long-term outcomes may be better than in many other conditions.

References:

1. Rodriguez-Roisin R, Vestbo J (2011). *Global strategy for the diagnosis, management and prevention of COPD, Global Initiative for Chronic Obstructive Lung Disease (GOLD).* Available at: <http://www.goldcopd.org>.
2. Murphy PB, Kumar A, Reilly C *et al.* Neural respiratory drive as a physiological biomarker to monitor change during acute exacerbations of COPD. *Thorax* 2011;**66**:602–8.
3. Davidson AC, Banham S, Elliott M *et al.* BTS/ICS guideline for the ventilatory management of acute hypercapnic respiratory failure in adults. *Thorax* 2016;**71**(suppl 2):ii1–35.
4. Brochard L, Mancebo J, Wysocki M *et al.* Noninvasive ventilation for acute exacerbations of chronic obstructive pulmonary disease. *N Engl J Med* 1995;**333**:817–22.
5. Scanlon PD, Connett JE, Waller LA *et al.* Smoking cessation and lung function in mild-to-moderate chronic obstructive pulmonary disease. The Lung Health Study. *Am J Respir Crit Care Med* 2000;**161**:381–90.

6. Pride NB. Smoking cessation: effects on symptoms, spirometry and future trends in COPD. *Thorax* 2001;**56**(suppl 2):ii7–10.
7. Nickol AH, Hart N, Hopkinson NS *et al*. Mechanisms of improvement of respiratory failure in patients with COPD treated with NIV. *Int J Chron Obstruct Pulmon Dis* 2008;**3**:453–62.
8. Barbas CS, de Matos GF, Pincelli MP *et al*. Mechanical ventilation in acute respiratory failure: recruitment and high positive end-expiratory pressure are necessary. *Curr Opin Crit Care* 2005;**11**:18–28.
9. Beck J, Gottfried SB, Navalesi P *et al*. Electrical activity of the diaphragm during pressure support ventilation in acute respiratory failure. *Am J Respir Crit Care Med* 2001;**164**:419–24.
10. Kallet RH, Diaz JV. The physiologic effects of noninvasive ventilation. *Respir Care* 2009;**54**:102–15.
11. Plant PK, Owen JL, Elliott MW. Early use of non-invasive ventilation for acute exacerbations of chronic obstructive pulmonary disease on general respiratory wards: a multicentre randomised controlled trial. *Lancet* 2000;**355**:1931–5.
12. Schettino GP, Tucci MR, Sousa R, Valente Barbas CS, Passos Amato MB, Carvalho CR. Mask mechanics and leak dynamics during noninvasive pressure support ventilation: a bench study. *Intensive Care Med* 2001;**27**:1887–91.
13. Mehta S, McCool FD, Hill NS. Leak compensation in positive pressure ventilators: a lung model study. *Eur Respir J* 2001;**17**:259–67.
14. Willson GN, Piper AJ, Norman M *et al*. Nasal versus full face mask for noninvasive ventilation in chronic respiratory failure. *Eur Respir J* 2004;**23**:605–9.
15. O'Driscoll BR, Howard LS, Davison AG. BTS guideline for emergency oxygen use in adult patients. *Thorax* 2008;**63**(Suppl 6):vi1–68.
16. Jolliet P, Tassaux D. Clinical review: patient-ventilator interaction in chronic obstructive pulmonary disease. *Crit Care* 2006;**10**:236.
17. Nava S, Ambrosino N, Bruschi C, Confalonieri M, Rampulla C. Physiological effects of flow and pressure triggering during non-invasive mechanical ventilation in patients with chronic obstructive pulmonary disease. *Thorax* 1997;**52**:249–54.
18. Ramsay M, Mandal S, Suh ES *et al*. Parasternal electromyography to determine the relationship between patient-ventilator asynchrony and nocturnal gas exchange during home mechanical ventilation set-up. *Thorax* 2015;**70**:946–52.
19. Fanfulla F, Delmastro M, Berardinelli A, Lupo ND, Nava S. Effects of different ventilator settings on sleep and inspiratory effort in patients with neuromuscular disease. *Am J Respir Crit Care Med* 2005;**172**:619–24.
20. Clini E, Sturani C, Rossi A *et al*. The Italian multicentre study on noninvasive ventilation in chronic obstructive pulmonary disease patients. *Eur Respir J* 2002;**20**:529–38.
21. NHS PrimaryCareCommissioning (2011). *Service specification for a home oxygen assessment and review service*. Available at: <https://www.networks.nhs.uk/nhs-networks/east-of-england-respiratory-programme/documents/Service%20Specification%20for%20a%20HOS%20Assessment%20and%20Review%20Service%20v2%201%2011%20October2011.pdf>.
22. Plant PK, Elliott MW. Chronic obstructive pulmonary disease • 9: Management of ventilatory failure in COPD. *Thorax* 2003;**58**:537–42.
23. [No authors listed]. Continuous or nocturnal oxygen therapy in hypoxemic chronic obstructive lung disease: a clinical trial. Nocturnal Oxygen Therapy Trial Group. *Ann Intern Med* 1980;**93**:391–8.
24. [No authors listed]. Long term domiciliary oxygen therapy in chronic hypoxic cor pulmonale complicating chronic bronchitis and emphysema. Report of the Medical Research Council Working Party. *Lancet* 1981;**317**:681–6.
25. Lloyd-Owen SJ, Donaldson GC, Ambrosino N *et al*. Patterns of home mechanical ventilation use in Europe: results from the Eurovent survey. *Eur Respir J* 2005;**25**:1025–31.

26. Windisch W HM, Storre JH, Dreher M. High-intensity non-invasive positive pressure ventilation for stable hypercapnic COPD. *Int J Med Sci* 2009;**6**:72–6.
27. Lin CC. Comparison between nocturnal nasal positive pressure ventilation combined with oxygen therapy and oxygen monotherapy in patients with severe COPD. *Am J Respir Crit Care Med* 1996;**154**:353–8.
28. Glenn WW, Hogan JF, Loke JS, Ciesielski TE, Phelps ML, Rowedder R. Ventilatory support by pacing of the conditioned diaphragm in quadriplegia. *N Engl J Med* 1984;**310**:1150–5.
29. National Institute for Health and Care Excellence (2010). *Chronic obstructive pulmonary disease in over 16s: diagnosis and management.* NICE guidelines CG101. Available at: <https://www.nice.org.uk/guidance/CG101>.
30. Godtfredsen NS, Lam TH, Hansel TT *et al.* COPD-related morbidity and mortality after smoking cessation: status of the evidence. *Eur Respir J* 2008;**32**:844–53.
31. Strassmann R, Bausch B, Spaar A, Kleijnen J, Braendli O, Puhan MA. Smoking cessation interventions in COPD: a network meta-analysis of randomised trials. *Eur Respir J* 2009;**34**:634–40.
32. Hoogendoorn M, Feenstra TL, Hoogenveen RT, Rutten-van Mölken MPMH. Long-term effectiveness and cost-effectiveness of smoking cessation interventions in patients with COPD. *Thorax* 2010;**65**:711–18.
33. Hui KP, Hewitt AB. A simple pulmonary rehabilitation program improves health outcomes and reduces hospital utilization in patients with COPD. *Chest* 2003;**124**:94–7.
34. Wijkstra P, Van Altena R, Kraan J, Otten V, Postma D, Koeter G. Quality of life in patients with chronic obstructive pulmonary disease improves after rehabilitation at home. *Eur Respir J* 1994;**7**:269–73.
35. Lacasse Y, Goldstein R, Lasserson TJ, Martin S (2006). Pulmonary rehabilitation for chronic obstructive pulmonary disease. *Cochrane Database Syst Rev* 2006;**4**:CD003793.
36. Hill NS. Pulmonary Rehabilitation. *Proc Am Thorac Soc* 2006;**3**:66–74.
37. Redelmeier DA, Bayoumi AM, Goldstein RS, Guyatt GH. Interpreting small differences in functional status: the six minute walk test in chronic lung disease patients. *Am J Respir Crit Care Med* 1997;**155**:1278–82.
38. Griffiths TL, Burr ML, Campbell IA *et al.* Results at 1 year of outpatient multidisciplinary pulmonary rehabilitation: a randomised controlled trial. *Lancet* 2000;**355**:362–8.
39. Costello R, Deegan P, Fitzpatrick M, McNicholas WT. Reversible hypercapnia in chronic obstructive pulmonary disease: a distinct pattern of respiratory failure with a favorable prognosis. *Am J Med* 1997;**102**:239–44.
40. Nizet TAC, van den Elshout FJJ, Heijdra YF, van de Ven MJT, Mulder PGH, Folgering HTM. Survival of chronic hypercapnic COPD patients is predicted by smoking habits, comorbidity, and hypoxemia. *Chest* 2005;**127**:1904–10.

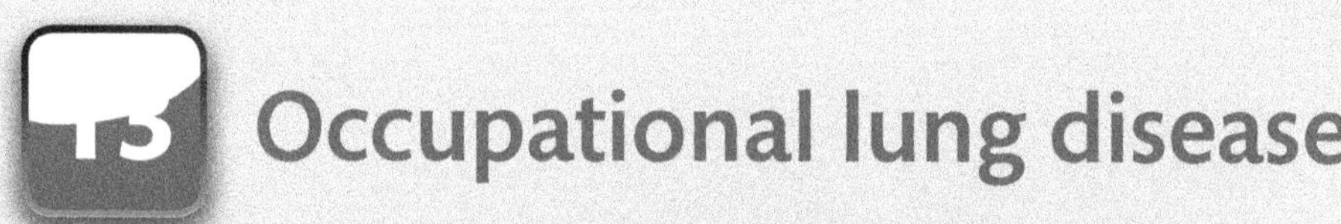

Occupational lung disease

Johanna Feary and Joanna Szram

Expert commentary Paul Cullinan

Case history 1

A 59-year-old man was referred by his GP to the respiratory clinic; he reported chest tightness and breathlessness which had been ongoing for over 10 years. He gave a past history of mild childhood asthma that resolved during his teenage years. His GP had diagnosed him with asthma recurrence at the age of 46 years; until recently, he had only needed occasional salbutamol to control his symptoms. Over the last 2 years, he had experienced worsening symptoms that he felt were related to his job; this had prompted referral to the chest clinic.

The patient had left school at 16 and attended a bakery college for 2 years. He then worked as a baker in a small family bakery for 10 years and subsequently in a variety of local supermarket chains for 19 years, for most of the past 15 years as a manager. He moved to his current employer, a large supermarket chain, as a bakery manager 12 years ago. He reported that, due to staff cutbacks, his role was downgraded to full-time baker about 2 years before attending clinic. Since moving back to the bakery, he had noticed a marked increase in his asthma symptoms. His specific tasks in the bakery included mixing dough; this process involved emptying large sacks of flour and smaller sachets of yeast and 'improver' into large mechanical mixers. He described visible dust in the air in the bakery; as far as he was aware, no respiratory protective equipment (RPE), e.g. masks, was advised (or available), and only limited local 'exhaust' ventilation (LEV) was present.

His asthma symptoms were characterized by breathlessness and chest tightness and occurred mostly in the evening, after a day at work. He was taking his salbutamol inhaler around four times a day, including at night when he was waking frequently due to asthma symptoms. He had noticed that his symptoms were less severe on days when he was not at work and had almost disappeared during a fortnight's holiday earlier in the year. On specific questioning, he reported that the worsening of his asthma symptoms had been predated by a 4-month history of sore, itchy eyes, as well as rhinorrhoea, sneezing, itching, and nasal congestion with associated anosmia. He had attributed these symptoms to hay fever, although they continued past the end of the usual grass pollen season. Over-the-counter nasal sprays had only partly improved these symptoms.

The patient was an ex-smoker with a 20-pack year history. His brother had been treated for asthma in childhood but had no symptoms in adulthood; there was no other relevant family history. The patient had a pet dog but denied any symptoms related to this or any other animals. He had a past medical history of osteoarthritis and had been taking a statin to treat high cholesterol for several years. He was not aware of any drug allergies.

Clinical tip Taking an occupational history in respiratory disease

Presenting symptoms

- Respiratory symptoms: nature, duration, onset, severity.
- Associated symptoms: upper respiratory tract (ENT), systemic.
- Temporal relationship to work: at work, after work, away from work/holidays.
- Relationship to current occupation: time from onset of exposure, change of activity/hours/task/role.

Occupational history

- From leaving school to present: dates/duration—occupational title and tasks.
- Current occupation: job role, tasks, hours, colleagues, environment.
- Exposures: substances used by individual/colleagues.
- Provision of occupational health/health and safety/RPE/ventilation/extraction.

Clinical examination and chest radiograph were normal. Blood tests were taken; full blood count and differential white cell count (WCC) were normal; his total serum IgE level was elevated (223 IU/ml). Spirometry showed an obstructive pattern with significant bronchodilator reversibility: FEV_1 2.35 L (68% predicted), FVC 4.20 L (102% predicted), with a significant 15% (350 mL) improvement in FEV_1 post-bronchodilator, a degree of variability strongly suggestive of asthma.

At this point, a diagnosis of occupational (bakers') asthma was suspected, and he was referred to the regional specialist occupational lung disease clinic for further assessment. Skin prick tests (SPTs) were positive to grass pollen (5 mm) and negative to other common aero-allergens. Work-specific SPTs to bakery allergens were positive to flour (3 mm) and negative to alpha amylase (an enzyme used commonly in the baking industry to improve texture and increase shelf life, described by bakers as an 'improver'), soy flour, and yeast (all 0 mm), with appropriate negative (saline) and positive (histamine) controls. Specific IgE to wheat flour was positive at 0.6 kU/L (normal range <0.35 kU/L).

The patient was asked to complete a detailed 4-week work-related peak flow diary, recording his best peak flow every 2–3 hours from waking until bedtime on both working days and days off (recording forms available to download at <www.lungsatwork.org.uk>). The results were plotted and demonstrated lower readings (with greater variability) on work days and improvement on days away from work (Figure 13.1). When he returned to clinic, non-specific bronchial provocation testing was carried out; his PC_{20} to histamine was 1.2 mg/mL, demonstrating significant bronchial hyper-responsiveness, supportive of asthma.

In order to establish definitively whether the patient's symptoms were attributable to occupational asthma (OA) due to flour or a work-related exacerbation of pre-existing asthma from dust irritation, he was admitted to the specialist challenge facility for a week. Single-blind specific provocation testing to flour was carried out; the patient was exposed to a concentration of 1% flour within lactose powder, using a dust-tipping technique (this mimics his workplace exposure, albeit with a shorter duration of exposure—up to a maximum of 20 minutes). This exposure resulted in symptoms identical to (but less severe than) those he experienced at work, accompanied by a significant drop in FEV_1 immediately after challenge (>15%, compared to baseline; Figure 13.2). These symptomatic and physiological responses were not seen following control challenge with lactose powder alone but were found to be reproducible on repeat testing with flour. His bronchial responsiveness to histamine fell from around 1 mg/mL to 0.2 mg/mL throughout successive testing.

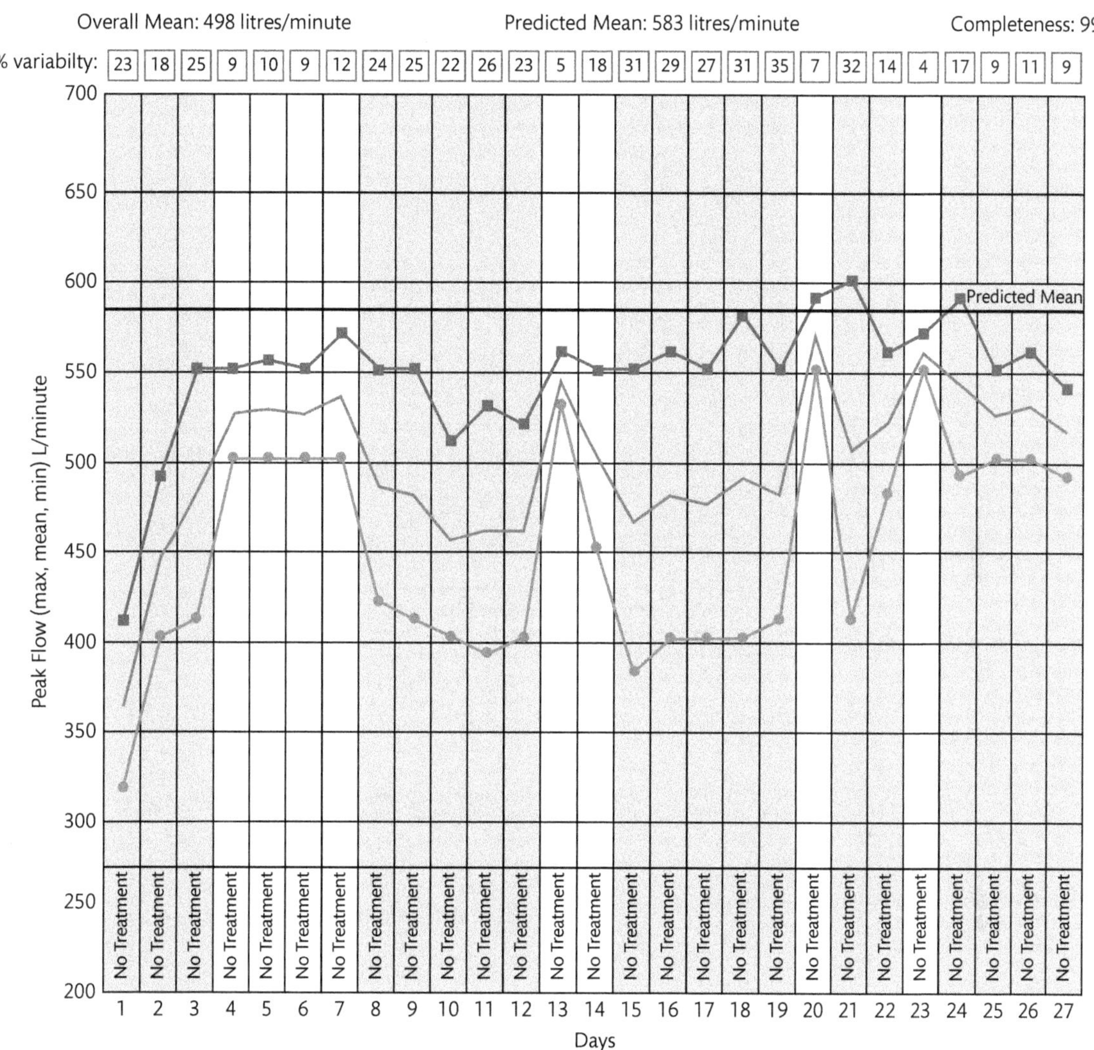

Figure 13.1 Peak flow record showing peak expiratory flow rate variability on work days, with improvement on non-work days.

Learning point Specific inhalation challenges

Methodology

- Single-blind (patient unaware of challenge type) control—in dust challenges, lactose powder is used.
- Challenges with small concentrations of the suspected agent (can be mixed with control substance) given on subsequent days; exposures occur for up to 20 minutes per challenge period. Subsequent concentration and exposure time vary according to previous responses.
- Symptoms and FEV_1 recorded at regular intervals before and after challenge (baseline, immediately after challenge, at 15-minute intervals for 1 hour, then hourly for 8–10 hours).
- Non-specific bronchial hyper-responsiveness (NSBHR), using histamine or methacholine, is measured immediately before and the morning after each specific challenge.
- Active challenges are repeated on at least two occasions to ensure reproducibility of response. Where necessary, a control challenge may also be repeated.

(Continued)

Indications for use (UK population)

- Patients in whom a diagnosis has not been reached following workplace peak flow recording.
- Patients with exposure to >1 potential respiratory sensitizing agent—to identify which, if any, is responsible for work-related symptoms.
- Where work-related symptoms are too severe and the employer considers the risk too high to justify workplace exposure for completion of serial peak flow measurements.
- Patients with no current exposure but the potential for future exposure—as work-relatedness cannot be measured.

Characteristic responses to specific inhalation challenge testing

- 'Immediate' or 'early' response with a drop in FEV_1 to 15% or more from baseline, recovering 1-2 hours after challenge.
- 'Late' reaction developing several hours after exposure and occasionally persisting for several hours, often with a concurrent measurable increase in NSBHR.
- 'Dual' (combined early and late) responses are common.
- Irritant and hypersensitivity responses can look similar in patients with significantly uncontrolled asthma.

NB. Very few centres in the UK offer specific inhalation challenge.

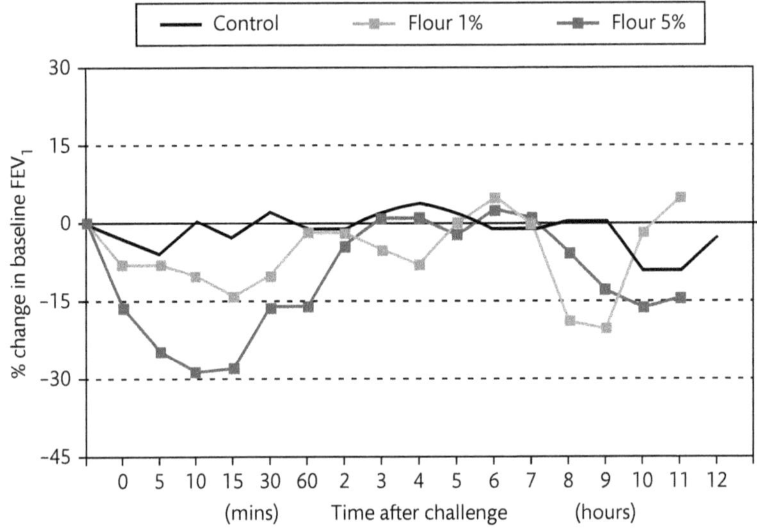

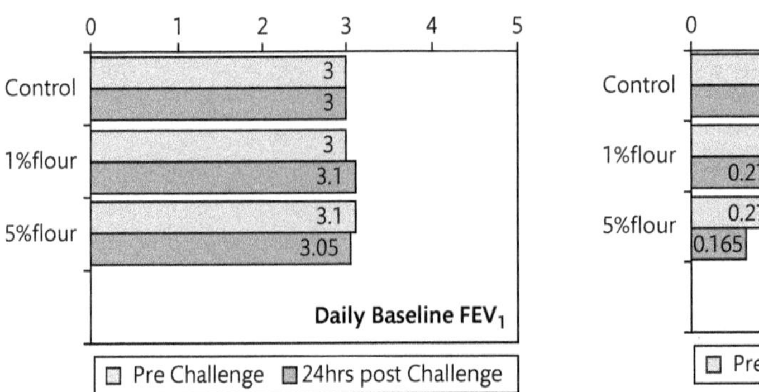

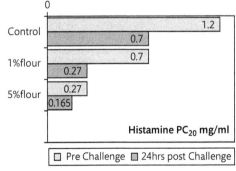

Figure 13.2 Specific inhalation challenge to flour, showing a significant drop in FEV_1 immediately after challenge.

On the basis of his clinical and occupational history, physiological and immunological testing, and specific provocation test results, a diagnosis of occupational (bakers') asthma and rhinitis was made. He was started on a combination corticosteroid and long-acting beta-agonist inhaler bd in order to stabilize his disease. After meeting with his line manager and the supermarket's occupational health department, he was redeployed to another section of the supermarket where he was no longer exposed to flour (the petrol station shop). His symptoms improved, in part, over the next 4 months, although he continued to require maintenance inhalers.

Learning point Agents causing occupational asthma

Bakers' asthma is one of the commonest forms of OA, occurring as a result of sensitization to flour amylase. Nearly 400 workplace substances have been identified as agents that may cause asthma, although some are responsible for very few cases. A list of frequently recognized substances, categorized according to molecular mass, is given in Table 13.1; in general, it is reasonable to assume that any airborne protein or highly reactive chemical has the potential to cause sensitization and subsequent disease. High-molecular mass (HMM) allergens (>2 kDa) are generally airborne proteins and result in an immune response characterized by the generation of specific IgE antibodies similar to that for common non-occupational allergens such as pollen. Atopic individuals have a higher innate susceptibility to developing sensitization to HMM allergens. Low-molecular mass (LMM) allergens (<2 kDa) are generally chemical agents; the precise immunological mechanism of disease is less clear but is thought to involve conjugation with a host protein (e.g. serum albumin) prior to becoming antigenic.

Discussion

OA is common at a population level and is under-recognized; it is estimated that 10–15% of new, recurrent, or deteriorating asthma in adulthood is related to the workplace environment [1, 2]. There are three distinct ways in which asthma and work can be related and which should, where possible, be differentiated.

Occupational asthma

OA arises *de novo* from the workplace as a result of airborne exposure to a sensitizing agent. A number of common high-risk industries are responsible for the majority of cases reported in the UK (Table 13.1). Figure 13.3 shows a suggested algorithm for the clinical management of a suspected case of occupational asthma.

The typical clinical course of OA is preceded by an asymptomatic, latent period (usually between 3 and 12 months) following the start of regular exposure, during which time sensitization to the culprit agent takes place. First exposure most commonly occurs in the context of a new job but can also be attributed to a new or increased exposure in a current position. Symptoms of allergic conjunctivitis and/or rhinitis are almost universal and normally precede the development of asthma symptoms by several months; importantly, not all patients with occupational rhinitis go on to develop asthma. Once OA has developed, symptoms occur during, or immediately after, periods of exposure at work, with improvement away from work. Variation in working hours can complicate this temporal relationship; in some cases, isolated 'late-phase' symptoms occur—these reactions are commoner with particular agents (mainly LMM 'chemicals'). Further diagnostic difficulty can occur if affected individuals are only assessed after a long history of symptomatic exposure, as there may be a delay, or even a lack of improvement, in symptoms during periods away from work.

Table 13.1 Frequently reported high- and low-molecular mass causes of occupational asthma

High-molecular mass (HMM) agents	
Occupational group	*Agent(s)*
Bakers and millers	Flour (wheat, barley, rye, oat, soya), fungal alpha amylase, egg and milk proteins
Laboratory technicians, research scientists, animal handlers	Small animal proteins (urine, dander, serum), insect proteins, other animal proteins, latex
Food processors	shellfish and fish proteins, cocoa proteins, enzymes, linseed, green coffee bean, castor bean, tea dust
Detergent powder manufacturers	Enzymes (protease, amylase, lipase, cellulase)
Health-care workers	Latex
Farmers, farm workers, and agriculturists	Animal urine, insect larvae, poultry feathers, fruit, vegetable and flower pollens, fungi, grain dust, mites, cow dander, cow beta-lactoglobulin
Florists, botanists	Pollens, weeping fig, spider mite, vine weevil
Low-molecular mass (LMM) agents	
Occupational group	*Agent(s)*
Spray painters	Hexamethylene diisocyanate, various amines
Solderers, electronic workers	Colophony fume, cyanoacrylates, toluene diisocyanate
Hairdressers	Persulfate salts, henna
Woodworkers	Hard wood dusts: western red cedar, iroko, mahogany
Pharmaceutical workers	Psyllium, ispaghula, methyldopa, penicillins
Health-care workers	Monomer acrylates, antibiotics, psyllium
Metal refiners, electroplaters	Complex platinum salts, hexavalent chromium, nickel
Food processors	Metabisulfite, chloramine-T
Textile/fabric workers	Reactive dyes, acacia gum
Chemical processors	Phthalic anhydride, trimellitic anhydride
Plastics workers	Diphenylmethane diisocyanate, monomer acrylates, polyamines

Work-exacerbated asthma

In contrast to OA, work-exacerbated asthma is caused by non-specific irritant exposures which can exacerbate symptom control in pre-existing or coincident asthma. Exacerbating factors can occur alone or in combination and include airborne irritants (e.g. general 'nuisance' dust, fumes), environmental conditions (e.g. cold, dry air), or physical work conditions (e.g. increased work of breathing due to exertion). Symptoms develop soon (often immediately) after first exposure to the irritant (i.e. there is no 'latency'). Work-exacerbated asthma is probably commoner than OA but is still under-reported; management entails cooperation between the worker and employer to control relevant exposures, where possible, use of RPE, and optimization of asthma treatment.

Irritant-induced asthma

'Irritant-induced' asthma (previously termed 'reactive airways dysfunction syndrome' (RADS) [3]) is, by convention, considered as occurring following very high (normally one-off) exposure to one or several respiratory irritants. It has a non-immunological mechanism, with most well-characterized cases resulting from single inhalation of agents such as chlorine or nitrogen oxides. Symptoms tend to develop rapidly following a defined, high-intensity exposure such as an accidental spill. In most cases, there is no preceding history of respiratory disease.

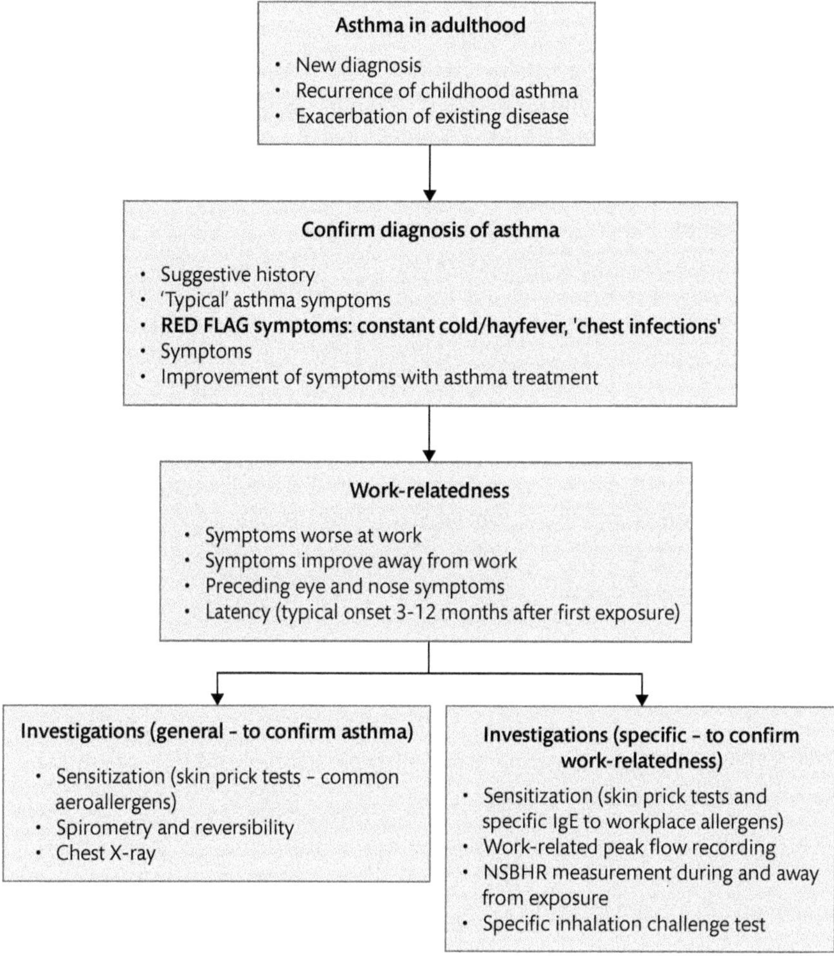

Figure 13.3 Suggested algorithm for the clinical management of a suspected case of occupational asthma.

Specific investigations

Immunological testing to demonstrate sensitization to putative HMM allergens (and some LMM compounds) may be carried out using SPTs with soluble antigen extracts or measurement of specific IgE in serum. Positive responses denote sensitization, not allergic disease. False negatives (to both SPT and specific IgE) are very uncommon for most HMM agents if the correct test reagents are used—for most LMM agents, there are no helpful immunological tests.

Lung function testing using serial peak flow (or FEV_1) measurements is a very sensitive method of detection of a work-related change [4–9], provided readings are made competently and frequently over a period of time that includes time at, and away from, work. Workers are asked to perform measurements every 2 hours from waking until sleep for a 4-week period; this technique usually has sufficient sensitivity to detect work-related variability [5, 10]. Records that include a period of absence from work (such as a holiday) are useful, particularly in more long-standing cases in which recovery of airway hyper-responsiveness often takes >2 days.

Non-specific bronchial responsiveness testing using histamine or methacholine has been used to demonstrate changes in airway reactivity before and after occupational exposure. This is a sensitive technique when performed by an experienced laboratory but is a labour-intensive process, requiring multiple visits to the hospital and is often impractical for both patient and clinician.

Specific inhalation challenge testing is the gold standard test for the diagnosis of OA and is carried out by specialist occupational lung disease services. Patients are exposed to putative allergens for short periods and at relatively low concentrations in carefully controlled laboratory conditions that aim as far as possible to recreate their work conditions. Measurements of lung function and airway reactivity are carried out before, during, and after provocation, and responses to workplace allergens are compared to non-allergenic control exposures [11]. In the UK, these tests are generally used only when simpler techniques have failed to provide a definitive answer or a diagnosis cannot be established by other means. In other countries, such as parts of Canada and Finland, testing is mandatory to ensure eligibility for state compensation. Challenge testing can be difficult if the culprit agent is not clearly identifiable, asthma control is too unstable (most centres ask patients to stop regular asthma therapy for several days before challenge), or if the patient has been away from workplace exposures for a prolonged period of time [12, 13].

Learning point Management and outcome of occupational asthma

It is possible to achieve 'cure' in OA or, failing that, to significantly minimize symptoms associated with persistent disease. This outcome is almost always only achieved by complete avoidance of the culprit allergen through a change in work environment, relocation to an area where no exposure will occur, or a change in occupation. Unfortunately, for some individuals, this may result in job loss and unemployment. Some individuals may prefer to use RPE, such as masks (which must be selected and worn appropriately and removed, stored, and maintained correctly,) in combination with taking standard asthma therapy, often as a temporary course of action, whilst relocation is being organized. This approach is seldom adequate in the long term and often does not control disease, as allergen exposure (albeit at very low dose) is still likely to occur. Treatment with inhaled steroids may improve prognosis [14], but outcome is variable, with a recent systematic review suggesting that only around a third of patients will recover completely from their asthma after complete avoidance of exposure [15]. Complete symptomatic recovery is less likely in those of older age at diagnosis (as with this case), with increasing duration of symptomatic exposure, and with reduction (rather than avoidance) of exposure [16–18]. Physiologically measurable recovery usually occurs in the first 2 years after avoidance of exposure [19].

Case history 1: Expert comment

So long as you remember to think about the disease (in every working adult with new or recurrent or difficult asthma), there are few technical difficulties in the diagnosis and management of workers with OA. Far trickier is juggling the health and economic needs of your patient, and, for this, you need a detailed understanding of their position and that of their employers. Making contact with the relevant occupational health service is usually very helpful, although far too few employees have such access. Finally, remember that making a diagnosis of OA in a patient who has not got it is generally disastrous. Current standards of care suggest referral to a respiratory specialist with a particular interest in occupational lung diseases [20].

Case history 2

A 27-year-old man was referred to a regional ILD clinic for a specialist opinion. He had been born 6 weeks premature and, at the age of 1 month, had had an acute respiratory illness, thought to be whooping cough, which necessitated a 4-week hospital admission. He had subsequent problems with persistent cough and frequent episodes of wheezing in infancy, but these resolved at around the age of 2 years. Thereafter, he was fit and well and, until recently, had attended a local gym on a regular basis. There was no other relevant past medical history; he took no regular or over-the-counter medications and denied illicit drug use. He drank minimal alcohol and was a lifelong never-smoker. He had worked as a laminator, manufacturing fibreglass panels since June 2006.

Two years before referral, at the age of 25, he attended his local hospital with an episode of acute severe breathlessness and right-sided subcostal pain. Clinical examination was normal, but he was tachypnoeic at rest, and ABGs, when breathing room air, showed a pO_2 of 61 mmHg and a pCO_2 of 42 mmHg. A chest radiograph was normal. A V/Q lung scan showed multiple matched defects, with a low probability for pulmonary thromboembolic disease. He was discharged without a formal diagnosis and was readmitted 2 days later with neck pain and swelling. On examination, he was found to have surgical emphysema affecting his neck; a CT thorax confirmed free gas in the mediastinum and pericardium, but no evidence of a pneumothorax; a barium meal did not show any evidence of oesophageal perforation. There were no extrathoracic symptoms or evidence of connective tissue disease (CTD). An echocardiogram showed mild tricuspid regurgitation, but no pulmonary hypertension (PH), and good left ventricular function. He was treated for possible asthma with a combined corticosteroid–long-acting beta-2-agonist inhaler and regular bronchodilators. His symptoms improved but did not resolve completely. Oxygen saturations on discharge were 95% on room air.

When he was seen 2 years later in the ILD clinic, a repeat CT thorax showed widespread mosaicism (Figure 13.4); lung function tests showed airflow obstruction, with evidence of gas trapping (Figure 13.5). Alpha-1-antitrypsin level was normal, and an auto-antibody screen was negative. A bronchoscopy and transbronchial biopsy to obtain tissue were non-diagnostic and complicated by a pneumothorax.

He was started on prednisolone 40 mg daily; after 4 weeks, a small improvement in FEV_1 from 1.3 L to 1.5 L was seen. He failed to attend a number of follow-up

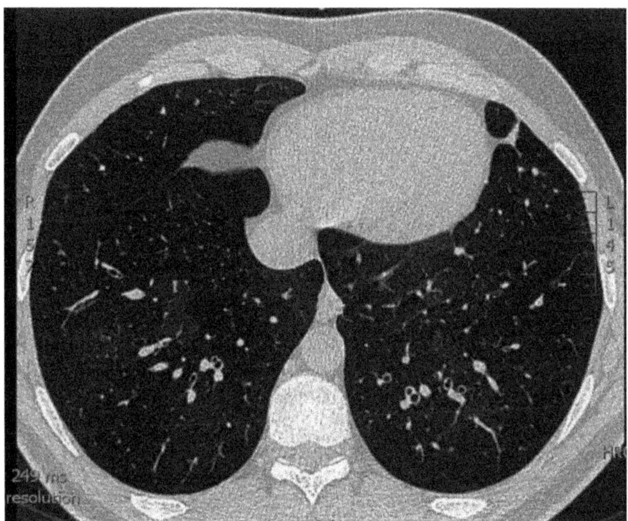

Figure 13.4 CT thorax showing widespread mosaicism.

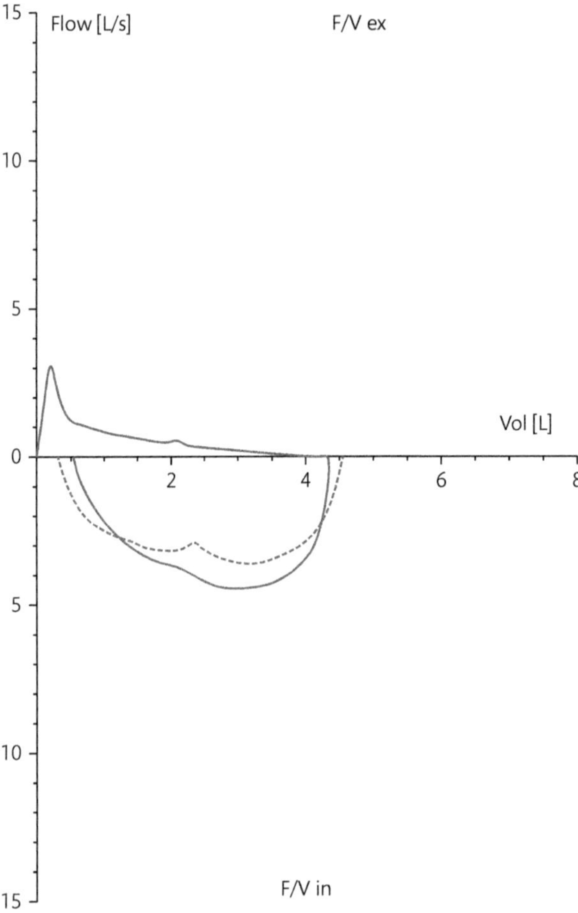

Figure 13.5 Lung function tests showing airflow obstruction and gas trapping.

appointments and was seen again 1 year later; at this time, an open lung biopsy was performed. Histology was reported as showing evidence of chronic airway inflammation with some evidence of intra-luminal fibrosis, in keeping with constrictive obliterative bronchiolitis (Figure 13.6). No definite changes of PH were seen in the pulmonary artery branches.

A further occupational history was sought at this time, and the patient was reviewed by an occupational lung disease specialist physician. Prior to his current employment, he had worked in a number of different jobs; none had involved any significant occupational exposures. He reported that, at the time of the onset of his symptoms, he was working as a laminator in the manufacture of wooden boats for a small local boat building company; he reported high intensity and duration of exposure to fibreglass, wood, and a variety of 'chemicals' felt by the specialist to be reactive in nature. He had never worn any form of RPE at work. He had started work in this job 1 year before the onset of his symptoms. Following this, he had been off work sick for 2 months and had been redeployed by the company to an office job. His symptoms had improved on removal from his previous work environment. To his knowledge, no other current employees had been unwell; he had no information

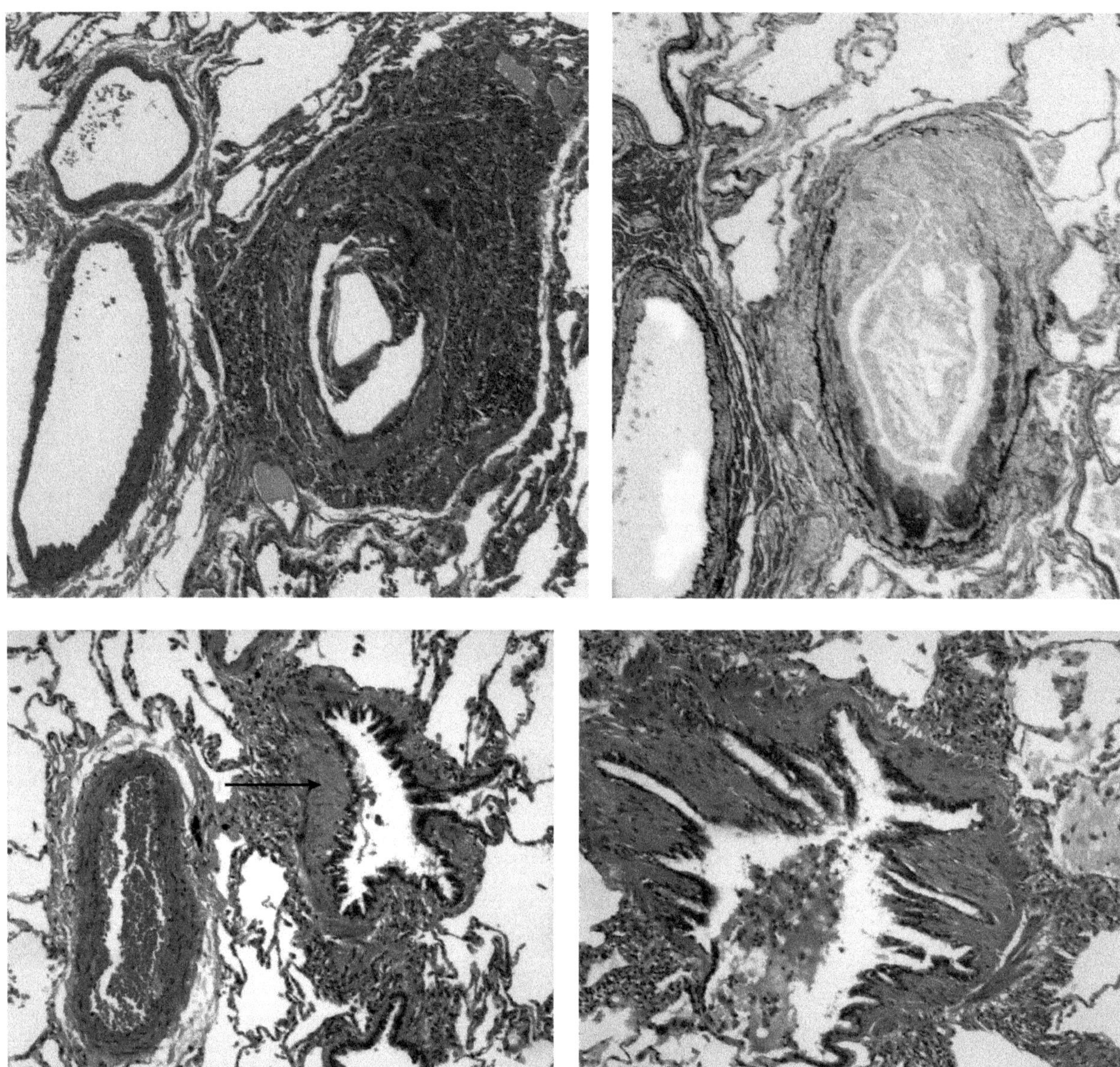

Figure 13.6 Histology from open lung biopsy showing chronic bronchiolitis with evidence of constriction. (a) A bronchiole showing narrowing of its lumen by a mixture of loose fibroblastic tissue and foreign body-type granulomatous inflammation (suggesting a localized response to an inhalation insult). (b) Elastic Van Gieson (EVG) stain confirming the destruction of airways wall with loss of elastin layers. (c) A separate airway showing a lesser extent of chronic inflammation with focal, more established fibrosis in the airway wall (arrow). (d) A further bronchiole showing more intense inflammation without narrowing but demonstrating the accumulation of macrophages and mucus, an indirect feature of adjacent obstruction.

regarding ex-employees at the same company. The company did not have any occupational health provision.

A diagnosis of obliterative bronchiolitis (OB) as a result of occupational exposure—thought to be due to exposure to either a chemical or fibreglass—was made, based on the following supportive evidence: the onset of symptoms within a year of regular exposure to the workplace, the absence of any other explanation for OB in this individual (aside from the history of childhood respiratory infection, the symptoms of which fully resolved by the age of 2, with a long period of subsequent good health), and the improvement of symptoms on removal from the work environment. In support of this occupational attribution, a small number of other cases have been reported in other boat builders in the UK [21].

He was managed with inhaled corticosteroids and bronchodilators, which continued to have some symptomatic benefit; he was advised to seek prompt treatment of any respiratory infections and to keep up-to-date with influenza and pneumococcal vaccinations. Due to his young age and severe airflow obstruction, an assessment for lung transplantation was also undertaken.

Discussion

A complete, thorough, and detailed occupational history should be taken in all cases of newly diagnosed respiratory disease and, in particular, where no other identifiable cause is present. The timing of symptoms relative to any employment changes (this can include job change, increased hours or intensity, differences in exposures and environment) is particularly important. Identification of any occupational factors that may be causal is vital; this can be very difficult in rare diseases. Sir Austin Bradford–Hill outlined a list of criteria suggestive of a causative role in disease in the 1950s [22].

Evidence base Bradford–Hill criteria for causation (attribution of disease)

A group of minimal conditions are necessary to provide adequate evidence of a causal relationship between an incidence and a consequence, established by the English epidemiologist Sir Austin Bradford–Hill (1897–1991) in 1965 [22].

The criteria are:

1. strength of association (relative risk, odds ratio);
2. consistency (repeated observation);
3. specificity (of relationship between exposure and response);
4. temporal relationship (cause to precede consequence);
5. biological gradient (dose–response relationship);
6. plausibility (biological plausibility);
7. coherence (with known natural history of disease);
8. experiment (reversibility);
9. analogy (is a similar response seen for similar or related exposures?).

A lifetime job history should be recorded, including the nature of the jobs, all reported exposures, the size of the organization (workforce, output), and the availability of environmental controls and whether personal protective equipment is worn. The health of colleagues and ex-employees should be asked about, if known. Access to company occupational health can be invaluable, but this should only be undertaken after gaining consent from the patient; smaller employers are less likely to have formal occupational health provision. Removal of exposure is often key, although, in some cases, disease progression appears to continue. Long-latency diseases are particularly hard to attribute to occupational causes, as the relevant exposures may have occurred over 40 years previously; a frequently quoted example is the relationship between asbestos exposure and mesothelioma.

Obliterative bronchiolitis

The majority of cases of OB occur in patients with chronic allograft rejection following a lung transplant or those with chronic graft-versus-host disease following a haematopoietic stem cell transplant. Other risk factors for OB include CTDs, severe or recurrent LRTIs (usually viral and occurring almost exclusively in childhood), chronic hypersensitivity pneumonitis (HP), and acute inhalation injuries from toxic fumes [23–24], as well as a number of distinct occupational exposures.

Prognosis, irrespective of the underlying aetiology, is poor, and, whilst the rate of decline is variable, most patients will deteriorate slowly and develop respiratory failure over the course of months to years. Various management strategies have been employed; these commonly include systemic corticosteroids, sometimes in combination with other immunosuppressive treatment. Long-term macrolide therapy has been used, with some success (possibly due to an immunomodulatory effect), but has not been tested in randomized clinical trials. Secondary bacterial infection often leads to irreversible deterioration, so prevention is a key priority, with vaccination, physiotherapy, and prophylactic or prompt antibiotic therapy.

Most recently, OB due to an occupational cause was identified in workers in a microwave popcorn factory in the US [25–34].

Evidence base Obliterative bronchiolitis in popcorn workers

Occupational OB was identified in a cluster of eight popcorn workers in the US in 2002 [25, 26]. A subsequent workplace survey at this plant found irreversible obstructive lung function at three times the rate expected in population controls; when limited to non-smokers, the rate was ten times that of a referent population. Subsequent investigations across the country revealed cases in at least ten other similar manufacturing plants [27–31]. The causative agent in the popcorn workers was found to be diacetyl, a volatile artificial 'butter' flavouring used in the manufacture of microwave popcorn. These studies showed a dose dependence, with a greater prevalence of disease in factories using larger quantities of diacetyl. Whilst other agents were considered as potentially causative agents, the available data suggested that the relationship between exposure and disease was strongest for diacetyl—with a further four cases identified in a diacetyl manufacturing company [32]. Animal and *in vitro* studies also supported the causative role of this agent [33, 34]. Unfortunately, in this cohort, removal from exposure failed to bring about improvement in the majority of cases.

Case history 2: Expert comment

Cases like this can pose all sorts of problems if you do not think clearly through them. Most patients will want to know if their job has made them ill. Often your answer can only be 'I'm not sure'; admitting and managing such uncertainty is not easy for many doctors. Often it is helpful to turn the question round: 'is it, in my opinion, safe for this patient to remain in their job?' When patients are seriously ill—as this man was—then a precautionary approach is probably appropriate. A wait-and-see stance may be appropriate in those with less severe disease. Again, contact with the patient's occupational health service usually helps; and other specialist advice is readily available. Finally, remember that you will need to be prepared to defend everything you put in writing, since it may later be read by a lawyer.

Other pneumoconioses are also described in novel circumstances or workplaces. ILD has been observed and described in nylon flock workers in Canada [35–37]. Fine fibres of nylon, known as 'flock', are used in clothing, upholstery, and blanket production; respirable fibres are generated during the process of adhesion of the flock to other fabrics. The radiological, pathological, and physiological features of the disease have most in common with HP—and improvement may occur on cessation of exposure. Recent clusters of silicosis cases in denim jean sandblasters [38], non-stick frying pan manufacturers in Turkey [39] and kitchen and bathroom surface manufacturers in Israel [40] have also been published, demonstrating novel exposures causing 'traditional' pneumoconioses.

Conclusion

Lung disease related to occupation can present in any general respiratory clinic, and many appear identical to disease due to non-occupational causes. Respiratory physicians should be aware of the potential of an occupational cause or contribution to lung disease and ensure that an appropriate occupational history is taken from patients presenting with respiratory disease for a specialist opinion.

A final word from the expert

There can be few trainees in respiratory medicine who need any **further** reminder to take a proper occupational history; nonetheless, it is always surprising how often it gets missed. In diseases of short latency—OA is a prime example—it is appropriate to concentrate on work done prior to, and at the time of, the first symptoms, remembering that occupational rhinitis often accompanies, and generally precedes, asthma. In diseases with a longer latency (silicosis, asbestos-induced diseases, and the like), a fuller employment history is required; starting from the end of school is often helpful. Learning to take a decent occupational history is not straightforward, and it is usually helpful to get some training from an experienced practitioner.

A characteristic history is, in most cases, just the start of the diagnostic process; rarely is it both possible and prudent to make a diagnosis of an occupational lung disease on the basis of a history alone. The consequences of an erroneous diagnosis can be disastrous; the costs of a 'false positive' may be especially high, since they often lead to an unnecessary termination in employment without any clinical improvement. In general, be wary about advising a patient to give up a job solely on health grounds; again, advice from an occupational physician or nurse advisor can be very helpful.

More so than in other branches of respiratory disease, occupational issues require you to answer two questions: (1) has my patient got their disease from their job and (2) what will be the consequences, to them and their employment, of that decision? Finally, remember that there are plenty of specialists around who are more than happy to advise.

References

1. Toren K, Blanc PD. Asthma caused by occupational exposures is common - a systematic analysis of estimates of the population-attributable fraction. *BMC Pulm Med* 2009;**9**:7.

2. Balmes J, Becklake M, Blanc P *et al.* American Thoracic Society Statement: Occupational contribution to the burden of airway disease. *Am J Respir Crit Care Med* 2003;**167**:787–97.
3. Brooks SM, Weiss MA, Bernstein IL. Reactive airways dysfunction syndrome (RADS). Persistent asthma syndrome after high level irritant exposures. *Chest* 1985;**88**:376–84.
4. Perrin B, Lagier F, L'Archeveque J *et al.* Occupational asthma: validity of monitoring of peak expiratory flow rates and non-allergic bronchial responsiveness as compared to specific inhalation challenge. *Eur Respir J* 1992;**5**:40–8.
5. Malo JL, Cote J, Cartier A, Boulet LP, L'Archeveque J, Chan-Yeung M. How many times per day should peak expiratory flow rates be assessed when investigating occupational asthma? *Thorax* 1993;**48**:1211–17.
6. Liss GM, Tarlo SM. Peak expiratory flow rates in possible occupational asthma. *Chest* 1991;**100**:63–9.
7. Leroyer C, Perfetti L, Trudeau C, L'Archeveque J, Chan-Yeung M, Malo JL. Comparison of serial monitoring of peak expiratory flow and FEV1 in the diagnosis of occupational asthma. *Am J Respir Crit Care Med* 1998;**158**:827–32.
8. Cote J, Kennedy S, Chan-Yeung M. Sensitivity and specificity of PC20 and peak expiratory flow rate in cedar asthma. *J Allergy Clin Immunol* 1990;**85**:592–8.
9. Bright P, Newton DT, Gannon PF, Pantin CF, Burge PS. OASYS-3: improved analysis of serial peak expiratory flow in suspected occupational asthma. *Monaldi Arch Chest Dis* 2001;**56**:281–8.
10. Blainey AD, Ollier S, Cundell D, Smith RE, Davies RJ. Occupational asthma in a hairdressing salon. *Thorax* 1986;**41**:42–50.
11. Pickering CA. Inhalation tests with chemical allergens: complex salts of platinum. *Proc R Soc Med* 1972;**65**:272–4.
12. Carroll KB, Secombe CJ, Pepys J. Asthma due to non-occupational exposure to toluene (tolylene) di-isocyanate. *Clin Allergy* 1976;**6**:99–104.
13. Cartier A, Malo JL, Forest F *et al.* Occupational asthma in snow crab-processing workers. *J Allergy Clin Immunol* 1984;**74**(3 Pt 1):261–9.
14. Malo JL, Cartier A, Cote J *et al.* Influence of inhaled steroids on recovery from occupational asthma after cessation of exposure: an 18-month double-blind crossover study. *Am J Respir Crit Care Med* 1996;**153**:953–60.
15. Rachiotis G, Savani R, Brant A, MacNeill SJ, Newman TA, Cullinan P. Outcome of occupational asthma after cessation of exposure: a systematic review. *Thorax* 2007;**62**:147–52.
16. Vandenplas O, Dressel H, Wilken D *et al.* Management of occupational asthma: cessation or reduction of exposure? A systematic review of available evidence. *Eur Respir J* 2011;**38**:804–11.
17. de Groene GJ, Pal TM, Beach J *et al.* Workplace interventions for treatment of occupational asthma. *Cochrane Database Syst Rev* 2011;**5**:CD006308.
18. Beach J, Rowe BH, Blitz S *et al.* Diagnosis and management of work-related asthma. *Evid Rep Technol Assess (Summ)* 2005;**129**:1–8.
19. Malo JL, Cartier A, Ghezzo H, Lafrance M, McCants M, Lehrer SB. Patterns of improvement in spirometry, bronchial hyperresponsiveness, and specific IgE antibody levels after cessation of exposure in occupational asthma caused by snow-crab processing. *Am Rev Respir Dis* 1988;**138**:807–12.
20. Fishwick D, Barber CM, Bradshaw LM *et al.* Standards of care for occupational asthma: an update. *Thorax* 2012;**67**:278–80.
21. Cullinan P.McGavin CR, Kreiss K, Nicholson AG. Obliterative bronchiolitis in fibreglass workers: a new occupational disease? *Occup Environ Med* 2013;**70**:357–9.
22. Bradford-Hill A. The environment and disease: association or causation? *Proc R Soc Med* 1965;**58**:295–300.
23. Ghanei M, Moqadam FA, Mohammad MM, Aslani J. Tracheobronchomalacia and air trapping after mustard gas exposure. *Am J Respir Crit Care Med* 2006;**173**:304–9.

24. Pipavath SJ, Lynch DA, Cool C, Brown KK, Newell JD. Radiologic and pathologic features of bronchiolitis. *AJR Am J Roentgenol* 2005;**185**:354–63.
25. Kreiss K, Gomaa A, Kullman G *et al.* Clinical bronchiolitis obliterans in workers at a microwave popcorn plant. *N Engl J Med* 2002;**347**:330–8.
26. [No authors listed]. From the Centers for Disease Control and Prevention. Fixed obstructive lung disease among workers in the flavour-manufacturing industry—Missouri, 2000–2002. *JAMA* 2002;**287**:2939–40.
27. Kanwal R. Bronchiolitis obliterans in workers exposed to flavouring chemicals. *Curr Opin Pulm Med* 2008;**14**:141–6.
28. Centers for Disease Control and Prevention (CDC). Fixed obstructive lung disease among workers in the flavor-manufacturing industry—California, 2004—2007. *MMWR Morb Mortal Wkly Rep* 2007;**56**:389–93.
29. Kanwal R, Kullman G, Piacitelli C *et al.* Evaluation of flavourings-related lung disease risk at six microwave popcorn plants. *J Occup Environ Med* 2006;**58**:149–57.
30. Kim TJ, Materna BL, Prudhomme JC *et al.* Industry-wide medical surveillance of California flavour manufacturing workers: cross-sectional results. *Am J Ind Med* 2010;**53**:857–65.
31. Lockey JE, Hilbert TJ, Levin LP *et al.* Airway obstruction related to diacetyl exposure at microwave popcorn production facilities. *Eur Respir J* 2009;**34**:63–71.
32. van Rooy FG, Rooyackers JM, Prokop M, Houba R, Smit LA, Heederik DJ. Bronchiolitis obliterans syndrome in chemical workers producing diacetyl for food flavorings. *Am J Respir Crit Care Med* 2007;**176**:498–504.
33. Harber P, Saechao K, Boomus C. Diacetyl induced lung disease. *Toxicol Rev* 2006;**25**:261–72.
34. Palmer SM, Flake GP, Kelly FL *et al.* Severe airway epithelial injury, aberrant repair and bronchiolitis obliterans develops after diacetyl instillation in rats. *PLoS One* 2011;**6**:e17644.
35. Centers for Disease Control and Prevention (CDC). Chronic interstitial lung disease in nylon flocking industry workers—Rhode Island, 1992—1996. *MMWR Morb Mortal Wkly Rep.* 1997;**46**:897–901.
36. Kern DG, Crausman RS, Durand KT, Nayer A, Kuhn C 3rd. Flock worker's lung: chronic interstitial lung disease in the nylon flocking industry. *Ann Intern Med* 1998;**129**:261–72.
37. Eschenbacher WL, Kreiss K, Lougheed MD, Pransky GS, Day B, Castellan RM. Nylon flock-associated interstitial lung disease. *Am J Respir Crit Care Med* 1999;**159**:2003–8.
38. Akgun M, Araz O, Akkurt I *et al.* An epidemic of silicosis among former denim sandblasters. *Eur Respir J* 2008;**32**:1295–303.
39. Köksal N, Kahraman H. Acute silicosis in teflon-coated pan manufacturing due to metal sandblasting. *Int J Occup Environ Health* 2011;**17**:210–13.
40. Kramer MR, Blanc PD, Fireman E *et al.* Artificial stone silicosis: disease resurgence among artificial stone workers. *Chest* 2012;**142**:419–24.

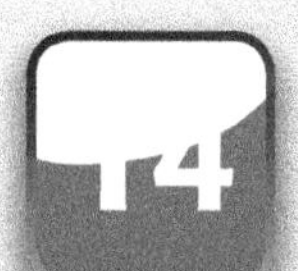

Pulmonary disease caused by non-tuberculous mycobacteria

Janet Stowell

Expert commentary Ronan Breen

Case history

A 62-year-old ex-smoker with severe COPD (FEV_1 1.0 L/minute, 33% predicted; FVC 1.8 L/minute, 47% predicted) presented with worsening dyspnoea, a cough productive of purulent sputum, and weight loss (8 kg in the last year). He had a history of asbestos exposure and had been treated for pulmonary TB of his right lung 20 years earlier. At this time, he received 6 months of quadruple therapy with rifampicin, pyrazinamide, isoniazid, and ethambutol. The organism was fully sensitive, and treatment adherence was satisfactory.

On examination, he looked pale and unwell. His chest was hyperexpanded, and crackles were audible in his right mid- and lower zones. His chest radiograph showed long-standing right upper zone scarring (Figure 14.1), with new consolidation in the right mid- and lower zones and increased volume loss (Figure 14.2).

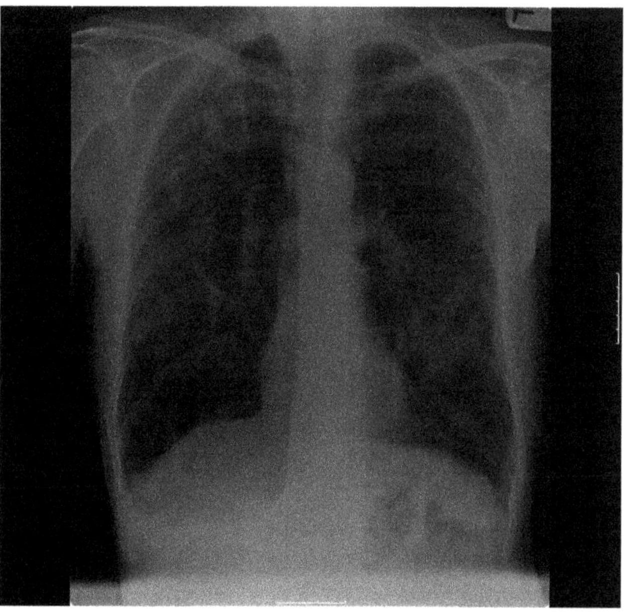

Figure 14.1 Pre-presentation chest radiograph.

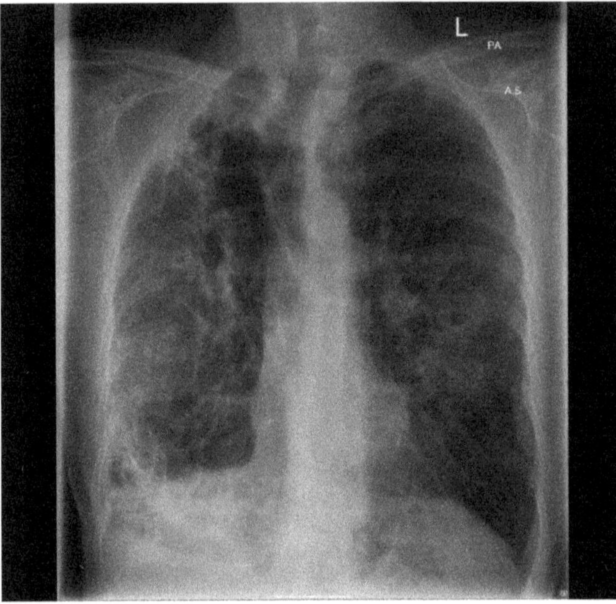

Figure 14.2 Presentation chest radiograph.

A HRCT scan of his chest revealed bilateral pleural plaques and extensive emphysema, with right apical scarring, traction bronchiectasis, and volume loss (long-standing) (Figure 14.3). The notable change was new peripheral consolidation in the right middle and lower lobes and a small pleural effusion (Figure 14.4).

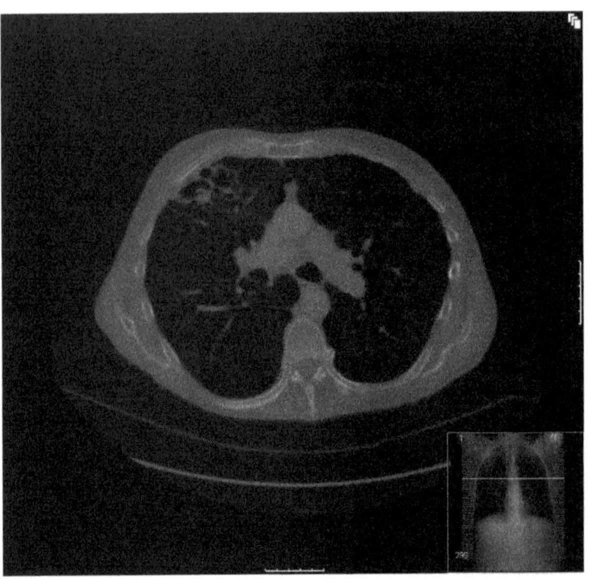

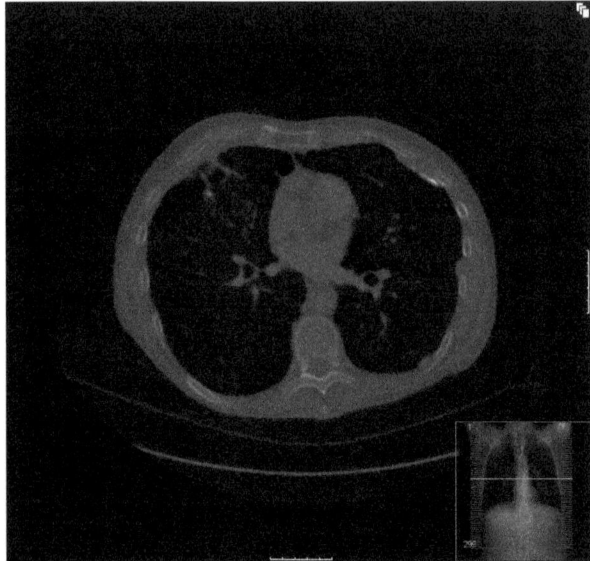

Figure 14.3 Representative slices from a HRCT scan pre-presentation.

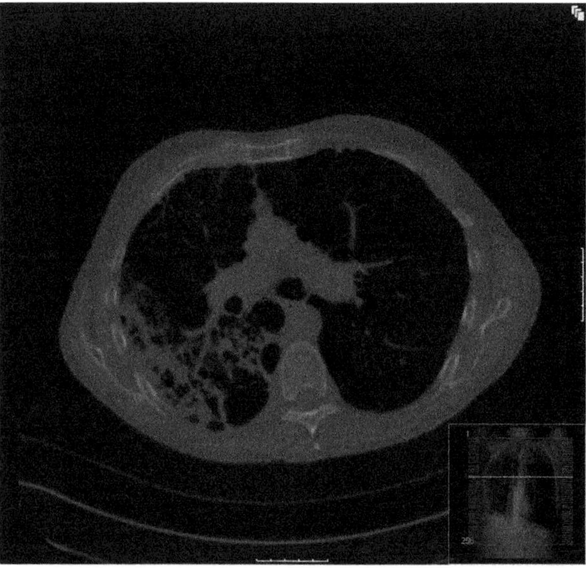

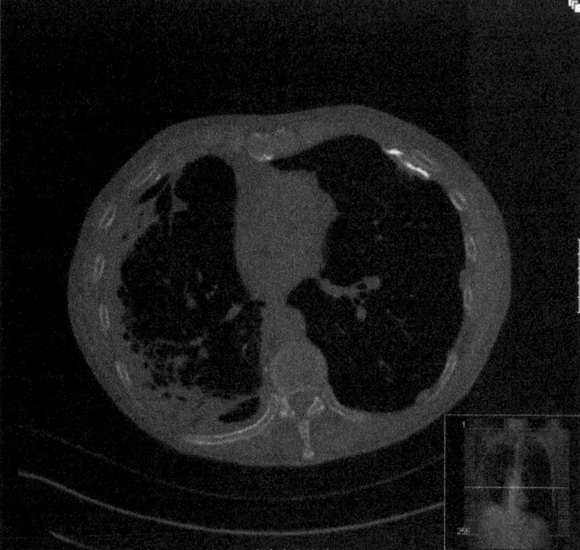

Figure 14.4 HRCT scan at presentation showing new peripheral right-sided consolidation.

Clinical tip Radiological changes in non-tuberculous *Mycobacterium* pulmonary disease

- Progressive consolidation with cavitation and fibrosis (fibrocavitary disease). Fibrocavitatory disease can look very similar to that caused by TB. There are subtle differences, but none of them sufficiently specific to exclude the diagnosis of TB on the basis of radiographic appearance.
- Multifocal bronchiectasis ± multiple small nodules (nodular/bronchiectatic disease).
- Pleural involvement from underlying areas of the lung is common, but pleural effusion is rare [1].
- Solitary nodules without cavitation may be seen. Often referred to as suspected lung cancer, these nodules show avidity on FDG-PET scanning. Surgical resection is usually curative.

Sputum was smear-positive for acid- and alcohol-fast bacilli (AAFB). TB nucleic acid amplification testing (NAAT) was negative for *Mycobacterium* TB (MTB) complex. Sputum grew *Mycobacterium malmoense* at 20 days. Immunoglobulins were normal, and HIV antibody test was negative.

Learning point Susceptibility to pulmonary disease caused by non-tuberculous mycobacteria

Non-tuberculous mycobacteria (NTM) (also called atypical or opportunistic mycobacteria) is a term used to distinguish environmental mycobacteria from mycobacteria that cause TB (*Mycobacterium tuberculosis*) and leprosy (*Mycobacterium leprae*). They can be isolated from soil, water (including tap water), dust, milk, and various animals and birds. Patients with pre-existing structural lung disease or deficient immune systems are more prone to infection than healthy individuals with a normal lung architecture. Defects in interferon gamma (IFN-γ) and IL-12 synthesis and response pathways have been shown to increase disease susceptibility in otherwise immunocompetent individuals [2, 3].

The patient who develops fibrocavitary NTM pulmonary infection is typically middle-aged and male, a smoker or an ex-smoker with COPD, and/or a history of previous TB and/or alcohol excess [1]. There is also a recognized association between nodular bronchiectatic disease and post-menopausal women with a low BMI and chest wall abnormalities (scoliosis or pectus excavatum) [4]. Fibronodular bronchiectasis has been called **Lady Windermere syndrome**, after the Oscar Wilde play [5]. It has

(Continued)

Learning point

NAAT is extremely useful in practice, as a negative result for MTB complex avoids unnecessary concern around infection control and the need for contact tracing.

been suggested that elderly women acquire the condition because they voluntarily suppress their cough, and infected secretions are retained in the right middle lobe and lingula. Most NTM infection complicating fibronodular bronchiectasis is due to *Mycobacterium avium* complex (MAC) which comprises *Mycobacterium avium* and *Mycobacterium intracellulare*, but it can be caused by other NTM, including *Mycobacterium abscessus* and *Mycobacterium kansasii* [6].

A syndrome indistinguishable from HP has also been described in patients exposed to NTM in solution, particularly associated with the use of hot tubs, a condition termed 'hot tub lung' [7]. These patients develop granulomatous lung disease due to colonization of NTM via inhalation of aerosolized inadequately sterilized water, which may recover by simply avoiding NTM exposure but, in some cases, requires treatment with antibiotics and/or steroids. This can also be seen in metal workers.

Learning point Key laboratory features of NTM

The significance of an NTM isolate is established by considering the specimen from which it came, the degree of growth, the identity of the organism, and the number of isolates. It follows that as much material as possible should be provided to the lab for NTM culture, with clear instructions to culture for mycobacteria [8]. The burden of organisms in clinical material is usually reflected by the number of organisms seen on microscopic examination of stained smears, so the extent of smear positivity can be used as a guide to disease burden. It is noteworthy, however, that negative smears do not necessarily mean that NTM are not present [1].

Specimens should be cultured in both liquid and solid media. Cultures in liquid media have a higher yield of mycobacteria and produce more rapid results, but solid media allow the observation of colony morphology, growth rates, and recognition of mixed infections and quantitation of the infecting organism [9]. Most NTM grow within 2-3 weeks on subculture. The rapidly growing mycobacteria (RGM) *M. fortuitum*, *M. abscessus*, and *M. chelonae* grow within 7 days.

NTM should be identified to the species level [9]. Methods of rapid species identification include commercial DNA probes (available for MAC, *M. kansasii*, and *M. gordonae*) and high-performance liquid chromatography (HPLC) [10]. Alternative methods (suitable for RGM) are DNA sequencing or PCR restriction endonuclease assay (PRA) [11]. The technique of DNA sequencing exploits the highly conserved, yet species-specific, nature of NTM 16S ribosomal DNA (rDNA). This is an approximately 1500-nucleotide sequence encoded by the 16S rDNA, which is a highly conserved gene with regions common to all organisms (conserved regions) and areas where nucleotide variation occur (variable regions). Sequence analysis focusses on two hypervariable regions (known as regions A and B) for species identification [12]. The PCR/PRA method combines PCR amplification of a 65-kDa heat shock protein in the genome of NTM with restriction enzyme digestion. The size of the restriction fragment is generally species-specific [11].

Chemotherapy with rifampicin and ethambutol (15 mg/kg) was started and continued for 24 months. The patient tolerated the tablets well and improved clinically, gaining weight and expectorating less sputum. His radiology markedly improved (Figure 14.5). His sputum became culture-negative 9 months into treatment and remained so on follow-up checks for 1 year post-completion of treatment.

Clinical tip

Assays of lymphocyte IFN-γ (production (ELISPOT) should not be used to diagnose active TB or NTM. The RD-1 genomic segment of **MTB**, which encodes the early secreted antigenic target 6-kDa protein (ESAT-6) antigen, is also present in *M. kansasii*, *M. marinum*, and *M. szulgai*. Therefore, exposure to these NTM could result in false-positive results [13] which complicate the clinical picture.

Learning point Burden of NTM disease

In the last 60 years, the prevalence of NTM disease in the developed world has increased. It is not clear whether there is a true increase in NTM disease in immunocompetent patients or whether the increase can be explained by greater awareness of NTM and an increased likelihood of specimens being collected for mycobacterial culture [14, 15]. Other explanations include reduced immunity to mycobacteria because of the reduced prevalence of TB and greater exposure to mycobacteria due

(Continued)

to changes in personal hygiene habits from bathing to showering (NTM are frequently present in tap water, resistant to chlorination and ozonization, and readily aerosolized in shower heads) [7]. The ageing population with chronic disease and the increased utilization of immunosuppression in a variety of conditions is also likely to be contributory.

In the last 15 years, the number of NTM species identified has more than doubled. Currently, >150 NTM species have been catalogued. The increase relates to improved microbiologic techniques for isolating NTM, in combination with important advances in molecular techniques, with the acceptance of 16S rRNA gene sequencing as a standard for defining new species [16].

Whilst the number of species of NTM now recognized is vast, those associated with human disease, particularly those affecting the lungs, constitute a relatively small group which exhibit geographical variation. *M. kansasii* is the commonest opportunistic mycobacterial pathogen in the Midlands and southern half of the UK; *M. malmoense* is the commonest in northern UK and Scotland, and *M. xenopi* predominates (37% of isolates) in the south-east of England. MAC is found in all parts of the UK but is particularly common in patients with HIV (CD4 <100) where it is responsible for >90% of the opportunistic mycobacterial infections [17]. Other (less common) organisms affecting the lungs are *M. abscessus*, *M. fortuitum*, *M. celatum*, *M. asiaticum*, and *M. sulgai*.

Expert comment

Although RGM are rare causes of clinical lung disease, positive isolates should prompt further sample collection and clinical review, as there may have been overgrowth of a more significant mycobacterium, e.g. MTB, or a culture of *M. abscessus* may be a clue to underlying cystic fibrosis.

Pulmonary physicians may also be consulted about non-pulmonary isolates as the 'mycobacterial expert'. Skin and soft tissue infections often after surgery may be seen with RGM, such as *M. fortuitum* and *M. chelonae*, or related to trauma whilst in water as with *M. marinum*. These infections may need a combination of surgery and drug therapy, and appropriate expert advice should be sought. Children may present with lymph node swelling due to *M. avium* or *M. malmoense*, and resection is usually curative.

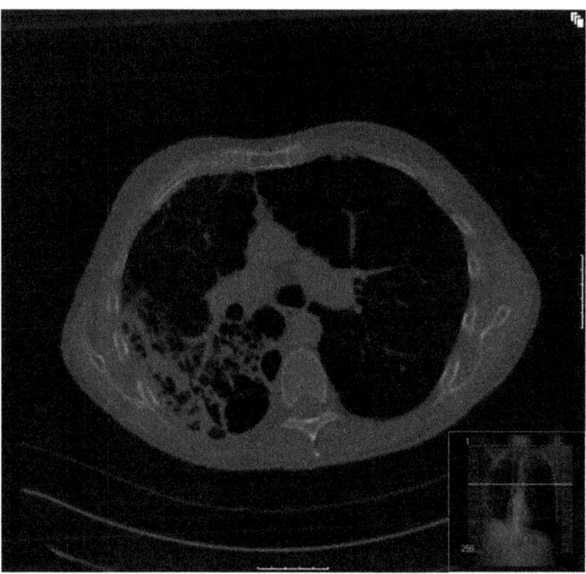

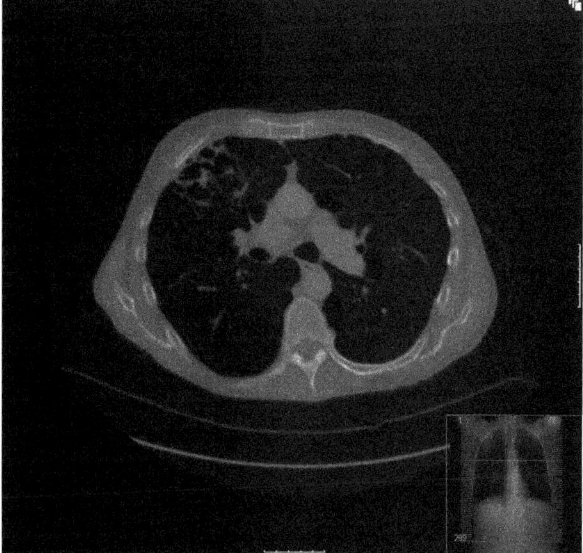

Figure 14.5 HRCT scan showing radiological improvement post-treatment. (a) Pre-treatment. (b) Post-treatment.

Learning point Approach to treatment of pulmonary disease caused by NTM

The choice of a therapeutic regimen for a specific patient depends on the goals of therapy for that patient. The most aggressive therapy (including an injectable agent) might be appropriate for patients with extensive disease or disease which has relapsed or for whom microbiologic and clinical improvement is important and feasible [1]. Less aggressive therapy might be appropriate for frail patients with multiple co-morbidities and the potential for problematic drug interactions, especially if they have more indolent disease.

Prior to the randomized trial of treatment for NTM pulmonary disease in HIV-negative patients, conducted by the BTS in 2000 [18], the literature consisted largely of retrospective reports of the results of various multidrug regimens given to small numbers of patients. These regimens were variably tolerated, and it was not clear which drugs were most efficacious for which organisms. Compounding uncertainty was the seemingly paradoxical lack of correlation between the clinical response and the results of *in vitro* sensitivity tests of single anti-mycobacterial drugs [19, 20]. However, synergy between rifampicin and ethambutol was reliably demonstrated, and regimens containing these two drugs were successful, despite *in vitro* resistance to each drug when tested singly against the organism [21–23].

Expert comment

Prior to commencing therapy against NTM infection, the physician and patient should undertake a careful evaluation of its appropriateness. This is most important when therapy is against organisms such as *M. xenopi* and MAC, for which treatment is lengthy and may not be curative and the health status may already be significantly impaired. ATS treatment criteria (see Discussion, p. 177) are a very helpful guide but should not be the sole criteria used, and fulfilment should not be seen to mandate treatment. Other aspects of care should be optimized such as nutrition, sputum clearance, management of gastro-oesophageal reflux by pharmacological and physical (e.g. sleeping more upright) measures, pulmonary rehabilitation, and smoking cessation. Where appropriate, assessment should also be made to ensure that clinical deterioration is not due to an alternative pathology such as malignancy.

Evidence base Rifampicin, ethambutol, and isoniazid versus rifampicin and ethambutol

The BTS prospective multinational trial investigated the role of isoniazid as a third agent. It compared the regimen of rifampicin, ethambutol, and isoniazid (REH) with the regimen of rifampicin and ethambutol (RE), given for 2 years to a total of 223 patients with *M. malmoense* (106), MAC (75), or *M. xenopi* (42).

Study findings:

1. the results of *in vitro* susceptibility tests do not correlate with the patient's response to chemotherapy;
2. REH and RE are tolerated better than previous regimens containing second- or third-line anti-mycobacterial drugs;
3. the addition of isoniazid reduces the failure of treatment and relapse rates for MAC and has a tendency to do so for *M. xenopi*, but the REH regimen showed a trend for higher death rates overall (8% versus 1% with RE);
4. treatment of *M. malmoense* with RE for 2 years appeared preferable to that with REH;
5. *M. xenopi* was associated with the greatest mortality (57% at 5 years); MAC was the most difficult to eradicate; *M. malmoense* had the most favourable outlook (42% alive and cured at 5 years).

The study concluded that isoniazid had little or no place in the treatment of *M. xenopi* or *M. malmoense*. It is of use in MAC if RE is failing to render the sputum culture negative [18].

Sixteen months on, from completion of anti-mycobacterial treatment, a routine chest radiograph showed patchy shadowing in the right lower zone (Figure 14.6).

The patient was not unwell, febrile, or productive of sputum, but his weight had fallen by 3 kg since his last review 4 months before. He underwent bronchoscopy, and

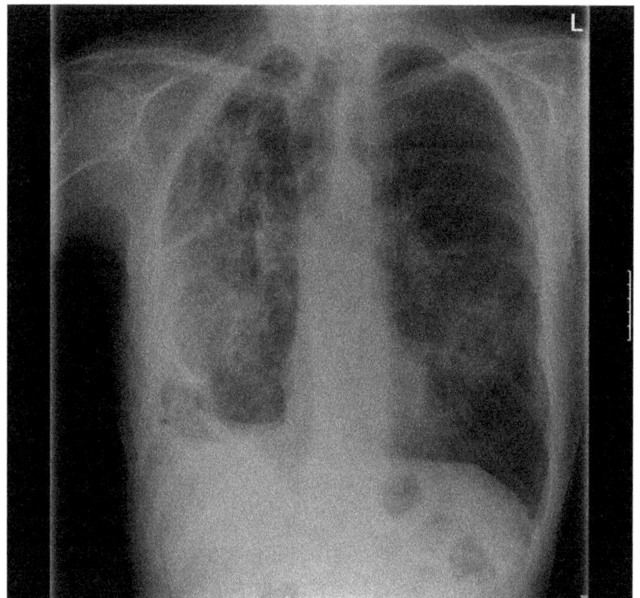

Figure 14.6 Chest radiograph showing new right-sided consolidation.

Expert comment

If a patient is non-productive of sputum, then it may be necessary to obtain respiratory samples by other means. Bronchoscopy is an excellent method of doing this, but sputum induction provides a cheaper and non-invasive alternative that may be better tolerated, especially if required to be repeated.

M. malmoense was again isolated from the bronchial washings. His cough recurred, productive of small amounts of purulent sputum. Treatment with rifampicin and ethambutol was recommenced. Four months into treatment, his weight loss continued, and a CT scan showed increased consolidation in the right lower lobe, with some of the previously noted bullae becoming thick-walled and containing fluid (Figure 14.7).

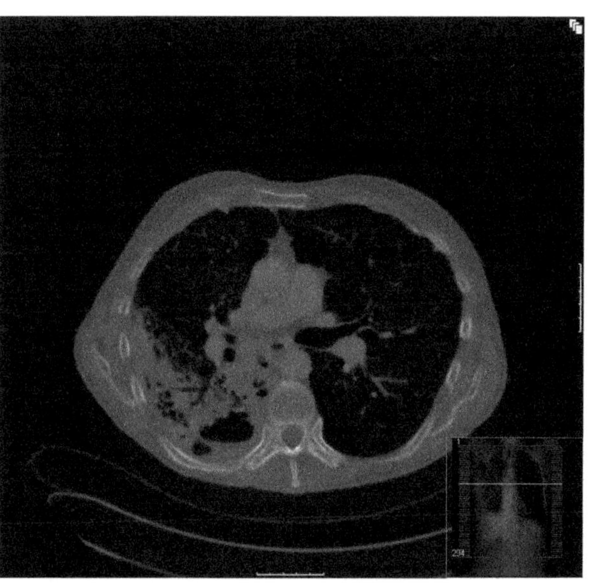

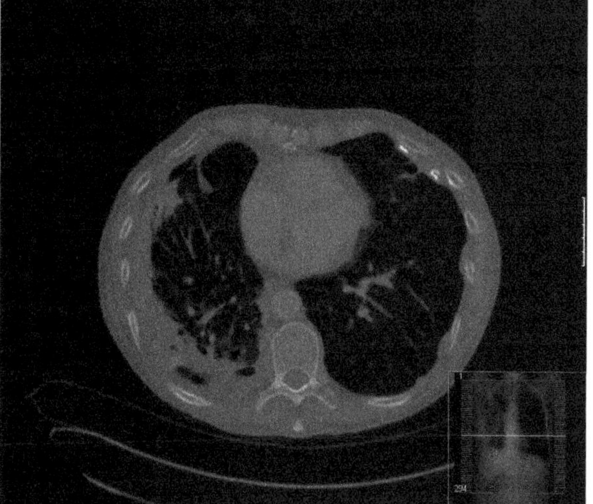

Figure 14.7 CT scan showing progression of consolidation.

Clarithromycin 500 mg bd was added to his existing treatment regimen of rifampicin and ethambutol.

Evidence base Clarithromycin versus ciprofloxacin as adjuncts to rifampicin and ethambutol

In 2008, the BTS published a further multicentre randomized trial assessing the value of clarithromycin and ciprofloxacin in the treatment of NTM pulmonary disease in HIV-negative patients. A regimen of 2 years of rifampicin, ethambutol, and clarithromycin (REClari) was compared with 2 years of rifampicin, ethambutol, and ciprofloxacin (RECipro) for pulmonary disease caused by MAC, *M. malmoense*, and *M. xenopi*. A group of patients was further randomized to receive immunotherapy with *M. vaccae* or to no immunotherapy. Any patient not improving at 1 year received supplementation with the drug not received in the original allocation of treatment.

Study findings: considering all three species taken together, there were no differences in outcome between the REClari and RECipro groups; 20% in each group were unable to tolerate the regimen allocated, ciprofloxacin being associated with more unwanted effects than clarithromycin (16% versus 9%). Immunotherapy did not improve outcome [24].

A further 4 months on this modified treatment regimen made no difference to his clinical condition. He exhibited worsening dyspnoea, productive cough, and weight loss (despite dietary supplementation with high-calorie drinks). His sputum remained positive for *M. malmoense*. His case was discussed with the cardiothoracic surgeons, but it was decided that his lung function was too poor to consider a lobectomy (FEV_1 0.9 L/minute, 30% predicted; FVC 1.6 L/minute, 42% predicted; with TLCO 35% predicted).

Clinical tip Role of surgery in NTM disease

Surgery is advocated for patients with localized disease who fail medical therapy and have adequate pulmonary reserve. If undertaken, the BTS recommends continuing chemotherapy for at least 18 months post-operatively. Post-operative morbidity and complications, including broncho-pleural fistula, haemorrhage, and empyema, can be problematic in these patients [25, 26]. However, there is evidence that timely surgical intervention in a carefully selected cohort of patients in a specialized centre, in which the thoracic surgeons have considerable experience with this type of challenging surgery, can bring about excellent results [27, 28]. There are currently no established criteria for patient selection.

A special circumstance that merits a mention is the surgical removal of a solitary pulmonary nodule caused by MAC. Data are sparse, but expert consensus is that, in the absence of other MAC-related disease radiographically, surgical resection of the solitary nodule is curative, with no antibiotic therapy necessary [1].

Over the next 3 months, he deteriorated further; his sputum increased in volume and purulence, and he became febrile, weak, and lethargic. Radiologically, there was marked deterioration. CT chest showed a thick-walled posterior right-sided cavity, extending almost the entire length of the thoracic cavity (Figure 14.8).

Sputum grew both *M. malmoense* and *Aspergillus fumigatus*. The serum IgE level was normal; there were no eosinophils in the sputum and no excess in the blood. Serum precipitins (IgG) for *Aspergillus* were positive.

Oral itraconazole was commenced, and anti-mycobacterial treatment with rifampicin, ethambutol, and clarithromycin continued. Clinical improvement was minimal. He continued to have fever and productive cough, and his weight had

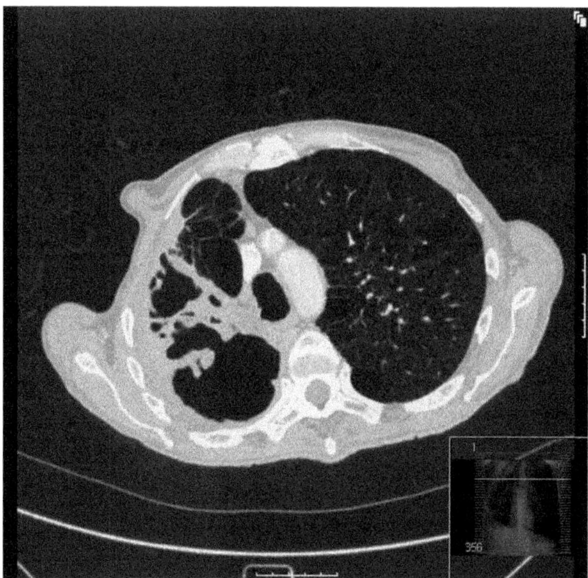
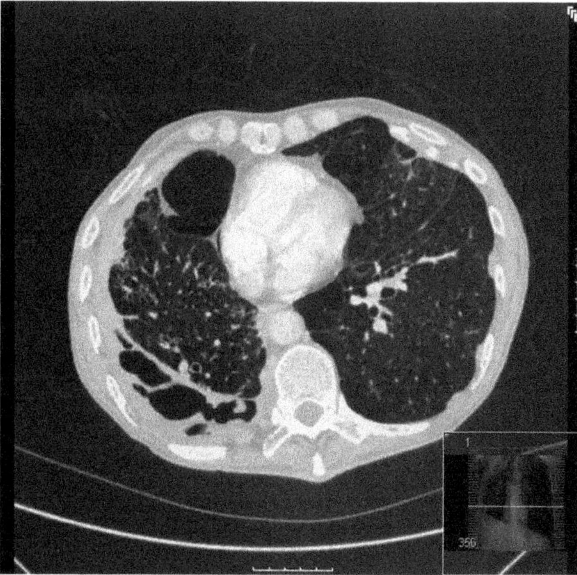

Figure 14.8 CT showing increased cavitating consolidation with a cavity containing soft tissue, suggestive of fungal disease.

dipped to 15 kg below his baseline. He was admitted to hospital for treatment with IV amphotericin. The dietician was consulted, and overnight feeding via a nasogastric tube was commenced.

Clinical tip Drug interactions

It is important to be aware of the pharmacological interaction between rifampicin and itraconazole which is complex. Itraconazole inhibits the CYP 450 hepatic enzyme system, resulting in increased levels of rifampicin, whilst rifampicin is a potent inducer of CYP 450 and has been shown to significantly lower itraconazole levels [29]. Individual patients behave differently when it comes to achieving therapeutic levels of individual drugs, and expert pharmacological advice should be sought in such cases. Rifabutin should be considered as an alternative to rifamycin, and other conazoles, such as voriconazole, may facilitate a more effective clinical response. LFTs should be carefully monitored at 4 weeks and 3-monthly thereafter, along with signs of ocular toxicity. Cardiomyopathy can rarely complicate treatment with conazoles, so a low threshold for echocardiography is advised if there are clinical concerns. IV amphotericin may also have a role in severe disease.

Ten days on, he was no better, so prednisolone was added (initially 1 mg/kg, then gradually weaned). This resulted in rapid clinical improvement; he became afebrile, and the sputum volume and purulence reduced. Over the next 2 weeks, he regained some strength and started to gain weight. He was discharged from hospital on maintenance treatment with rifampicin, ethambutol, clarithromycin, itraconazole, and prednisolone and monitored closely in the outpatient clinic.

Six months on, he is doing well, gaining weight and coughing infrequently. He is mildly productive of non-purulent sputum in the mornings, which continues to grow *M. malmoense*, but is culture-negative for *A. fumigatus*.

Expert comment

Treating both NTM and *Aspergillus* concurrently can be extremely challenging, and expert advice should be sought. Patients with fibrocavitatory disease may often have serological and microbiological evidence of colonization with *Aspergillus*, but this should not be taken as evidence of the need to treat without clear clinical and radiological evidence. In most cases, treatment of NTM will remain the clinical priority, although, as in this case, the converse can occur, and effective treatment of the predominant infection should not be compromised unnecessarily.

Clinical tip Regimens for use in HIV-negative patients with pulmonary disease due to opportunistic mycobacteria

See Table 14.1.

Table 14.1 Regimens for use in HIV-negative patients with pulmonary disease due to opportunistic mycobacteria

NTM	Regimen	Duration
M. kansasii	Isoniazid 300 mg daily PLUS Rifampicin 600 mg daily PLUS Ethambutol (15 mg/kg) daily	Until sputum culture negative for at least 1 year
M. malmoense	Optimal chemotherapy is not known	Unknown
M. xenopi	Optimal chemotherapy is not known	Unknown
M. avium complex (MAC)	**Nodular or bronchiectatic pulmonary disease:** Clarithromycin 500–1000 mg PO three times a week or azithromycin 500 mg PO three times a week PLUS Rifampicin 600 mg PO three times a week or rifabutin 200 mg three times a week PLUS Ethambutol 25 mg/kg PO three times a week **Fibrocavitary MAC lung disease or severe nodular or bronchiectatic disease*:** Clarithromycin 500–1000 mg PO daily or azithromycin 250 mg PO daily PLUS Rifampicin 600 mg PO daily or rifabutin 150–300 mg daily PLUS Ethambutol 15 mg/kg PO daily	Until sputum culture negative for at least 1 year

* Consider streptomycin or amikacin as a fourth agent for the first 8 weeks.
Based on the 2007 ATS guidelines [1].

Clinical tip Drug toxicity and monitoring

Ototoxicity and vestibular toxicity due to aminoglycosides are usually irreversible. Patients who receive streptomycin or amikacin MUST be warned about the signs and symptoms of toxicity (unsteady gait, tinnitus, and hearing impairment) at the start of therapy and again on subsequent visits, with discontinuation or decrease in dosage or frequency if signs suggestive of toxicity occur. Baseline audiometry testing, together with repeat interval testing whilst receiving parenteral aminoglycoside, should be performed. Baseline liver and renal function should be documented and checked at 4 weeks and 3-monthly thereafter.

Discussion

This case illustrates a typical presentation of NTM disease in a male ex-smoker with COPD. Despite adhering to 24 months' dual therapy (rifampicin and ethambutol), he experienced a protracted clinical course. He had a period of >1 year of culture-negative sputum but then relapsed, necessitating recommencement of dual therapy and the addition of a macrolide. He continued to decline; his sputum grew *A. fumigatus*, and a secondary diagnosis of chronic invasive aspergillosis was made. He was started on antifungal treatment. Clinical improvement finally came about with the addition of oral steroids.

This case demonstrates a level of complexity greater than many cases of pulmonary NTM encountered in routine clinical practice in HIV-negative patients, but it is certainly not on its own. Each presentation must be evaluated thoroughly on an individual basis. Minimum evaluation should include:

1. a chest radiograph or, in the absence of cavitation, a chest HRCT scan;
2. three or more sputum specimens for acid-fast bacilli (AFB) smear and mycobacterial culture;
3. exclusion of other disorders such as TB [1]. The ATS microbiologic criteria for diagnosis are: positive culture results from at least two separate expectorated sputum samples, or one bronchial wash/BAL, or transbronchial or other lung biopsy with mycobacterial histopathologic features (granulomatous inflammation or AFB) in the context of culture-positive sputum or BAL [1].

Diagnosis must be firmly established, and appropriate treatment planned. Response to treatment must be monitored at timely intervals, and careful surveillance arranged to detect drug interactions/toxicity which may warrant a change in drug regimen.

An important take-home point from this case is that failure to respond to antimycobacterial treatment, or a relapse during treatment, may be caused by concomitant infection with *Aspergillus*. The clinician should remain vigilant for the possibility of *Aspergillus* co-infection during NTM treatment, but, as discussed earlier, this diagnosis should be very carefully considered due to the difficulty of combining treatment.

There are data showing that the prevalence of *Aspergillus*-related lung disease is higher in patients with bronchiectasis and NTM than in patients with bronchiectasis and no evidence of NTM (higher rate of positive *Aspergillus* serology and radiological features of *Aspergillus*-related disease) [30]. Lung disease associated with *Aspergillus* can manifest in a number of ways. Aspergillomas may originate in large cavity lesions of inactive *M. kansasii* infection and may complicate pulmonary disease caused by *M. xenopi*. Chronic airway invasive aspergillosis (chronic necrotizing pulmonary aspergillosis (CNPA) or semi-invasive aspergillosis) is an alternative presentation seen in patients with *M. malmoense* and MAC.

It is of interest that treatment with corticosteroids had such a positive impact on the recovery of this patient, although there was no evidence of ABPA. One possible explanation for this is that a local hypersensitivity reaction contributes to tissue destruction and is suppressed by steroid treatment.

HIV disease and opportunistic mycobacterial disease

HIV-positive patients with NTM infections usually have more disseminated disease. Disease confined to the lungs is rare (<5% of cases) [10]; cavitatory disease is unusual (<5% of cases), and haemoptysis is less common. Apical scarring or upper lobe

Expert comment

Although NTM complicating HIV infection has become much less common with the widespread and early use of ART, this may change due to the high rates of smoking and accelerated emphysema reported in many HIV treatment cohorts predisposing to fibrocavitatory NTM disease. Presentation with NTM, even in an elderly patient with COPD, may still provide an opportunity to identify undiagnosed HIV, and testing should be offered routinely.

involvement occurs in <10%. The chest radiograph typically shows diffuse interstitial or reticulonodular infiltrate (50% of cases) or alveolar infiltrate (20%) [31].

Progressive weakening of the immune system with blood CD4 counts <100 cells/microlitre predisposes to disseminated mycobacterial disease, which is mostly caused by MAC [1]. *M. kansasii* follows MAC as the second most frequent cause of disseminated mycobacteriosis in AIDS patients (3% of cases). *M. kansasii* pulmonary disease also occurs, late in the course of HIV infection, when immunosuppression is advanced. Untreated disease can be rapidly fatal [32].

Restoring immunocompetence is key to the success of NTM treatment. Effective ART may clear NTM, without the need for more specific therapy, or unmask the presence of NTM as part of the immune restoration inflammatory syndrome (IRIS). MAC-related IRIS is very well described and should be suspected in IRIS-related complications which follow commencement of antiretroviral therapy. The choice of anti-mycobacterial regimens needs consideration, given the established interactions between rifamycins, macrolides, and protease inhibitors. Adverse effects leading to premature discontinuation of treatment are much commoner in the HIV-positive patient cohort [1]. Expert advice should be sought when treating difficult cases, because discontinuation often results in recurrence of disease and bacteraemia [33].

A final word from the expert

NTM isolation in clinical isolates and associated disease continue to increase. Many cases are clinically challenging, and the involved physician should ideally have an interest in this area and be able to carefully consider each case to decide whether treatment will be beneficial and, if started, what the aims of such therapy are. Clinical decisions should not just focus on anti-mycobacterial drugs, as other aspects of care should be optimized prior to, and during, NTM treatment. It should also be remembered that observation may be appropriate, even when treatment criteria have been fulfilled. Treating physicians will often need to access expertise in radiology, microbiology, pharmacology, and surgery and benefit from discussing difficult cases with an experienced colleague. The views of both the patient and carers should also be paramount, as treatment may be both toxic and non-curative. In a patient population that is frequently burdened with co-morbidities, even when therapy is aiming for cure, its appropriateness in individual cases should be carefully and frequently reviewed.

References

1. David EGriffith, Aksamit T, Brown-Elliott BA *et al.*; ATS Mycobacterial Diseases Subcommittee; American Thoracic Society; Infectious Disease Society of America. An Official ATS/IDSA Statement: diagnosis, treatment and prevention of nontuberculous mycobacterial diseases. *Am J Respir Crit Care Med* 2007;**175**:367–416.
2. Dorman SE, Holland SM. Interferon-gamma and interleukin-12 pathway defects and human disease. *Cytokine Growth Factor Rev* 2000;**11**:321.
3. Casanova JL, Abel L. Genetic dissection of immunity to mycobacteria: the human model. *Annu Rev Immunol* 2002;**20**:581–620.
4. Iseman MD, Buschman DL, Ackerson LM. Pectus excavatum and scoliosis: thoracic anomalies associated with pulmonary disease caused by *Mycobacterium avium* complex. *Am Rev Respir Dis* 1991;**144**;914.

5. Reich JM, Johnson RE.*Mycobacterium avium* complex pulmonary disease presenting as an isolated lingular or middle lobe pattern: the Lady Windermere syndrome. *Chest* 1992; **101**:1605–9.
6. Dhillon SS, Watanakunakorn C. Lady Windermere syndrome: middle lobe bronchiectasis and *Mycobacteriumavium* complex infection due to voluntary cough suppression. *Clin Infect Dis* 2000;**30**:572–5.
7. Stephen K Field, Robert L Cowie. Lung disease due to the more common nontuberculous mycobacteria. *Chest* 2006;**129**:1653–65.
8. [No authors listed]. Management of opportunistic mycobacterial infections: Joint Tuberculosis Committee Guideline 1999. Subcommittee of the Joint Tuberculosis Committee of the British Thoracic Society. *Thorax* 2000;**55**:210–18. 2000.
9. National Committee for Clinical Laboratory Standards (2003). *Susceptibility testing of mycobacteria, nocardiae, and other aerobic actinomycetes. Approved Standard*. Document No. M24-A. Wayne, PA: National Committee for Clinical Laboratory Standards.
10. Butler WR, Guthertz LS. Mycolic acid analysis by high performance liquid chromatography for identification of *Mycobacterium species. Clin Microbiol Rev* 2001;**14**:704–26.
11. Telenti A, Marchesi F, Balz M, Bally F, Bottger EC, Bodmer T. Rapid identification of mycobacteria to the species level by polymerase chain reaction and restriction enzyme analysis. *J Clin Microbiol* 1993;**31**:175–8.
12. Tortoli E. Impact of genotypic studies on mycobacterial taxonomy: the new mycobacteria of the 1990s. *Clin Microbiol Rev* 2003;**2**:319–54.
13. Andersen P, Munk ME, Pollock JM *et al*. Specific immune based diagnosis of tuberculosis. *Lancet* 2000;**356**:1099–104.
14. Kilby JM, Gilligan PH, Yankaskas JR *et al*. Nontuberculous mycobacteria in adult patients with cystic fibrosis. *Chest* 1992;**102**:70–5.
15. Barker AF. Bronchiectasis. *N Engl J Med* 2002;**346**:1383–93.
16. Tortoli E. Impact of genotypic studies on mycobacterial taxonomy: the new mycobacteria of the 1990s. *Clin Microbiol Rev* 2003;**2**:319–54.
17. Grange JM, Yates MD. Infections caused by opportunistic mycobacteria: a review. *J R Soc Med* 1986;**79**:226–9.
18. Research Committee of the British Thoracic Society. First randomised trial of treatments for pulmonary disease caused by *M avium intracellulare, M malmoense* and *M xenopi* in HIV negative patients: rifampicin, ethambutol and isoniazid versus rifampicin and ethambutol. *Thorax* 2001;**56**:167–72.
19. Banks J, Jenkins PA, Smith AP. Pulmonary infection with *Mycobacterium malmoense*: a review of treatment and response. *Tubercle* 1985;**66**:197–203.
20. Banks J, Hunter AM, Campbell IA *et al*. Pulmonary infection with *Mycobacterium xenopi*: review of treatment and response. *Thorax* 1984;**39**:376–82.
21. Heifets LB. Synergistic effect of rifampicin, streptomycin, ethionamide and ethambutol on *Mycobacterium intracellulare. Am Rev Respir Dis* 1982;**125**:43–8.
22. Banks J, Jenkins PA. Combined versus single antituberculosis drugs on the in vitro sensitivity patterns of nontuberculous mycobacteria. *Thorax* 1987;**42**:838–42.
23. Hoffner SE, Svenson SB, Kallenius G. Synergistic effects of anti-mycobacterial drug combinations on *Mycobacterium avium* complex determined radiometrically in liquid medium. *Eur J Clin Microbiol* 1987;**6**:530–5.
24. Jenkins PA, Campbell IA, Banks J, Gelder CM, Prescott RJ, Smith AP. Clarithromycin vs ciprofloxacin as adjuncts to rifampicin and ethambutol in treating opportunistic mycobacterial lung diseases and an assessment of *Mycobacterium vaccae* immunotherapy. *Thorax* 2008;**63**:844.
25. Pomerantz M, Madsen L, Goble M *et al*. Surgical management of resistant *Mycobacterium tuberculosis* and other mycobacterial pulmonary infections. *Ann Thorac Surg* 1991;**52**:1108–12.

26. Shiriaishi Y, Nakajima Y, Takasuna K *et al.* Surgery for *Mycobacterium avium* complex lung disease in the clarithromycin era. *Eur J Cardiothorac Surg* 2002;**21**:314–18.
27. Van Ingen J, Verhagen AF, Dekhuijzen PN *et al.* Surgical treatment of non-tuberculous mycobacterial lung disease: strike in time. *Int J Tuberc Lung Dis* 2010;**14**:99–105.
28. Mitchell JD, Bishop A, Cafaro A, Weyait MJ, Pomerantz M. Anatomic lung resection for non-tuberculous mycobacterial disease. *Ann Thorac surg* 2008;**85**:1887–92.
29. Strolin Benedetti M. Inducing properties of rifabutin, and effects on the pharmacokinetics and metabolism of concomitant drugs. *Pharmacol Res* 1995;**32**:177–87.
30. Kunst H, Wickremasinghe M, Wells A, Wilson R. Nontuberculous mycobacterial disease and *Aspergillus*-related lung disease in bronchiectasis. *Eur Respir J* 2006;**28**:352–7.
31. Modilevsky T, Sattler FR, Barnes PF. Mycobacterial disease in patients with human immunodeficiency virus infection. *Arch Intern Med* 1989;**149**;2001–5.
32. Horsburgh CR Jr, Selick RM. The epidemiology of disseminated non-tuberculous mycobacterial infection in the acquired immunodeficiency syndrome (AIDS). *Am Rev Respir Dis* 1989;**139**:4–7.
33. Kemper CA, Havlir D, Bartock AE *et al.* Transient bacteraemia due to *Mycobacterium avium* complex in patients with AIDS. *J Infect Dis* 1994;**170**:488–93.

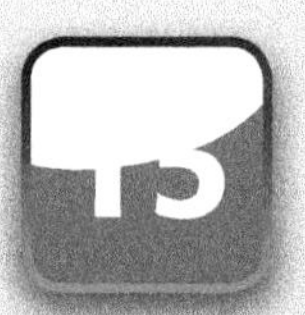

Oxygen: risks as well as benefits

Rory Mc Dermott

Expert commentary Craig Davidson

Case history

A 77-year-old ex-smoker presented to his GP with a 2-week history of increasing shortness of breath, a cough productive of purulent sputum, and wheeze. He had a long-standing diagnosis of COPD, and, despite having commenced his rescue pack of steroids and antibiotics, he was now breathless on minimal exertion. He had used his salbutamol nebulizer with increasing frequency over the past 24 hours and was breathless following the short walk into the surgery. His oxygen saturation was 81%, and respiratory rate 26 breaths/minute. The GP arranged for urgent transfer to hospital by ambulance, and, in transit, the paramedics administered oxygen-driven salbutamol nebulizers, followed by oxygen via a non-rebreathe reservoir mask at a flow rate of 10 L/minute. On arrival at the hospital, his respiratory rate was 18 breaths/minute; he appeared sleepy; oxygen saturations were 99%, and he had a temperature of 38.5°C.

Clinical tip Pulse oximetry

- Central cyanosis is an unreliable sign, as its perception varies between observers, and detection is affected by the presence of anaemia or polycythaemia. It is generally detected by most observers when the amount of deoxygenated haemoglobin is above 5 g/L. This corresponds to an oxygen saturation of 67% [1].
- Oximetry relies upon the detection of different relative absorptions of light by oxyhaemoglobin and deoxyhaemoglobin (spectrophotometry).
- The accuracy of oximetry is limited and reduced below 80% saturation. Inaccurate readings may also be caused by poor peripheral perfusion (low cardiac output or intense vasoconstriction) and probe movement.
- Pulse oximetry is unreliable in carbon monoxide poisoning and in the presence of significant methaemoglobinaemia. Carboxyhaemoglobin and methaemoglobin absorb light at the same wavelength as oxyhaemoglobin (660 nm), so that clinically significant hypoxia may exist despite an apparently 'normal' oxygen saturation.

A CXR revealed clear, hyperexpanded lung fields, with a marginally enlarged cardiothoracic ratio. The ECG demonstrated a sinus tachycardia at 105 beats/minute, with a right heart strain pattern. Blood tests were consistent with an infective process (Table 15.1), with a raised CRP and WCC. Antibiotics, nebulized bronchodilators, IV fluids, and oral steroids were started.

An ABG was performed (Table 15.2), and, in view of the results demonstrating a raised $PaCO_2$ with a high PaO_2, the non-rebreathe mask was removed, and he was placed on nasal cannulae at an oxygen flow rate of 2 L/minute. The oxygen saturation stabilized at 92%.

Table 15.1 **Admission blood test results**

Bloods	Value (normal range)
Haemoglobin	12.8 g/dL (12–16)
WCC	16.3×10^9/L (4–11)
Neutrophils	12.3×10^9/L
Platelets	263×10^9/L (135–420)
Sodium	137 mmol/L (135–145)
Potassium	4.6 mmol/L (3.5–5)
Urea	6.9 mmol/L (1.7–8.3)
Creatinine	107 micromoles/L (42–102)
CRP	97 mg/L (0–6)

Table 15.2 **Arterial blood gas results**

ABG	Admission (10 L/ minute oxygen via non-rebreathe mask)	Repeat ABG in ED (2 L/minute oxygen via nasal cannulae)	Following morning (3 L/minute oxygen via nasal cannulae)	Outpatient clinic (room air)
pH	7.30	7.36	7.32	7.39
$PaCO_2$ (kPa)	9.9	8.0	8.7	6.0
PaO_2 (kPa)	29.3	10.4	11.1	8.4
Lactate (mmol/L)	1.3	1.2	1.2	0.9
Base excess (mmol/L)	7	7	6.8	3
HCO_3^- (mmol/L)	31	31.5	32	27

Learning point Arterial-alveolar oxygen gradient

The A-a gradient, or **(ideal) alveolar-arterial oxygen difference**, is a sensitive measure of ventilation-perfusion (V/Q) mismatch [2], comparing the measured arterial PO_2 (PaO_2) against a calculated 'ideal' value—'the value the lung would have if there was no V/Q mismatching and the respiratory exchange ratio (R) remained the same' [3]. It allows identification of gas exchange deficits in what may otherwise appear to be normal ABG samples, especially when breathing a high known FiO_2. V/Q mismatch accounts for hypoxia in the majority of patients.

The 'ideal' alveolar PO_2 (PAO_2) is calculated using the simplified alveolar gas equation:

$$PAO_2 = FiO_2 - PACO_2/R$$

where R is the respiratory exchange ratio, usually 0.8. $PACO_2$ and $PaCO_2$ are practically interchangeable, as the amount of CO_2 in the alveoli is almost the same as in blood. Calculating the FiO_2 is straightforward, as the normal atmospheric pressure is 101 kPa; therefore, 21% oxygen translates to an FiO_2 of 21 kPa approximately. Similarly, breathing 35% O_2 gives an FiO_2 of 35 kPa. It is, however, difficult to know the exact FiO_2, unless using a fixed percentage of inspired oxygen mask.

For a normal young adult with a PaO_2 of 13 kPa, a $PaCO_2$ of 5 kPa on breathing air, the A-a gradient is:

$$PAO_2 - PaO_2 = [FiO_2 - (PaCO_2/0.8)] - PaO_2$$

$$= [21 - (5/0.8)] - 13$$

$$= 2 \text{ kPa}$$

An A-a gradient of 2 kPa represents the V/Q mismatch that normally occurs in the lung due to regional variation in ventilation and perfusion in the upright position. The V/Q mismatch increases with age, and the normal A-a difference in older persons can be up to 4 kPa.

A gradual decline in exercise tolerance was noted over the past few years, to the extent he now struggled with activities of daily living. He had recently been prescribed nebulized high-dose bronchodilators. He required antibiotics and steroids on a number of occasions over the previous 12 months.

On examination, he showed evidence of respiratory distress with hyperinflation; chest expansion was reduced, and auscultation revealed generally poor air entry, with widespread expiratory wheeze. There was pitting oedema of the ankles, and his JVP was elevated. He had a notable CO_2 flap and a bounding pulse.

The working diagnosis was that of acute hypercapnic respiratory failure (AHRF) due to an acute exacerbation of COPD itself precipitated by infection. The patient was transferred to the medical ward without an initial care plan in place. The repeat ABG performed in the ED showed an improvement in the acid–base balance, but persisting hypercapnia (Table 15.2). Crucially, although the medical clerking outlined that the patient was in AHRF, the oxygen prescription was not filled in on the drug chart.

Expert comment

This case highlights the real danger of 'reflex' administration of high-concentration oxygen in acute care, including in transport to hospital. Before applying high-concentration oxygen, all health-care staff need to ask themselves whether the patient in front of them could be at risk of hypercapnic respiratory failure (and not just if they might have COPD). The presence of AHRF increases the mortality of an acute exacerbation of COPD to at least 20% and carries a high risk of recurrence and a median survival of 1 year. Failure to recognize AHRF results in the making of inadequate care plans, increasing the risk to the patient even further.

The following morning, the patient was receiving nasal oxygen at 3 L/minute, and pulse oximetry showed an oxygen saturation of 95%. The nursing documentation was unclear as to when the oxygen flow rate had been increased or why. The absence of an oxygen prescription was highlighted by the pharmacist. A further ABG was performed. This showed an increase in the $PaCO_2$ and a persisting respiratory acidosis. The oxygen flow rate was reduced to 2 L/minute, and an oxygen prescription completed, indicating a target of 88–92%. The HDU team was alerted to the potential need for respiratory support. The oxygen saturation was 91% on this flow rate, and a repeat ABG on the lower flow rate showed resolution of the respiratory acidosis.

Clinical tip

It is recommended that patients who are at risk of hypercapnia have an ABG immediately on arrival in the ED in order to guide their management.

The patient made a rapid recovery and was discharged on the third day by the respiratory service, with a COPD bundle and an oxygen alert card and an outpatient follow-up appointment.

Expert comment

It is fortunate that harm was not caused through poor management in this case. There were clear indications for considering NIV on admission, and the lack of an oxygen prescription and the need for medical review and additional ABGs to be performed overnight are serious omissions. I would have expected the consultant leading the ward round to have used the opportunity for educating the team on these matters and ensuring completion of an adverse event report.

Expert comment

Up to 30% of patients with accelerated discharge following an acute exacerbation of COPD subsequently deteriorate and require readmission. There is increasing evidence to justify domiciliary visiting and/or regular phone contact during this risk period. Referral to a pulmonary rehabilitation service and/or involvement of the community team is also important. Although smoking cessation was not relevant in this case (he had not smoked for 10 years), this is a vital aspect of care and even

(Continued)

Clinical tip

Assessment for LTOT should be done during a period of clinical stability. Occasionally, oxygen is prescribed to facilitate discharge from hospital, but an early review is required to assess if oxygen is still required.

Clinical tip

If he had met the criteria for LTOT with a PaO_2 of <8 kPa (in light of the PH revealed by echocardiography at his follow-up appointment), he would need a further ABG to ensure the $PaCO_2$ did not rise significantly.

more important if home oxygen is being considered. Another aspect raised by this case is the need to initiate conversations about advance care planning. Even though NIV was not employed on this occasion, it is highly likely to be needed in the future.

One result of the raised awareness of the dangers of uncontrolled oxygen therapy has been a change in the training and advice given to ambulance crews who are now encouraged to risk-assess and to use targeted oxygen saturations and ideally mains-powered nebulizers, instead of being oxygen-driven. There is some preliminary evidence to suggest this has reduced the incidence of oxygen-induced AHRF. In a survey carried out in London, the receiving area in hospital is now the more likely place for inappropriate oxygen use. Although oxygen alert cards have been recommended, a universal precaution to target 88–92% is now regarded as a better approach to risk avoidance, partly as cards are often not understood or not carried by patients at times of crisis, but also because non-COPD patients who are nevertheless at risk, e.g. chronic asthma, cystic fibrosis, kyphoscoliosis, and neuromuscular disease involving the respiratory muscles, will not be so identified.

On review in clinic, the patient had made a good recovery from his infection but remained short of breath in activities of daily living. PFTs showed a severe obstructive deficit, with an FEV_1/FVC of <55%. His FEV_1 was 35% predicted and transfer factor 40%. An echocardiogram revealed moderate PH.

Pulse oximetry revealed an oxygen saturation of 92%, and an ABG was performed to assess the partial pressure of oxygen (Table 15.3). LTOT was not indicated, as the measured PaO_2 was >8 kPa (Table 15.3) [4, 5]. The oxygen saturation fell to a nadir of 89% during a walking test, and he found no appreciable symptomatic benefit when exercising with oxygen.

He subsequently attended a pulmonary rehabilitation course, resulting in an increased tolerance of higher levels of exercise.

Table 15.3 BTS and ATS guidelines

	BTS guidelines	ATS guidelines
LTOT indicated	PaO_2 ≤7.3 kPa*	PaO_2 ≤55 mmHg
LTOT indicated in presence of PH, peripheral oedema, or secondary polycythaemia (haematocrit >55%)	PaO_2 >7.3 but <8 kPa	PaO_2 56–59 mmHg

* Assessed breathing air during a period of clinical stability.
Adapted from British Thoracic Society and American Thoracic Society Guidelines [4, 5].

Discussion

Physiology

Oxygen in alveolar air diffuses down a concentration gradient across the enormous capillary bed of the lungs (surface area of up to 100 m^2). The transit time of blood in the alveolar capillary is around 0.75 s, and, under normal sea level conditions, full equilibration occurs by 0.25 s.

Oxygen is transported in the blood in two forms. The vast majority is transported to the tissues bound to red blood cells in the form of oxyhaemoglobin. A much smaller portion is dissolved in the blood, and its volume is directly proportional to the partial pressure of oxygen in the blood.

Learning point Oxygen dissociation curve

- The relationship between the partial pressure of oxygen in the blood and oxygen saturations is non-linear.
- The oxyhaemoglobin dissociation curve shows a steep drop in saturation below an oxygen tension of 8 kPa.
- Above this level, binding of oxygen to haemoglobin is avid, which facilitates effective transport of oxygen to the tissues. Quite large changes in the PaO_2 result in small changes in saturation.
- At lower PaO_2 values, as exist in vital organs and other tissues, the affinity for oxygen falls, and this aids 'offloading' of oxygen.
- The oxygen dissociation curve is shifted to the right by a variety of metabolic factors, including a fall in pH, high temperature, and raised CO_2 levels (the Bohr effect). These favour a greater delivery of oxygen to oxygen-starved tissues at times of physiological stress (Figure 15.1).

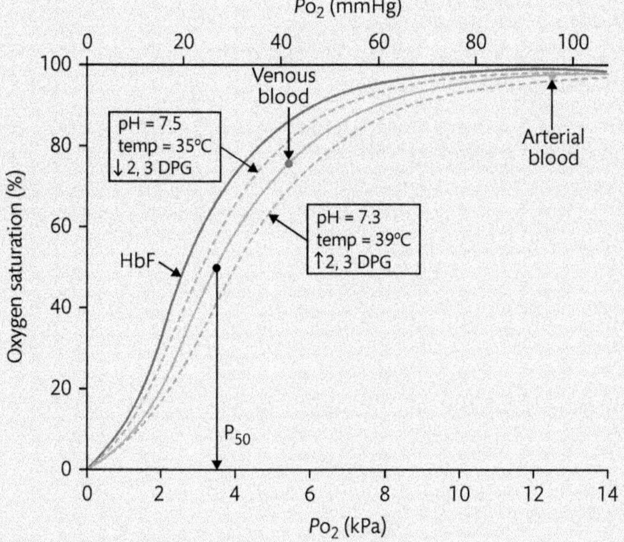

Figure 15.1 Oxygen dissociation curve.

Source: Thomas, C and Lumb, A, Physiology of Haemoglobin, Contin Educ Anaesth Crit Care Pain (2012) 12 (5): 251-256.

The oxygen content of arterial blood (CaO_2) and delivery to tissues (DO_2) are closely controlled. As in the above case, when the PaO_2 falls, a number of compensatory mechanisms engage to ensure adequate tissue oxygenation. Carotid body chemoreception stimulates an increase in alveolar ventilation and cardiac output. The presence of acidosis and fever also leads to a shift in the dissociation curve, favouring oxygen unloading. In acute or chronic lung disease, local hypoxic conditions arising from, for instance, pneumonia or bronchial obstruction result in pulmonary arterial vasoconstriction that shunts blood to alveolar units where gas exchange is better [6]. If hypoxaemia is sustained, erythropoietin stimulates an increase in haemoglobin production. An increase in capillary density is a further compensatory mechanism. This long-term adaptation is best seen in dwellers at high altitude.

Normal resting oxygen saturations may vary between individuals, based on a number of factors: age, health status (e.g. chronic lung pathology, congenital cardiac disease), ethnicity, and acclimatization to altitude. The brain is vulnerable to hypoxic damage, particularly when exposed to sudden drops in oxygen tension. However, the precise degree of hypoxaemia that causes neuronal damage is not well established, as anaemia and/or a reduced cardiac output will also contribute to tissue anoxia. It is generally accepted that an arterial saturation above 88% is unlikely to result in tissue injury in the absence of shock. Hypoxaemia commonly refers to a PaO_2 of <8 kPa (60 mmHg) [7], and a number of observational studies have recognized poorer outcomes for intensive care patients if exposed to blood oxygen levels below this [8–11].

Correcting hypoxaemia is a vital basic component of the management of all critically ill patients. Accepted guidelines advocate the administration of high-flow oxygen, using a flow rate of 10–15 L/minute and a reservoir bag attached to a non-rebreathe mask [12, 13]. This includes cases of cardiac arrest and resuscitation in cardiogenic shock, severe sepsis, major trauma, and anaphylaxis. Oxygen delivery to tissues needs to be optimized to meet the increased tissue oxygen demands, and, to do so, careful attention must be paid to a number of factors, including circulating volume and haemoglobin.

Learning point Optimizing oxygen delivery (DO_2)

DO_2 is a true assessment of tissue hypoxia but is difficult to measure. The worked example below demonstrates how appropriate fluid management in a critically ill, hypoxic patient significantly contributes to oxygen delivery to the tissues.

The delivery of oxygen to tissues is regulated by the quantity of haemoglobin (Hb), the level to which it is oxygen-saturated (SaO_2), and the cardiac output.

Each g/dL of haemoglobin carries 1.34 mL of oxygen when fully saturated (i.e. SaO_2 = 100%).

Therefore, let us imagine our patient above presenting in a critically unwell state with anaemia (Hb 10 g/dL), SaO_2 of 92%, and hypovolaemia (cardiac output 4 L/minute or 40 dL/minute) which will deliver 368 × 1.34 mL of oxygen to the tissues, i.e. 493 mL of O_2/minute.

$$(10 \times 0.92 \times 40 = 368)$$

Increasing the oxygen saturations to 98% allows delivery of 392 × 1.34 mL of oxygen, i.e. 525 mL of O_2/minute.

$$(10 \times 0.98 \times 40 = 392)$$

However, if the cardiac output were to increase to 5 L/minute (50 dL/minute), there is a bigger increase in the delivery of oxygen to the tissues (460 × 1.34 mL of oxygen, i.e. 616 mL of O_2/minute).

$$(10 \times 0.92 \times 50 = 460)$$

Clearly, you can see how our patient, if critically unwell, would be best served with high-flow oxygen **and** fluid resuscitation in order to maximize tissue delivery of oxygen.

Expert comment

The risk that excessive oxygen may precipitate hypercapnic respiratory failure is not confined to advanced COPD. As previously noted, at-risk patients include those with obesity hypoventilation syndrome, cystic fibrosis, neuromuscular conditions, and chest wall deformity. Recent studies suggest that this risk may also apply to patients with acute asthma and CAP [18, 19].

Oxygen has the potential to cause harm, and it should not be viewed as an innocuous therapy. The ability to precipitate or worsen hypercapnic respiratory failure is a well-documented complication of hyperoxaemia [14] and is demonstrated in the case above. Indeed, excessive oxygen therapy has been shown to directly affect the clinical outcomes of COPD patients in hospital, leading to an increased need for ventilatory support and increased mortality [15, 16]. Austin *et al.* reported an RCT which demonstrated a 2- to 4-fold increase in mortality in COPD exacerbations treated with high-flow oxygen, compared with titrated oxygen therapy (target saturation of 88–92%) [17].

The primary mechanism responsible for the adverse effect of high-concentration oxygen is worsening of V/Q mismatch. Hypoxic pulmonary vasoconstriction is inhibited, and poorly ventilated alveoli will remain overperfused [20]. The Haldane effect (decreased CO_2 buffering by oxyhaemoglobin), absorption atelectasis, and a reduction of respiratory drive may contribute to the risk of hypercapnic respiratory failure.

Expert comment

Given the ubiquity of oxygen use in hospitals and ambulances and the clear evidence of the potential harm of uncontrolled oxygen use, the BTS issued a guideline for emergency oxygen use in adult patients [21]. This was subsequently endorsed by the National Patient Safety Authority in a report detailing a number of serious clinical incidents involving inappropriate oxygen therapy [22]. The BTS has also promoted the importance of 'hospital oxygen champions' to locally drive the importance of oxygen prescription and its safe use and to reduce waste. Many hospitalized patients receive oxygen routinely, and much of this use is without benefit, is wasteful, and promotes the misbelief that oxygen treatment is without harm.

The guideline for emergency oxygen use makes the case that oxygen should be used as a treatment for hypoxaemia, and not breathlessness. Whilst most patients should be given oxygen therapy to maintain saturations between 94% and 98%, it recommends a target saturation of 88–92% in those at risk of hypercapnic respiratory failure, including ALL patients with COPD (as this risk is difficult to quantify). This can be delivered either by controlled oxygen delivery devices, e.g. Venturi masks, or low-flow nasal cannulae. (The latter, though 'uncontrolled', have the attraction of being better accepted by patients.)

Oxygen should be prescribed on the drug chart. The prescribing of fixed doses of oxygen is discouraged. Instead, the prescription should reflect the appropriate oxygen target saturation, along with advice on the initial oxygen delivery device. An important caveat exists. In a clinical emergency, it is essential that oxygen is not withheld, pending a prescription. Unfortunately, clinical practice has been slow to follow the guidelines. The 2013 BTS emergency oxygen audit highlighted that, of the 6214 patients receiving oxygen therapy, only 55% had any sort of oxygen prescription [23].

Oxygen therapy needs to be monitored. Oxygen saturations should be regularly checked, and nursing staff empowered to adjust the oxygen flow rate or change to a different delivery device, as necessary, to achieve saturations within the targeted range. BTS audits have shown that the oxygen saturation is only recorded by nursing staff on 20% of occasions. Furthermore, 23% of documented oxygen saturations were above the prescribed target saturation. Whilst these compliance figures are disappointing, it is encouraging to note that prescribing practice has improved, as only 10% of patients had a specified target range and 5% of drug rounds included an oxygen check in 2008.

Approximately one-third of all ambulance patients receive supplementary oxygen. There is strong evidence to favour the use of controlled oxygen in the pre-hospital setting for patients with a known or presumed diagnosis of COPD. The Joint Royal Colleges Ambulance Liaison Committee (JRCALC) in the UK has recognized this risk and published guidelines in accordance with the BTS [24].

An established diagnosis of COPD may not have been made or be available or known by the patient. The BTS has therefore suggested that anyone over 50 years of age with a smoking history and/or a history of long-standing breathlessness should be assumed to have COPD, and a lower oxygen saturation of 88–92% targeted. Supplying oxygen alert cards to patients known to be at risk of CO_2 retention (including patients with a history of type 2 respiratory failure requiring NIV) may further help to prevent excessive oxygenation during ambulance transfer, and there have been some encouraging reviews of their success in practice [25].

Expert comment

The expert believes universal precautions are a more sure way of avoiding oxygen-induced patient harm (see main text). Insisting on the prescribing of oxygen on hospital prescription charts is, with paper records, problematic, despite the importance that would accrue from doing so. The best examples lead staff to choose the most appropriate mask or flow rate and to guide oxygen removal when no longer required, but they are cumbersome, and frequent changes result in frequent chart changes, unsurprisingly unpopular with all staff. Electronic charting may be the answer.

The creation of oxygen champions may help spread the educational message, but senior medical and management support is needed to change practice. All oxygen harm incidents should be reported, as the risk management process can be a powerful lever in driving change. It is notable that committed respiratory physicians can make an enormous difference to individual hospital practice.

Learning point Oxygen delivery systems

Delivery systems for oxygen should be matched to patient need. A completed oxygen prescription will state the appropriate initial delivery device for each patient.

1. Nasal cannulae are a comfortable option recommended for most patients. They are better tolerated than masks and allow patients to eat and converse conveniently. The FiO_2 depends on the minute volume (MV), the flow rate, and the amount of oxygen entrainment (less when mouth-breathing). It should be used at a flow rate of 1–2 L/minute. Above this flow rate, oxygen enrichment is less predictable, and the risk of higher concentration increases, should the MV fall, e.g. during sleep, or should CO_2 narcosis develop.
2. The so-called 'simple' face masks used with a flow rate of 5–10 L/minute can deliver an FiO_2 of 0.35–0.5. Rebreathing may occur below 5 L/minute, as the CO_2 is inadequately 'washed out' of the mask. They are **only** suitable for patients with type 1 respiratory failure, as the inspired oxygen concentration is unreliable, and there is a real risk of precipitating hypercapnic respiratory failure. Many hospitals have abandoned the use of these masks.
3. Venturi (or fixed-performance) masks are used to deliver a controlled oxygen concentration. They are specifically aimed at patients with type 2 respiratory failure. A jet of oxygen entrains a predictable stream of air through the base of the Venturi valve (the Bernoulli effect). Accurate oxygen concentrations can be delivered, independent of the ventilatory minute volume and flow rate (although a minimum flow rate is required). Rebreathing is not a problem.
4. Non-rebreathe reservoir masks at a flow rate of 10–15 L/minute can provide an FiO_2 above 60% and should be used in the management of patients in shock.

Oxygen has traditionally been used in the management of acute coronary syndromes and is endorsed in both Advanced Care Life Support and European Society of Cardiology guidelines [12, 26] The evidence base was small studies performed in the 1930s [27].

We now know that hyperoxaemia causes a significant reduction in coronary blood flow [28] and may decrease the cardiac output and increase the systemic vascular resistance in patients with acute myocardial infarction and congestive cardiac failure [29]. Rawles *et al.* first reported the potential harm from hyperoxaemia in acute myocardial infarction [30], but subsequent trials have been inconsistent. A Cochrane review highlighted the need for more trial evidence [31].

Similar uncertainty surrounds the role of oxygen in acute stroke. Hypoxia in the first few hours after a stroke is associated with an increased risk of death [32]. The routine use of oxygen is, however, controversial following the publication of a quasi-randomized study by Ronning *et al.* [33]. This study showed a 1-year mortality of

18% in mild to moderate strokes given oxygen and 9% in the group given air (odds ratio 0.45, 95% CI 0.23–0.90; p = 0.023). Conversely, in the case of severe strokes, the oxygen group showed a tendency towards an improved 1-year survival. It is postulated that the presence of reactive oxygen species may cause reperfusion injury in the ischaemic brain. The BTS guidelines, which were approved by the cardiac and neurology colleges, recommend that oxygen should be administered only to hypoxic patients with a target saturation of 94–98% (or lower if there is a risk of hypercapnic respiratory failure).

Further questioning of oxygen therapy in the ICU has been raised in recent years. Hyperoxaemia in mechanically ventilated patients has been reported as an independent risk factor for in-hospital mortality [9]. In this study, a U-shaped mortality risk was seen, suggesting significant harm associated with both hypoxia and hyperoxaemia. Further large retrospective observational studies have suggested that hyperoxaemia may be associated with adverse outcomes in patients admitted to the ICU after resuscitation from cardiac arrest [8]. This may again be caused by hyperoxia increasing reperfusion injury.

Long-term oxygen therapy

Chronic hypoxia may lead to PH, often revealed by episodes of right heart failure during acute illness. LTOT was shown in both the Nocturnal Oxygen Therapy Trial (NOTT) [34] and the Medical Research Council (MRC) trial [35] to improve mortality and quality of life in COPD patients with resting hypoxia. These trials did not control for smoking or its cessation that might be expected to have been greater in those treated by LTOT.

Evidence base Report of the Medical Research Council Working Party: long-term domiciliary oxygen therapy in chronic hypoxic cor pulmonale complicating chronic bronchitis and emphysema

- Conducted in 1981 across three centres in the UK [35].
- Patients with hypoxia (mean PaO_2 of 6.8 kPa) and severe COPD randomized to oxygen 15 hours/day versus no oxygen.
- Mean age of 57 years, with severe airflow obstruction (average FEV_1 of 0.7 approximately), hypercapnia (average $PaCO_2$ of 7.3 kPa), and a mean pulmonary artery pressure of 34 mmHg.
- Well-matched groups followed for 5 years.
- A total of 19 of the 42 oxygen-treated patients died versus 30 of the 45 control patients.
- Difference was most marked in the small group of females (RR death 6.1 in favour of oxygen).
- Secondary end point of oxygen therapy seemed to stabilize the pulmonary artery pressure, as the control group continued to rise at 2.7 mmHg per year.

Evidence base Nocturnal Oxygen Therapy Trial (NOTT)

- Performed in North America and Canada [34] at around the same time as the MRC trial.
- A total of 203 patients enrolled.
- Randomized to use of continuous oxygen therapy (mean of 17.7 hours/day) versus overnight oxygen (12 hours).
- Similar patient profile to that of MRC, followed for 19.3 months.
- Annual mortality was 21% in the overnight oxygen group and 11% in the continuous oxygen group.
- Slight decrease in pulmonary artery pressure in the continuous oxygen group at 6 months.

Statistics from the UK Department of Health and the RCP in 2011 indicated that 85,000 people were prescribed home oxygen at a cost of £110 million. The report claimed that in up to 43% of the cases, oxygen either was not used as prescribed or was of no clinical benefit [36]. LTOT is primarily prescribed in order to prolong life, and current recommendations advise a minimum of 15 hours/day (and up to 24 hours/day) at a rate that will increase the resting saturations above 90% [37].

LTOT may improve the patient's pulmonary haemodynamics and quality of life (largely due to effects on cognition and sleep). Assessment for LTOT should take place during a period of clinical stability [38]. Those patients prone to hypercapnia with oxygen may need to be considered for NIV, in combination with LTOT, especially when sleep is disordered or there are frequent admissions with AHRF.

Unfortunately, over 50% of LTOT patients in the UK continue to smoke. That this is a failure of message delivery is evidenced by the figure only being 15% in Canada. All smokers receiving LTOT should be counselled that the clinical benefit of LTOT is likely to be limited by raised carboxyhaemoglobin levels due to continued cigarette smoke exposure. Smoking cessation should always be encouraged. Individual risk assessment are required in all patients with domiciliary oxygen who continue to smoke, as two in three domestic fires in homes with LTOT occur as a result of smoking.

A final word from the expert

Oxygen therapy is an essential element of resuscitation of the critically ill patient, but all health-care staff need to appreciate that it can also be harmful and that indiscriminate use will cause patient loss of life and is also hugely wasteful. Safe prescribing and administration of oxygen has the potential to improve patient outcome and should be prioritized in all clinical settings, including pre-hospital care. Educating health-care staff and employing universal precautions offers the best way of changing practice, but clinical champions are needed to drive change.

The evidence base for LTOT is old and unreliable, but unlikely to be repeated. Of much greater importance than prescribing an uncertain treatment, that many patients fail to use properly, are measures to support patients to take more exercise and to reduce or stop smoking. Clinicians need to better recognize when hypercapnic respiratory failure is a risk and put in place arrangements to better manage AHRF when it occurs.

References

1. Grace RF. Pulse oximetry. Gold standard or false sense of security? *Med J Aust* 1994;**160**:638–44.
2. Mellemgaard K. The alveolar-arterial oxygen difference. Size and components in normal man. *Acta Physiol Scand* 1966;**67**:10–20.
3. West JB (2013). *Pulmonary Pathophysiology: The Essentials*, eighth edition. Baltimore: Lippincott, Williams & Wilkins.
4. Qaseem A, Snow V, Shekelle P *et al.* Clinical Efficacy Assessment Subcommittee of the American College of Physicians. Diagnosis and management of stable chronic obstructive pulmonary disease: a clinical practice guideline from the American College of Physicians. *Ann Intern Med* 2007;**147**:633–8.

5. Hardinge M, Annandale J, Bourne S *et al.* British Thoracic Society Guidelines for home oxygen use in adults. *Thorax* 2015;**70**:i1–43.
6. von Euler US, Liljestrand G. Observations on the pulmonary arterial blood pressure in the cat. *Acta Physiol Scand* 1946;**12**:301–20.
7. Slutsky AS. Consensus conference on mechanical ventilation. Part I. European Society of Intensive Care Medicine, the ACCP and the SCCM. *Intensive Care Med* 1994;**20**:64–79.
8. Bellomo R, Bailey M, Eastwood GM *et al.* Arterial hyperoxia and in-hospital mortality after resuscitation from cardiac arrest. *Crit Care* 2011;**15**:R90.
9. Eastwood G, Bellomo R, Bailey M *et al.* Arterial oxygen tension and mortality in mechanically ventilated patients. *Intensive Care Med* 2012;**38**:91–8.
10. Kilgannon JH, Jones AE, Shapiro NI *et al.* Association between arterial hyperoxia following resuscitation from cardiac arrest and in-hospital mortality. *JAMA* 2010;**303**:2165–71.
11. De Jonge E, Peelen L, Keijzers PJ *et al.* Association between administered oxygen, arterial partial oxygen pressure and mortality in mechanically ventilated intensive care unit patients. *Crit Care* 2008;**12**:R156.
12. Resuscitation Council UK (2015). *Adult advanced life support.* Available at: <https://www.resus.org.uk/resuscitation-guidelines/adult-advanced-life-support/>.
13. Dellinger RP, Carlet JM, Masur H *et al.* Surviving Sepsis Campaign Management Guidelines Committee. Surviving Sepsis Campaign guidelines for management of severe sepsis and septic shock. *Crit Care Med* 2004;**32**:858–73.
14. Murphy R, Driscoll P, O'Driscoll R. Emergency oxygen therapy for the COPD patient. *Emerg Med J* 2001;**18**:333–9.
15. Roberts CM, Stone RA, Buckingham RJ, Pursey NA, Lowe D; National Chronic Obstructive Pulmonary Disease Resources and Outcomes Project implementation group. Acidosis, non-invasive ventilation and mortality in hospitalised COPD exacerbations. *Thorax* 2011;**66**:43–8.
16. Plant PK, Owen JL, Elliott MW. One year period prevalence study of respiratory acidosis in acute exacerbations of COPD: implications for the provision of non-invasive ventilation and oxygen administration. *Thorax* 2000;**55**:550–4.
17. Austin MA, Wills KE, Blizzard L, Walters EH, Wood-Baker R. Effect of high flow oxygen on mortality in chronic obstructive pulmonary disease patients in prehospital setting: randomised controlled trial. *BMJ* 2010;**341**:c5462.
18. Perrin K, Wijesinghe M, Healy B *et al.* Randomised controlled trial of high concentration versus titrated oxygen therapy in severe exacerbations of asthma. *Thorax* 2011;**66**:937–41.
19. Wijesinghe M, Perrin K, Healy B, Weatherall M, Beasley R. Randomized controlled trial of high concentration oxygen in suspected community-acquired pneumonia. *J R Soc Med* 2012;**105**:208–16.
20. Wagner PD, Laravuso RB, Uhl RR *et al.* Continuous distributions of ventilation-perfusion ratios in normal subjects breathing air and 100 per cent oxygen. *J Clin Invest* 1974;**54**:54–68.
21. O'Driscoll BR, Howard LS, Davison AG. BTS guideline for emergency oxygen use in adult patients. *Thorax* 2008;**63**(Suppl 6):vi1–68.
22. National Patient Safety Agency (2009). *Oxygen safety in hospitals. Rapid Response Report.* Available at: <http://www.nrls.npsa.nhs.uk/resources/?entryid45%20=+62811&entryid45=62811&q=0%C2%ACOxygen+safety+in+hospitals%C2%AC>.
23. British Thoracic Society (2013). *Emergency oxygen audit 2013.* Available at: <https://www.brit-thoracic.org.uk/document-library/audit-and-quality-improvement/audit-reports/bts-emergency-oxygen-audit-report-2013/>.
24. Joint Royal Colleges Ambulance Liaison Committee (2016). *UK ambulance services clinical guideline S2016.* Bridgwater: Class Professional Publishing. Available at: <http://www.jrcalc.org.uk/guidelines/>.
25. Tooley C, Ellis D, Greggs D *et al.* Too much of a good thing? Oxygen alert cards are helpful for COPD patients at risk of oxygen toxicity. *Thorax* 2006;**61**(Suppl II):112.

26. Van de Werf F, Ardissino D, Betriu A *et al*; Task Force on the Management of Acute Myocardial Infarction of the European Society of Cardiology. Management of acute myocardial infarction in patients presenting with ST-segment elevation. *Eur Heart J* 2003;**24**:28–66.
27. Levy RL, Barach AL. The therapeutic use of oxygen in coronary thrombosis. *JAMA* 1930;**94**:1363–5.
28. Farquhar H, Weatherall M, Wijesinghe M *et al*. Systematic review of studies of the effect of hyperoxia on coronary blood flow. *Am Heart J* 2009;**158**:371e7.
29. Thomson AJ, Webb DJ, Maxwell SR *et al*. Oxygen therapy in acute medical care. *BMJ* 2002;**324**:1406–7.
30. Rawles JM, Kenmure AC. Controlled trial of oxygen in uncomplicated myocardial infarction. *BMJ* 1976;**1**:1121–3.
31. Cabello JB, Burls A, Emparanza JI, Bayliss S, Quinn T. Oxygen therapy for acute myocardial infarction. *Cochrane Database Syst Rev* 2010;**6**:CD007160.
32. Rowat AM, Dennis MS, Wardlaw JM. Hypoxaemia in acute stroke is frequent and worsens outcome. *Cerebrovasc Dis* 2006;**21**:166–72.
33. Ronning OM, Guldvog B. Should stroke victims routinely receive supplemental oxygen? A quasi-randomised control trial. *Stroke* 1999;**30**:2033–7.
34. [No authors listed]. Continuous or nocturnal oxygen therapy in hypoxemic chronic obstructive lung disease: a clinical trial. Nocturnal Oxygen Therapy Trial Group. *Ann Intern Med* 1980;**93**:391–8.
35. [No authors listed]. Long term domiciliary oxygen therapy in chronic hypoxic cor pulmonale complicating chronic bronchitis and emphysema. Report of the Medical Research Council Working Party. *Lancet* 1981;**1**:681–6.
36. Duncan P, Okosi O. Reviewing home oxygen services. *Nursing Times* 2011;**107**:24–5.
37. Hardinge M, Annandale J, Bourne S *et al*. British Thoracic Society Guidelines for home oxygen use in adults *Thorax* 2015;**70**:i1–43.
38. Guyatt GH, Nonoyama M, Lacchetti CH *et al*. A randomized trial of strategies for assessing eligibility for long-term domiciliary oxygen therapy. *Am J Respir Crit Care Med* 2005;**172**:573–80.

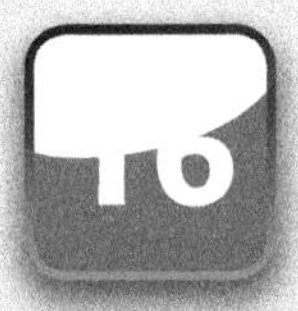

CASE 16

Water on the lung: a rare cause of a transudative effusion and new options for palliation

Lucy Schomberg

Expert commentary Nick Maskell

Case history

A 78-year-old Caucasian lady presented acutely with increased breathlessness and cough. Her past medical history included hypertension, hypercholesterolaemia, chronic kidney disease (baseline creatinine of 150 micromoles/mL (45–120 micromoles/mL)), and peripheral vascular disease. She was a smoker, having accrued a 60-pack year history, and she drank a bottle of brandy per week. Her medication history included amlodipine 10 mg od, atenolol 50 mg od, bumetanide 3 mg od, clopidogrel 75 mg od, doxazosin 4 mg od, mirtazapine 15 mg od, pravastatin 10 mg od, and ranitidine 150 mg bd.

On examination, she required 2 L of oxygen to maintain saturations of 95%; her blood pressure was 110/49; there was pedal oedema and reduced air entry in the right base. Her chest radiograph (Figure 16.1) demonstrated a right-sided pleural effusion.

She attended for pleural ultrasound, and a large hypoechogenic effusion was visualized on the right, with no pleural fluid on the left. A 12-French Seldinger chest drain was inserted on the right and attached to an underwater seal. The aspirated fluid had the appearance of water, compatible with a suspected transudative effusion. Over the course of the following days, 3 L of fluid was drained, with significant symptomatic improvement.

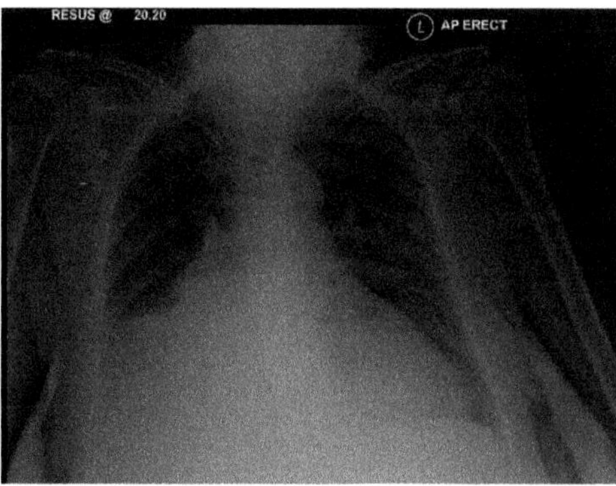

Figure 16.1 Initial chest radiograph demonstrating a new right-sided effusion.

Expert comment

A chest drain insertion is a very reasonable first step in her management. Some centres, including ours, may have opted for a diagnostic and therapeutic pleural aspiration initially. We would also ensure she had stopped her clopidogrel for at least 5 days, unless she was unable to wait due to the severity of her symptoms. This helps to minimize the risk of a bleeding complication.

Clinical tip The appearance of effusions on ultrasound

With increasing experience, it is possible to identify whether an effusion is exudative or transudative by appearances on ultrasound alone.

Exudative effusions often have an echogenic swirling pattern or septations due to the proteinaceous material. Transudative effusions often appear anechoic. However, if the transudative effusion is chronic, or repeated aspirations performed, the appearances can mimic those of an exudative effusion.

Learning point Emergence of thoracic ultrasound

In 2008, the National Patient Safety Agency issued a Rapid Response Report, highlighting the dangers of chest drain insertion, after 12 deaths and 15 cases of serious harm were reported from January 2005 to March 2008 [1]. This has led to new BTS guidelines being published in 2010 on pleural procedures and thoracic ultrasound which focus on the importance of the right person doing the right intervention at the right time, along with advocating ultrasound guidance for all pleural procedures for pleural fluid [2].

The Royal College of Radiologists have produced a second edition of the Ultrasound Training Recommendations for Medical and Surgical Specialties in 2012 which has altered the requirements for level 1 competency prior to independent practice. Along with the knowledge base of physics, anatomy, and pathology, each clinician needs to be supervised performing at least five scans per week for a minimum of 3 months [3].

Evidence base Safer thoracocentesis: an old lesson learnt anew

Grogan and colleagues performed a prospective randomized study in 1990 which demonstrated the increased safety of ultrasound-guided thoracocentesis [4]. Patients with a pleural effusion greater than half the hemidiaphragm, evident on chest radiography, and with no contraindications were randomized to three groups: (1) needle catheter, (2) needle without catheter, and (3) ultrasound-guided needle without catheter. The doctors underwent a didactic teaching session and were observed by the authors to ensure competence.

A total of 52 patients were randomized over 20 months. Twenty-six (50%) had a complication, either minor (patient discomfort or no fluid aspirated) or major (pneumothorax). Only three minor (16%) and no major complications occurred in group 3, whilst, in groups 1 and 2, there were seven (39%) and three (20%) major complications and 11 (61%) and three (20%) minor complications, respectively. Excluding mild to moderate pain, ultrasound-guided procedures had significantly fewer complications (0 of 19), compared to needle catheter (9 of 18; $p = 0.003$) and needle only (5 of 15; $p = 0.01$).

In our patient, the initial presumption was that this would represent a malignant effusion, but the pleural fluid characteristics listed in Table 16.1 demonstrated a transudative effusion by Light's criteria. The cytology was benign, and there was no microbiological evidence for infection. The challenge was to determine the cause of this patient's pleural effusion and the subsequent management.

Expert comment

It is always worth remembering that approximately 5% of malignant pleural effusions (MPEs) are transudates. Therefore, if the clinical history is very much in keeping with a malignant process, one should not be put off arranging a full set of investigations, just because the pleural fluid protein and LDH levels are at the transudate end of the spectrum.

In this case, I agree with the plan of trying to exclude the common causes of transudative pleural effusions—cardiac, hepatic, or renal. In our centre, echocardiograms are often difficult to obtain quickly and sometimes, due to poor views, contain only limited information. I find a serum N-terminal prohormone of brain natriuretic peptide (NT-proBNP) very useful, as the result is back the next day, and a normal level will exclude a cardiac cause for the effusion due to its very high negative predicted value.

Table 16.1 Pleural fluid

Pleural fluid protein	5 g/L
Pleural fluid glucose	4.6 mmol/L
Pleural fluid LDH	31 IU/L
Serum protein	52 g/L (60–80 g/L)
Serum glucose	5.9
Serum LDH	120 IU/L (140–280 IU/L)

Learning point Light's criteria

Establishing a cause for a pleural effusion can be very challenging, and determining whether an effusion is a transudate or an exudate is the first step. Light's criteria provide a clinically useful method, as if one or more of the criteria are met, the patient has an exudative effusion [5].

- pleural fluid protein/serum protein > 0.5;
- pleural fluid LDH/serum LDH >0.6;
- pleural fluid LDH > two-thirds the upper limit of normal for serum.

However, 15% of transudates are misclassified as exudates using Light's criteria (often only just meeting the criteria for an exudate). If the protein level is >40 g/L or the pleural fluid LDH is greater than the upper limit for serum LDH, the effusion is an exudate [6]. Another calculation which is useful in difficult-to-diagnose effusions is a difference between the serum albumin and pleural fluid albumin of >12 g/L [7]. Taken on its own, it misclassifies 13% of exudates as transudates, but, used in combination with Light's criteria, it can confirm a transudative effusion if there is doubt over the classification.

She underwent an echocardiogram which demonstrated a preserved left ventricle, and therefore the effusion was not felt to be caused by congestive cardiac failure. In light of her alcohol history, liver function testing and an ultrasound of the liver were arranged. The ultrasound demonstrated fatty change, and there was no ascites present. Her LFTs revealed a reduced albumin of 21 g/L (35–50 g/L) and an elevated cholesterol, suggesting the possibility of nephrotic syndrome. She had significant proteinuria on urine dipstick, and her protein:creatinine ratio was raised.

She was referred to the nephrologists who diagnosed nephrotic syndrome on the basis of hypoalbuminaemia, peripheral oedema, and proteinuria, although the cause of this was unclear, and diuresis was commenced. In light of her co-morbidities, a renal biopsy was not performed.

The patient had significant peripheral oedema, but the right leg was more tender than the left, and a thrombosis was suspected, as she was at high risk of thromboembolic disease. A deep vein thrombosis was visualized on Doppler ultrasound, and long-term anticoagulation was commenced, initially as IV heparin but subsequently as subcutaneous low-molecular-weight heparin.

Learning point Nephrotic syndrome

Diagnostic criteria [8]:

- proteinuria >3–3.5 g/24 hours or spot urine protein:creatinine ratio >300–350 mg/mmol;
- serum albumin <25 g/L;
- clinical evidence of peripheral oedema;
- severe hyperlipidaemia is often present.

(Continued)

Nephrotic syndrome can either be primary/idiopathic or secondary. The increased glomerular permeability leads to a loss of large molecules (mainly albumin) and the resulting proteinuria and peripheral oedema. Nephrotic syndrome can present with breathlessness due to several factors, including pleural effusions or thromboembolic disease.

There is an increased risk of venous and arterial thrombotic disease, most commonly manifesting as lower limb deep vein thrombosis. There are no RCTs regarding the screening for thromboembolic disease or when to anticoagulate. Anticoagulation brings its own challenges, as often IV heparin is required as a result of a reduced estimated glomerular filtration rate (eGFR), and procedures, such as a renal biopsy or, as in this case, a thoracocentesis, require meticulous planning.

The most important part of the management of nephrotic syndrome is determining the cause and treating this, if possible, and referral to the nephrologists is highly recommended. Along with this, a low-sodium diet, fluid restriction, and diuresis are often the mainstay of treatment, along with recognizing and treating complications such as thromboembolic disease and infection.

One possibility was membranous nephropathy due to an occult cancer, and therefore cross-sectional imaging was performed. This revealed a nodule in the left upper lobe. She was not able to tolerate a bronchoscopy, and her FEV_1 of 0.60 L (45% predicted) precluded her from a percutaneous biopsy. Therefore, a PET scan was arranged (Figure 16.2) to help add weight to the diagnosis of malignancy. The PET scan demonstrated a left upper lobe nodule, 1.6 cm by 1.7 cm, with a standardized uptake value (SUV) of 10, which was highly suspicious for a bronchogenic carcinoma.

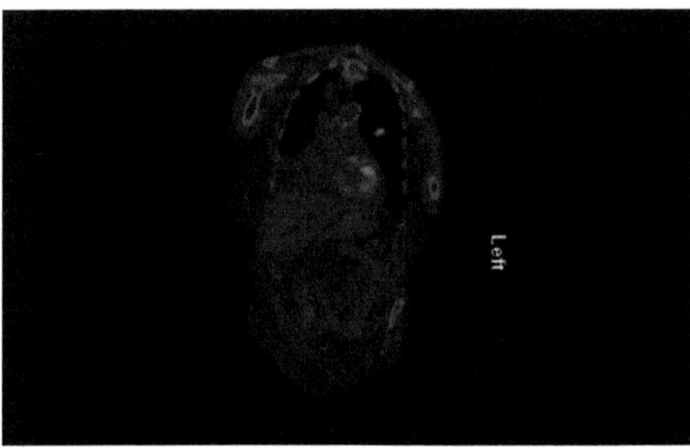

Figure 16.2 PET scan.

A radiological diagnosis of left-sided lung cancer was made, following discussion in the lung cancer multidisciplinary meeting, which presented with a paraneoplastic nephrotic syndrome, complicated by a large right-sided pleural effusion.

Learning point Nephrotic syndrome and lung cancer

The association between nephrotic syndrome and cancer has been known for over 40 years; although rare, it is important to be aware of this complication. A retrospective study in 1966 of 101 patients demonstrated an incidence of cancer in 10.9%, much greater than the expected incidence [9]. The commonest pathology on renal biopsy was membranous glomerulonephritis. The mechanism of pathogenesis is believed to be due to the products of the tumours, and not related to the stage of the cancer [10].

(Continued)

Paraneoplastic nephrotic syndrome has been linked with adenocarcinoma [11], squamous cell carcinoma [12, 13], and small cell carcinoma [14–16] of the lung.

The prognosis of lung cancer complicated by nephrotic syndrome depends on the treatment options for the underlying lung cancer. There are reports of improvement or resolution of the nephrotic syndrome following thoracic surgery [11], chemotherapy, and radiotherapy [12].

Paraneoplastic nephrotic syndrome can predate the malignancy [17], and therefore a high index of suspicion is vital. Management of the underlying malignancy is paramount.

Evidence base Membranous nephropathy and cancer

Lefaucheur *et al.* reviewed 240 cases with membranous nephropathy in the Paris region [17]. There was a 10% prevalence of cancer, of which a third was lung cancer. The cancer-associated membranous nephropathies were compared with matched controls with idiopathic membranous nephropathy (randomization was performed after stratifying by age and gender).

Patients with cancer-associated membranous nephropathy were older ($p < 0.001$) and more likely to be heavy smokers ($p < 0.01$), compared to controls, and were found to have a greater number of inflammatory cells infiltrating the glomeruli ($p = 0.001$).

The right-sided effusion recurred over the following weeks, causing significant dyspnoea, and further drainage was performed on several occasions, with one repeat sample for cytology. This provided temporary relief but required repeated visits to the hospital and interruptions in her anticoagulation.

Clinical tip Clotting, anticoagulants, and antiplatelet—safe or not?

The BTS guidelines [2] recommend non-urgent pleural aspirations, and chest drain insertions should be avoided until the INR is <1.5. The advice of your local haematologist should be sought if a procedure is essential and the patient has abnormal coagulation.

However, this can sometimes cause delays in procedures, especially relevant if the patient has significant symptoms. There is limited evidence that performing ultrasound-guided procedures on anticoagulants or antiplatelets does not lead to an excessive bleeding risk.

A review of 33 thoracocentesis performed on anticoagulants (warfarin, unfractionated or low-molecular-weight heparin, or a combination) demonstrated a 6% complication rate (two of 33), neither of which required intervention [18].

Clinical tip Pleural fluid cytology

Sixty per cent of malignant effusions can be diagnosed by cytology. The yield for sending >2 samples is very low, and a volume of between 40 and 60 mL is recommended [19].

This presented the problem of managing a lady with nephrotic syndrome, causing a recurrent right-sided transudative effusion probably caused by an underlying bronchogenic cancer, which was unable to be histologically confirmed, and who required long-term anticoagulation.

The recurrent effusion significantly impacted on her quality of life due to the breathlessness and repeated hospital attendances and procedures. She did not wish for further hospital stays or surgical procedures such as a thoracoscopy or VATS. Therefore, after a full and frank discussion with the patient, a tunnelled pleural catheter (TPC) was inserted as a palliative measure. This now requires weekly drainage, performed by the district nurses in her home, and her symptoms have dramatically improved. The hope is that a spontaneous pleurodesis will occur, allowing the removal of the catheter.

Expert comment

TPCs are being increasingly used in managing MPEs, with patients benefiting from ambulatory care and community-based treatment. Although physicians have been traditionally worried about using TPCs in chronic benign diseases, because of the risk of introducing infection to the pleural space, the risks do not appear to be significantly higher than in those with MPEs. A recent large series published in *Thorax* [30] had an overall infection rate of only 2%.

Discussion

Many pleural effusions are relatively easy to diagnose, but there remains a cohort of patients where reaching a unifying diagnosis can be incredibly challenging. The BTS guidelines offer a systematic approach, shown in Figure 16.3 [19], which can be complemented by in-depth state-of-the-art reviews on pleural disease management [6]. A full review of this is beyond the scope of this chapter.

The classical teaching for managing transudative effusions is to treat the underlying cause. The commonest causes for persistent transudative effusions are: congestive heart failure, cirrhosis, nephrotic syndrome, urinothorax, and CSF leaking into the pleura [6]. In practice, this means working closely across specialties to ensure optimal medical and surgical management. However, large and recurring transudative effusions can be particularly challenging to manage. This is especially pertinent in the older population, with multiple co-morbidities preventing invasive treatment of either the underlying cause or the effusion itself.

The optimal management of non-MPEs is controversial [20]. Nephrotic syndrome is associated with pleural effusions in 20% of cases [21], and there is very limited evidence for treatment of nephrotic-associated effusions [22]. The options range from repeated aspirations, inpatient chest drain insertion and medical pleurodesis [23], thoracoscopy with talc poudrage, or VATS and pleurodesis to the insertion of a pleurovenous or pleuroperitoneal shunt [24]. In this case, these options were not suitable due to patient choice, and therefore a TPC was considered.

Learning point Medical or surgical pleurodesis—the evidence in non-malignant effusions

There is limited evidence for medical pleurodesis in non-malignant effusions, with a reported success rate of 80% (20 of 25). The following criteria are recommended in patient selection:

(a) the effusion should be symptomatic;
(b) the lung should not be trapped;
(c) the effusion is refractory to medical management.

In hepatic hydrothorax [25], a surgical approach via VATS has been utilized, with varying degrees of success, and should be considered on a patient-by-patient basis. This can be used as a bridge to transplantation or as a palliative measure.

TPCs are increasingly used in MPEs, and there is literature on their use from 1986 [26]. Insertion is a relatively simple outpatient procedure which takes 20–30 minutes, performed by ultrasound guidance under light sedation with a local anaesthetic. A catheter is placed within the pleural cavity and tunnelled under the skin, with a cuff placed midway, with the aim to reduce infection and the risk of displacement. The pleural space can be drained intermittently via a valve, either by a member of the community team or, after appropriate training, the patient or their next of kin.

The aim of inserting a TPC in MPEs is to provide palliation of symptoms attributable to a pleural effusion, to decrease visits to the hospital, to reduce the number of procedures, to have minimal complications, and to improve quality of life. A systematic review based on 1370 patients, limited by poor-quality data, suggested the use of TPCs for MPEs showed improved symptoms and was not associated with major

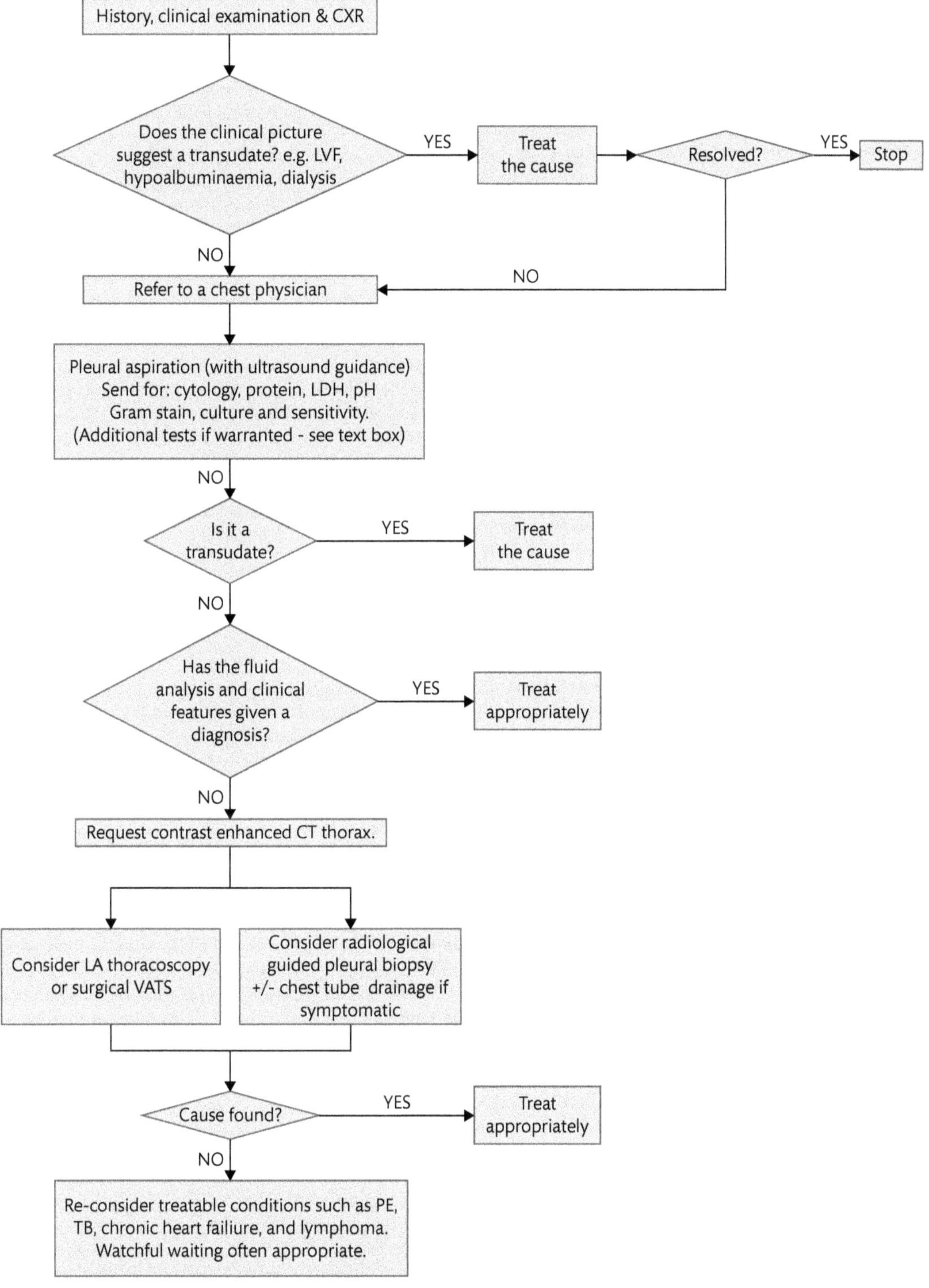

Figure 16.3 Diagnostic algorithm for the investigation of a unilateral pleural effusion.

Source: Hooper C, Lee YC, Maskell N. Investigation of a unilateral pleural effusion in adults: British Thoracic Society pleural disease guideline 2010. Thorax 2010 August;65(20100800).

complications [27]. One welcome effect of TPCs is spontaneous pleurodesis, and this was seen in 46% (430 of 943).

Evidence base The TIME2 RCT

There is little robust evidence for the use of TPCs. This trial compared outpatient TPC insertion with inpatient chest drain insertion and talc slurry pleurodesis in 106 patients with MPE across the UK. The primary end point was dyspnoea at 42 days.

Dyspnoea improved in both groups, but there was no statistically significant difference between the two groups at 42 days, and therefore TPCs cannot be recommended as superior on the basis of this trial.

The TPC patients had a statistically shorter hospital stay (0 days versus 4 days; $p < 0.001$) and a reduced need for further pleural procedures (3 versus 12; $p = 0.03$), but a higher rate of adverse events (27 versus 7; $p = 0.02$).

The secondary end points demonstrated potential benefits of TPCs, but the increased complication rate must be taken into consideration when discussing the options with patients [28].

The aims for patients with MPE are applicable to patients with difficult-to-manage transudative effusions, who often have a significantly reduced life expectancy. A recent review of the literature focussing on the insertion of TPCs in non-malignant effusions [29] concluded that they seem safe and effective.

The use of TPCs in five large UK centres was reviewed by Bhatnagar *et al.* [31]. They found 57 cases of TPC inserted for non-malignant effusions from 2007 to 2013, with the majority inserted after 2011. Patients underwent a median of three pleural procedures prior to insertion of a TPC, indicating the challenging nature of these effusions. However, 89% did not need any further pleural procedures following the TPC insertion. Eighty-four per cent had no complications, and 16% had a combination of suspected pleural infection (2%), skin infection (7%), fluid loculation (7%), drain site leakage (2%), pain (4%), blockage (2%), acute renal failure (4%), and mechanical failure of the drain (2%). A third of these patients had a hepatic hydrothorax, and these achieved a statistically significant lower rate of spontaneous pleurodesis ($p = 0.03$).

One of the concerns with recommending TPCs is the complication rate (ranging from 4% to 60%), including empyemas. The infection risks appear to be directly related to the time the catheter remains *in situ*, and therefore new developments include the possibility of outpatient pleurodesis with a talc slurry inserted via the TPC. A trial is currently recruiting to investigate this further in malignant disease, and the messages from this may help inform further management of non-malignant effusions.

Clinical tip Consent for insertion of TPCs

The main complications seen with TPCs are infections, including empyemas, along with drain displacement, drain occlusion, or pain around the site of entry [27,30, 31]. Therefore, consent should include these complications, along with bleeding, visceral injury, and pneumothorax [2]. Renal failure was seen in 4% of patients in a review of five centres in the UK [30], and therefore it is recommended for these patients to have their serum electrolytes and renal function checked regularly if a TPC has been inserted.

A final word from the expert

This case highlights several challenges in managing pleural disease, including making the correct diagnosis. An awareness of the rarer, but serious, causes of pleural effusions, including the link between lung cancer and nephrotic syndrome, is vital. Managing refractory non-malignant effusions in the older population with underlying co-morbidities can be incredibly difficult, and the emergence of another treatment option, in the form of the TPC, provides a potential solution which should be considered on a case-by-case basis. Large-scale randomized trials are needed to aid decision-making in the setting of refractory non-malignant effusions where management of the underlying condition has been optimized.

References

1. National Patient Safety Agency (2008). *Risks of chest drain insertion. Rapid Response Report. NPSA/2008/RRR003*. Available at: <http://www.nrls.npsa.nhs.uk/resources/?entryid45=59887>.
2. Havelock T, Teoh R, Laws D, Gleeson F. Pleural procedures and thoracic ultrasound: British Thoracic Society pleural disease guideline 2010. *Thorax* 2010;**65** (Suppl 1):61–76.
3. Royal College of Radiologists (2012). *Ultrasound training recommendations for medical and surgical specialties*, second edition. Available at: <https://www.rcr.ac.uk/sites/default/files/publication/BFCR%2812%2917_ultrasound_training.pdf>.
4. Grogan DR, Irwin RS, Channick R *et al*. Complications associated with thoracentesis. A prospective, randomized study comparing three different methods. *Arch Intern Med* 1990;**150**:873–77.
5. Light RW, Macgregor MI, Luchsinger PC, Ball WC Jr. Pleural effusions: the diagnostic separation of transudates and exudates. *Ann Intern Med* 1972;**77**:507–13.
6. Light RW. Update: management of the difficult to diagnose pleural effusion. *Clinical Pulmonary Medicine* 2003;**10**:39–46.
7. Burgess LJ, Maritz FJ, Taljaard JJ. Comparative analysis of the biochemical parameters used to distinguish between pleural transudates and exudates. *Chest* 1995;**107**:1604–9.
8. Hull RP, Goldsmith DJ. Nephrotic syndrome in adults. *BMJ* 2008;**336**:1185–9.
9. Lee JC, Yamauchi H, Hopper J Jr. The association of cancer and the nephrotic syndrome. *Ann Intern Med* 1966;**64**:41–51.
10. Lien YH, Lai L. Pathogenesis, diagnosis and management of paraneoplastic glomerulonephritis. *Nat Rev Nephrol* 2011;**7**:85–95.
11. Coltharp WH, Lee SM, Miller RF, Averbuch MS. Nephrotic syndrome complicating adenocarcinoma of the lung with resolution after resection. *Ann Thorac Surg* 1991;**51**:308–9.
12. Yoshida K, Maruta T, Yamada K, Kojima Y, Soejima T, Sugimura K. A case of squamous cell lung cancer with paraneoplastic nephrotic syndrome treated with radiotherapy. *J JASTRO* 2003;**15**:291–5.
13. Ebert B, Shaffer K, Rennke H. Some unusual paraneoplastic syndromes. Case 4. Paraneoplastic nephrotic syndrome in a patient with lung cancer. *J Clin Oncol* 2003;**21**:2624–5.
14. Boon ES, Vrij AA, Nieuwhof C, Van Noord JA, Zeppenfeldt E. Small cell lung cancer with paraneoplastic nephrotic syndrome. *Eur Respir J* 1994;**7**:1192–3.
15. Usalan C, Emri S. Membranoproliferative glomerulonephritis associated with small cell lung carcinoma. *Int Urol Nephrol* 1998;**30**:209–13.

16. Grivaux M, Renault D, Gallois JC, Barbanel C, Blanchon F. [Small cell lung cancer revealed by extramembranous glomerulonephritis]. *Rev Mal Respir* 2001;**18**:197–9.
17. Lefaucheur C, Stengel B, Nochy D *et al*. Membranous nephropathy and cancer: epidemiologic evidence and determinants of high-risk cancer association. *Kidney Int* 2006;**70**:1510–17.
18. Schoonover GA. Risk of bleeding during thoracentesis in anticoagulated patients. *Chest* 2006;**130**:141S.
19. Hooper C, Lee YC, Maskell N. Investigation of a unilateral pleural effusion in adults: British Thoracic Society pleural disease guideline 2010. *Thorax* 2010;**65**(Suppl 1):4–17.
20. Sudduth C, Sahn S. Pleurodesis for nonmalignant pleural effusions. Recommendations. *Chest* 1992;**102**:1855–60.
21. Cavina C, Vichi G. Radiological aspects of pleural effusions in medical nephropathy in children. *Ann Radiol Diagn (Bologna)* 1958;**31**:163–202.
22. Jenkins PG, Shelp WD. Recurrent pleural transudate in the nephrotic syndrome. *JAMA* 1974;**230**:587–8.
23. Glazer M, Berkman NBC, Lafair JS, Kramer MR. Successful talc slurry pleurodesis in patients with nonmalignant pleural effusion: report of 16 cases and review of the literature. *Chest* 2000;**117**:1404–9.
24. Artemiou O, Marta GM, Klepetko W, Wolner E, Muller MR. Pleurovenous shunting in the treatment of nonmalignant pleural effusion. *Ann Thorac Surg* 2003;**76**:231–3.
25. Ferrante D, Arguedas MR, Cerfolio RJ, Collins BG, van Leeuwen DJ. Video-assisted thoracoscopic surgery with talc pleurodesis in the management of symptomatic hepatic hydrothorax. *Am J Gastroenterol* 2002;**97**:3172–5.
26. Leff RS, Eisenberg B, Baisden CE, Mosley KR, Messerschmidt GL. Drainage of recurrent pleural effusion via an implanted port and intrapleural catheter. *Ann Intern Med* 1986;**104**:208–9.
27. Van Meter ME, McKee KY, Kohlwes RJ. Efficacy and safety of tunneled pleural catheters in adults with malignant pleural effusions: a systematic review. *J Gen Intern Med* 2011;**26**:70–6.
28. Davies HE, Mishra EK, Kahan BC *et al*. Effect of an indwelling pleural catheter vs chest tube and talc pleurodesis for relieving dyspnea in patients with malignant pleural effusion: the TIME2 randomized controlled trial. *JAMA* 2012;**307**:2383–9.
29. Miller SM, Prakash B, Bellinger C, Chin Robert Jr. To TPC or not to TPC? Tunneled pleural catheters in nonmalignant pleural effusions. *Clinical Pulmonary Medicine* 2012;**19**:232–6.
30. Bhatnagar R, Reid ED, Corcoran JP *et al*. Indwelling pleural catheters for non-malignant effusions: a multicentre review of practice. *Thorax* 2014;**69**:959–61.
31. Schneider T, Reimer P, Storz K *et al*. Recurrent pleural effusion: who benefits from a tunneled pleural catheter? *Thorac Cardiovasc Surg* 2009;**57**:42–6.

CASE

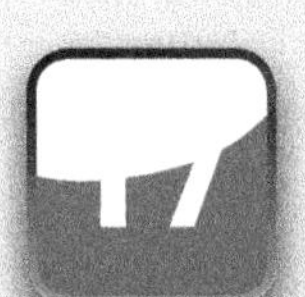

Pulmonary vasculature

Sophie Vergnaud and David Dobarro

Expert Commentary John Wort

Case history

A 16-year-old girl presented to her local district general hospital with a 12-month history of exertional breathlessness. She was previously well, with no past medical history. In the preceding year, she had noticed a gradual reduction in exercise tolerance. She had previously enjoyed an active lifestyle, running and dancing regularly, but was now experiencing significant New York Heart Association (NYHA) grade III breathlessness. Simultaneously, she had developed pain and stiffness in her hips, knees, ankles, and hands and ulceration of her fingertips, and she described symptoms consistent with Raynaud's phenomenon. She denied any drug use, recreational or otherwise, and had not taken diet pills. She did not smoke or drink alcohol. There was no significant family history.

Expert comment

The NYHA breathlessness score is designed to relate a patient's symptoms to everyday activities and their quality of life. Although designed for patients with heart failure, it is often used for patients with PH, along with the WHO classification. NYHA grade III relates to marked clinical limitations; the patient may be comfortable at rest, but less-than-ordinary activity leads to breathlessness, fatigue, or palpitations. Clearly, this history is already very concerning. The patient is likely to have a systemic rheumatological condition that is either affecting her lungs or heart, or both.

Physical examination revealed an appropriately developed 16-year-old girl of slim build. Her JVP was elevated at 3 cm, and her systemic blood pressure was 98/60, with a regular heart rate of 90 beats/minute. Her lungs were clear to auscultation. There was a loud pulmonary component of the second heart sound, with a left parasternal heave.

Learning point Basic pulmonary physiology

The pulmonary circulation is a high-flow, high-compliance, low-resistance system. This means it can adjust to alterations in flow, with little change in resistance. Its purpose is to deliver unoxygenated blood from the right ventricle to the alveolar capillary network during each cardiac cycle for gas exchange and oxygenation, before returning to the left atrium. Because of the effect of gravity, blood flows more easily to the bases of the lungs, leaving little or no flow to apical capillaries. At the apices, therefore, ventilation exceeds perfusion, and, at the bases, perfusion exceeds ventilation.

(Continued)

With increased pulmonary flow or increased pulmonary vascular resistance (PVR), capillaries may be recruited to participate in gas exchange. Because pulmonary capillaries are so compliant, if alveolar pressure exceeds that in the capillaries, the capillary will narrow or collapse.

Pulmonary artery walls contain smooth muscle cells. The tone of this vascular smooth muscle determines the radius of the vessel, and hence its resistance.

Pulmonary vessels constrict in response to reduced alveolar ventilation and hypoxia. Within the lung, this causes increased resistance and redistribution of blood flow to areas that are better ventilated.

Pulmonary vessels dilate in response to nitric oxide. Nitric oxide is produced by nitric oxide synthase in the vascular endothelium in response to increased blood flow, thereby reducing resistance. Pulmonary vessels also dilate in response to prostacyclin production in the lung, as these are vasodilators.

Clinical tip When to suspect pulmonary arterial hypertension (PAH)

Early symptoms of PH are often non-specific. Whilst the commonest symptom is breathlessness, other symptoms may include fatigue, weakness, and abdominal distension. Chest pain is thought to occur in 41% of patients, in the absence of coronary artery disease, and proposed to be caused by right ventricular and ischaemia or extrinsic compression of the left main coronary artery by a dilated pulmonary trunk [1]. Severity of symptoms is related to prognosis, and presentation with syncope is ominous, as it reflects a low cardiac output. Onset is often insidious, with an average delay of 18 months from onset of symptoms to diagnosis for PAH. This interval has not changed in 10 years [2].

Clinical signs may be subtle until advanced stages of disease:

- tachypnoea;
- peripheral cyanosis progressing to central cyanosis;
- raised JVP with prominent 'a' wave from increased force of atrial contraction or a large 'v' wave in severe tricuspid regurgitation;
- right ventricular heave;
- loud pulmonary component of the second heart sound;
- right ventricular third heart sound;
- tricuspid regurgitation;
- pulmonary regurgitation;
- right heart failure.

Any patient with unexplained exertional breathlessness in the absence of obvious cardiac or respiratory disease should raise the possibility of PAH.

She was referred to, and reviewed by, the local rheumatologists who diagnosed diffuse cutaneous systemic sclerosis (DcSSc), with U3 RNP antibody positive and Raynaud's phenomenon. She was found to have myopathy on muscle biopsy and widespread telangiectasia causing epistaxis. She was started on prednisolone, methotrexate, and folic acid.

Learning point Causes of pulmonary hypertension

PH is not a final diagnosis, but a haemodynamic and pathophysiological condition (defined as an increase in mean pulmonary arterial pressure (PAP) >25 mmHg at rest on right heart catheterization (RHC)) [3] that should prompt further investigation into the underlying cause. The clinical classification of PH has undergone several changes over the years. The most recent is the 2013 classification (fifth World Symposium in Nice, France) summarized below (Box 17.1) [4].

(Continued)

Pulmonary arterial hypertension (PAH) is characterized by the presence of pre-capillary PH in the absence of other causes such as heart disease, lung disease, or chronic thromboembolic disease.

Idiopathic (previously termed 'primary') PAH (IPAH) is extremely rare, and its incidence is just 1–2 per million per year (female:male sex ratio = 2.3:1) [5]. It most commonly occurs between the ages of 20 and 45. It is pathologically indistinguishable from PAH associated with other conditions, particularly CTDs. Of these, it most commonly complicates the clinical course of systemic sclerosis. It occurs in 15–20% of cases of systemic sclerosis, in the absence of ILD, and doubles in mortality, with a median survival of 4 years from diagnosis.

Expert comment

Although the age range of 20–45 years is traditionally held to be true, it appears that, in the last 10 years, the age of patients referred with IPAH is increasing. In fact, in the UK, the median age is well over 50. In keeping with this, patients have increasing numbers of co-morbidities such as ischaemic heart disease, diabetes, renal dysfunction, and sleep-disordered breathing.

Box 17.1 Updated clinical classification of pulmonary hypertension (Dana Point 2013)

1. Pulmonary arterial hypertension
   - 1.1 Idiopathic PAH
   - 1.2 Heritable PAH
     - 1.2.1 BMPR2
     - 1.2.2 ALK-1, ENG, **SMAD9**, **CAV1**, **KCNK3**
     - 1.2.3 Unknown
   - 1.3 Drug- and toxin-induced
   - 1.4 Associated with:
     - 1.4.1 Connective tissue disease
     - 1.4.2 HIV infection
     - 1.4.3 Portal hypertension
     - 1.4.4 Congenital heart diseases
     - 1.4.5 Schistosomiasis

1'. Pulmonary veno-occlusive disease and/or pulmonary capillary haemangiomatosis

1'' Persistent pulmonary hypertension of the newborn (PPHN)

2. Pulmonary hypertension due to left heart disease
   - 2.1 Left ventricular systolic dysfunction
   - 2.2 Left ventricular diastolic dysfunction
   - 2.3 Valvular disease
   - 2.4 **Congenital/acquired left heart inflow/outflow tract obstruction and congenital cardiomyopathies**
3. Pulmonary hypertension due to lung diseases and/or hypoxia
   - 3.1 Chronic obstructive pulmonary disease
   - 3.2 Interstitial lung disease
   - 3.3 Other pulmonary diseases with mixed restrictive and obstructive pattern
   - 3.4 Sleep-disordered breathing
   - 3.5 Alveolar hypoventilation disorders
   - 3.6 Chronic exposure to high altitude
   - 3.7 Developmental lung diseases
4. Chronic thromboembolic pulmonary hypertension (CTEPH)
5. Pulmonary hypertension with unclear multifactorial mechanisms
   - 5.1 Haematologic disorders: chronic haemolytic anaemia, myeloproliferative disorders, splenectomy
   - 5.2 Systemic disorders: sarcoidosis, pulmonary histiocytosis, lymphangioleiomyomatosis
   - 5.3 Metabolic disorders: glycogen storage disease, Gaucher's disease, thyroid disorders
   - 5.4 Others: tumoural obstruction, fibrosing mediastinitis, chronic renal failure, **segmental pulmonary hypertension**

BMPR, bone morphogenic protein receptor type II; CAV1, caveolin-1; ENG, endoglin; HIV, human immunodeficiency virus; PAH, pulmonary arterial hypertension.

Fifth World Symposium on Pulmonary Hypertension, Nice 2013. Main modifications to the previous Dana Point classification are in **bold**.

Source: Simonneau G, Gatzoulis MA, Adatia I, Celermajer D, Denton C, Ghofrani A, Gomez Sanchez MA, Krishna Kumar R, Landzberg M, Machado RF, Olschewski H, Robbins IM, Souza R. Updated clinical classification of pulmonary hypertension. J Am Coll Cardiol. 2013 Dec 24;62(25 Suppl):D34–41.

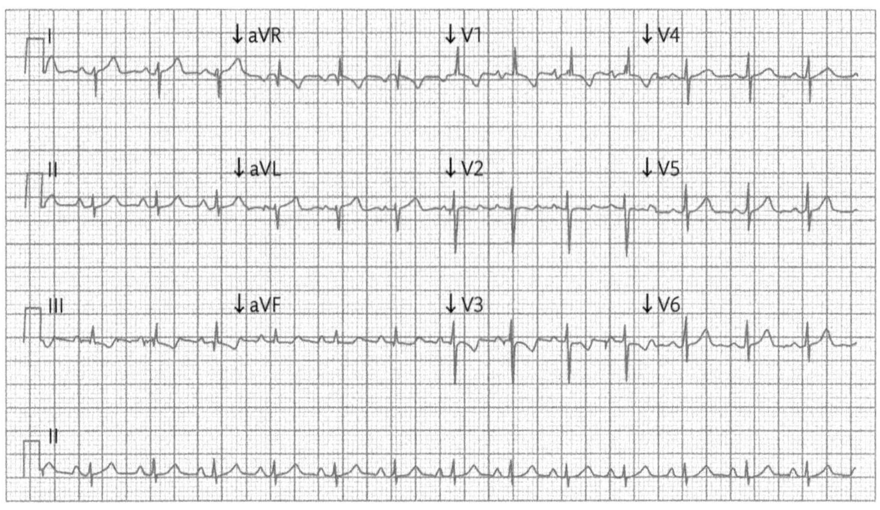

Figure 17.1 ECG showing right ventricular strain.

A CXR showed an enlarged cardiac silhouette and normal lung fields. Her ECG showed sinus rhythm, right axis deviation, incomplete right bundle branch block, a normal PR interval, but with p *pulmonale*, and asymmetric inverted T waves in V1–V3 and lead III, suggesting right ventricular strain (Figure 17.1).

PFTs revealed a restrictive defect with FEV_1, FVC, and TLCO all 70% predicted. A CT scan of the chest showed no evidence of pulmonary fibrosis, normal-sized pulmonary arteries, an increased cardiac silhouette, and a mild pericardial effusion. A V/Q scan ruled out a PE.

A transthoracic echocardiogram showed a raised right ventricular end-systolic pressure of 67 mmHg, a dilated right atrium and right ventricle, right ventricular dysfunction, and a normal left heart size and function.

Expert comment

The normal picture of a patient with PAH is to have near normal FEV_1 and FVC, although, as stated, a restrictive pattern has been described. However, it is more usual to have a mild reduction in TLCO or KCO. Significantly reduced gas transfer is associated with a worse prognosis. It also raises the possibility of another pathology such as associated lung disease or pulmonary veno-occlusive disease.

Expert comment

There are several ways of measuring right ventricular dysfunction. One commonly used measure is the tricuspid annular plane systolic excursion, or TAPSE. It gives an indication of the longitudinal function of the right ventricle. Ideally, the TAPSE should be >2 cm. A TAPSE of <1.5 cm is associated with a worse prognosis.

Clinical tip Investigating pulmonary hypertension in the district general hospital

Blood tests: thrombophilia screen, auto-antibody screen (excluding systemic sclerosis is particularly important); consider HIV and hepatitis serology, haemoglobinopathy screen, thyroid function, NT-proBNP/BNP (useful in diagnosis and monitoring) [6].

Spirometry: to exclude other causes of breathlessness. In PH, the pattern normally seen is a normal FEV_1/FVC ratio, sometimes with a restrictive pattern, and reduced TLCO/KCO. Young patients with PH may have normal spirometry.

CXR: may show prominence of the pulmonary arteries, enlarged cardiac chambers, pulmonary oedema, pleural effusions, or evidence of underlying parenchymal lung disease.

ECG: may reveal sinus tachycardia or signs of right heart strain such as right axis deviation, right ventricular hypertrophy, right bundle branch block, or right atrial enlargement such as prominent peaked P waves in the right precordial and inferior leads. It is abnormal in 80–90% of symptomatic cases [7] but is inadequate as a screening tool, with a sensitivity of 55% and a specificity of 70%. A normal ECG does not exclude PH.

Transthoracic echocardiogram: is the most useful non-invasive investigation and best screening investigation for PH [8]. It can detect the presence of underlying intracardiac shunts, left or right heart

(Continued)

disease, and valvular abnormalities and allows the estimation of right ventricular end-systolic pressure (RVESP) by Doppler echocardiography [9].

HRCT or CT pulmonary angiogram (CTPA): to exclude underlying lung disease, mosaic perfusion defects, and pulmonary artery filling defects.

V/Q lung scan: may be normal in IPAH or may reveal large perfusion defects in chronic thromboembolic disease.

Cardiac MRI: is useful for imaging the right ventricle and pulmonary circulation and for ruling out other conditions that may mimic PH.

Abdominal ultrasound: may be helpful in diagnosing portal hypertension, thus raising the suspicion of porto-pulmonary hypertension.

She was referred to her nearest specialist PH centre for further investigation where she had a RHC, which confirmed PAH. Her PAP was 49/21, with a mean of 34 mmHg, a PCWP of 9 mmHg, a cardiac output of 5.9 L/minute, and a PVR of 340 dynes/s/cm^5 (4.25 Wood units, WU).

Clinical tip Referring to specialist centres

Who to refer?

- All patients with suspected PH for which there is no obvious cause.
- Patients with PH secondary to hypoxic lung disease, or patients with cardiac disease but excessive symptoms or an estimated pulmonary artery systolic pressure of >60 mmHg on echocardiography.
- Symptomatic patients with a condition that is associated with PH.

All patients should have an ECG, a CXR, a transthoracic echocardiogram, a V/Q scan, and/or a CTPA and spirometry. They should be seen by a local respiratory physician or cardiologist. Referrals should not be delayed for further investigations when it is clear that PH may be the dominant problem.

Source: Consensus statement on the management of pulmonary hypertension in clinical practice in the UK and Ireland. *Thorax* 2008;**63**(Suppl II):ii1–ii41.

Learning point Further investigations in the specialist setting

Further investigations are aimed at confirming the diagnosis, clarifying the clinical group of PH and the specific aetiology within the PAH group, and evaluating the functional and haemodynamic impairment [3].

- The **6MWT**, as per the ATS guidelines, has a well-recognized role in monitoring progress and prognosis in PH [10,11]. A normal distance is >500 m. A low 6MWT is predictive of poor survival.
- **RHC** remains the only way of confirming and prognosticating the diagnosis of PH. The diagnosis is made if the **mean PAP exceeds >25 mmHg** [12]. The PCWP should also be measured and is an approximation of the left atrial pressure. A PCWP of >15 mmHg indicates left ventricular disease. Measurement of right ventricular function is important in determining prognosis, and indicators of poor prognosis are: (i) elevated right atrial pressure (>10 mmHg), (ii) elevated right ventricular end-diastolic pressure (>10 mmHg), (iii) reduced mixed venous oxygen saturations (SvO_2 <63%), and (iv) reduced cardiac output (<2.5 L/minute).
- **Vasoreactivity studies** determine which patients will respond favourably to long-term vasodilator therapy with calcium channel blockers (only indicated in patients with a diagnosis of IPAH). Administration of inhaled nitric oxide, adenosine, or IV epoprostenol at the time of RHC, resulting in a fall in mean PAP of at least 10 mmHg to below 40 mmHg, with either an increase or no change in cardiac output suggests a positive response to vasodilator therapy [8]. Approximately 10% of patients with IPAH are acute responders, but, of these, just 50% are chronic responders to calcium channel blockers [13].

Expert comment

Although there is no mention of the right atrial pressure or venous oxygen saturation, however, at this moment, the cardiac output is well preserved, which is a good prognostic sign, and the PVR is only mildly raised.

Expert comment

Actually, patients with pulmonary veno-occlusive disease are more likely to have a normal PCWP, which should more correctly be expressed as pulmonary artery wedge pressure. Another way of measuring the left atrial pressure is to measure the left ventricular end-diastolic pressure (LVEDP), but this would require catheterization of the left side of the heart.

Evidence base Super-1

Randomized, double-blind study comparing sildenafil versus placebo over 12 weeks in 278 patients with IPAH, CTD, and congenital heart disease across all functional classes III/IV. Results showed significant improvement in functional class and haemodynamics [14].

Expert comment

During follow-up in a patient with PAH, there are various parameters that can be used to decide on a satisfactory response. These include an improvement in functional class to I or II, a 6MWT of >380–440 m, normalization of right ventricular function (and size) on echocardiography and RHC, and a reduction of BNP to normal. Many of these targets may not be achievable, but they must remain active goals.

Treatment with sildenafil, a phosphodiesterase-5 inhibitor, was approved by the primary care trust, and she was started on sildenafil 20 mg tds, uptitrated to 50 mg tds, with only mild side effects.

Three months later, her breathlessness had improved slightly, with some increase in her exercise tolerance on the flat and a slight improvement in her 6MWT to 370 m from 300 m. However, she experienced syncope on moderate exertion, upgrading her to WHO class IV symptoms. On repeat RHC, her mean PAP had risen to 43 mmHg, with an increase in PVR to 460 dynes/s/cm^5 and a drop in cardiac output to 5.2 L/minute. Approval was sought and granted for additional treatment with the selective endothelin A (ET_A) receptor antagonist sitaxentan (since withdrawn worldwide due to hepatic toxicity). She was started on this and referred to the local heart and lung transplant hospital for assessment. Warfarin was held off due to her telangiectasia and risks of epistaxis and gastrointestinal haemorrhage. IV prostanoids were discussed but deferred due to the patient's wishes.

Six months into her treatment with sitaxentan, her repeat RHC showed some improvement, with a drop in her mean PAP down to 30 mmHg and PVR to 290 dynes/s/cm^5. Her 6MWT had improved to 400 m. She continued on her combined therapy, with slow and gradual increases in her dose of sildenafil. Over the next 6 months, things remained stable, with no further deterioration.

Clinical tip Assessing and monitoring disease

The European Society of Cardiology suggests a 9-point approach to assessing and monitoring disease severity, stability, and prognosis (Table 17.1) [3]:

1. clinical evidence of right ventricular failure;
2. rate of progression of symptoms;
3. syncope;
4. WHO functional class;
5. 6MWT;
6. CPET;
7. BNP/NT-proBNP plasma levels;
8. echocardiographic findings;
9. haemodynamics.

Table 17.1 Parameters with established importance for assessing disease severity, stability, and prognosis in PAH (European Society of Cardiology guidelines)

Better prognosis	Determinants of prognosis	Worse prognosis
No	Clinical evidence of right ventricular failure	Yes
Slow	Rate of progression of symptoms	Rapid
No	Syncope	Yes
I, II	WHO functional class	IV
Longer (>500 m)	6MWT	Shorter (<300 m)
Peak oxygen consumption >15 mL/minute/kg	CPET	Peak oxygen consumption <12 mL/minute/kg
Normal or near normal	BNP/NT-proBNP plasma levels	Elevated and rising
No pericardial effusion TAPSE >2 cm	Echocardiography	Pericardial effusion TAPSE <1.5 cm
RAP <8 mmHg and CI ≥=2.5 L/minute/m^2	Haemodynamics	RAP >15 mmHg and CI ≤=2.0L/min/m^2

The Task Force for the Diagnosis and Treatment of Pulmonary Hypertension of the European Society of Cardiology (ESC) and the European Respiratory Society (ERS), endorsed by the International Society of Heart and Lung transplantation (ISHLT): Guidelines for the diagnosis and treatment of pulmonary hypertension. European Heart Journal 2009; 30:2493–2537.

Over the following year, her condition gradually worsened, both symptomatically and on haemodynamic monitoring. She was treated with a course of iloprost by the rheumatologists for finger ulceration, and she was started on mycophenolate mofetil, which was gradually increased before stopping methotrexate altogether. Sitaxentan was withdrawn due to worldwide concerns over drug-related hepatotoxicity, and she was changed to another ET_A receptor antagonist bosentan. She was also commenced on warfarin. Despite no symptomatic improvement with bosentan, she remained reluctant to progress to treatment with IV prostanoids. Instead, she was recruited into a trial using cicletanine, a diuretic that had shown promise in animal studies for PH.

Evidence base

- **BREATHE-1** (Rubin *et al.*, 2002) [15]: randomized, double-blind study comparing bosentan versus placebo over 16 weeks in 213 patients with functional class III/IV PAH. Showed significant improvement in time to clinical worsening.
- **BREATHE-2** (Humbert *et al.*, 2004) [16]: randomized, double-blind study comparing the addition of bosentan to epoprostenol versus placebo + epoprostenol at the start of therapy, over 16 weeks in 33 patients with functional class III/IV IPAH and CTD. Showed non-significant trends in favour of combination therapy, but no end points reached.
- **EARLY** (Galiè *et al.*, 2008) [17]: randomized, double-blind study comparing early use of bosentan versus placebo over 6 months in 185 patients with functional class II PAH. Showed significant improvement in time to clinical worsening and reduction in NT-proBNP levels in the bosentan group, compared to placebo. No improvement in mortality.

The patient's condition continued to deteriorate 4 months into the cicletanine trial. Her syncopal episodes became more frequent and her breathlessness much more limiting, and she reported episodes of exertional chest pain. She lost her confidence leaving the house alone and stopped being able to exercise. The cicletanine trial was stopped worldwide because of lack of efficacy, so her cicletanine was stopped, and she was started on digoxin and spironolactone for the developing signs of right heart failure (ankle oedema, elevated JVP, and positive hepatojugular reflex).

On review in clinic, she was unable to complete the 6MWT, managing a distance of only 130 m. A repeat RHC showed that her mean PAP had increased to 58 mmHg and PVR to over 1000 dynes/s/cm^5, and her cardiac output was down to 4 L/minute, with a cardiac index of 2.3 L/minute/m^2.

She was admitted for IV epoprostenol and showed a gradual improvement, as illustrated by her NT-proBNP trend (Figure 17.2).

The NT-proBNP dropped to 73 from a peak of 402 pmol/L, correlating with her admission for IV epoprostenol and mirroring the related fall in her 6MWT (Figure 17.3).

Since commencing epoprostenol, her 6MWT has improved to 263 m. She continues on IV therapy, uptitrating slowly, with a target of between 20 and 40 ng/kg/minute, in combination with sildenafil and bosentan, with moderate and gradual improvement. She has been referred back to the local transplant centre for review and consideration for transplantation. It is important to note that she has had no more syncopal episodes for the last 5 months.

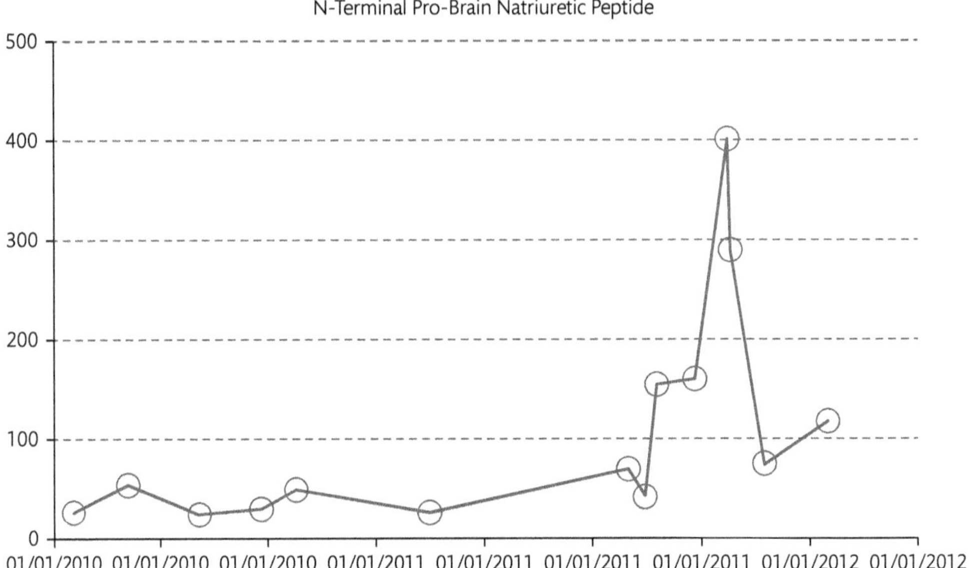

Figure 17.2 NT-proBNP measurements over disease duration.

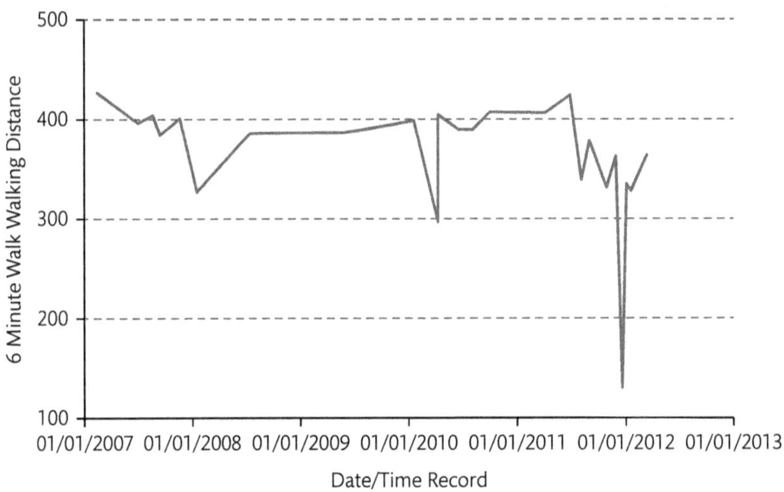

Figure 17.3 6-minute walk measurements over disease duration.

Discussion

This patient demonstrated a classical history and typical signs of PH, from her early presentation to her progression of symptoms with syncope and right heart failure. The presence of telangiectasia in this patient is also interesting, as it has been proposed as a potential clinical marker of PH in scleroderma [18]. PH should always be considered and actively excluded in any patient with scleroderma due to its high prevalence (approximately 20% in this population in the absence of ILD) [19]. ILD should also be actively excluded, as its prevalence can be up to 90% in this group [20] and is associated with poorer prognosis.

This case highlights the diagnostic and therapeutic approach for patients presenting with PH and the impact that patient choice and patient factors have on the treatments given. It also demonstrates that, due to the limited proven therapies available for PH, enrolment in clinical trials is often part of the therapeutic approach in treating these patients.

Current treatment strategies

Patients with PH should be managed in specialist centres, and care should be delivered by an MDT, including respiratory physicians, cardiologists, transplant physicians, cardiothoracic surgeons, radiologists, specialist nurses, and palliative care specialists. The aims of treatment are to improve symptoms and quality of life, increase exercise capacity, and improve prognosis.

Anticoagulation

Anticoagulation is recommended in patients with IPAH, heritable PAH, and PAH due to anorexigens, as these are the only group where evidence (albeit retrospective and single-centred [21–23]) has shown survival benefit. In associated forms of PAH the potential benefits should, however, be weighed against the risks of haemorrhage, especially in patients with CTD-associated PAH and porto-pulmonary hypertension. Therefore the role of anticoagulation in PAH remains a matter of discussion. Lifelong anticoagulation is indicated in CTEPH.

Oxygen therapy

Increased alveolar oxygenation reduces PVR, thus implying that oxygen therapy should be beneficial in PH. Acute oxygen administration has been demonstrated to reduce PVR in both hypoxic and non-hypoxic patients with PH, although there are no randomized controlled studies to confirm the benefits of long-term oxygen supplementation. The current advice is that oxygen should be prescribed as per the BTS Working Group on Home Oxygen Services for 15 hours/day when PaO_2 is persistently <8 kPa [25]. Where daytime oxygenation is satisfactory, nocturnal oxygenation should be assessed, and oxygen prescribed to correct oxygen saturations <90% [8]. Ambulatory oxygen can also be prescribed as per BTS guidelines [25] if there is evidence of correctible desaturation of <4% to <90% during the 6MWT. Supplementary oxygen therapy has also been recommended for air travel [25].

Supportive medical therapy

Particular attention should be paid to:

- family planning and high risks of pregnancy;
- maintaining physical activity;
- optimal treatment of heart failure and arrhythmias;
- immunizations against pneumococcal pneumonia and influenza.

Calcium channel blockers

Patients with IPAH and a positive vasodilator response at RHC should be offered long-term treatment, such as diltiazem, amlodipine, or nifedipine, titrated as allowed by the blood pressure. Only 54% [13] (of the 10% that are acute positive responders) will maintain a long-term response to vasodilators, with significant improvement in prognosis and symptoms.

Expert comment

A recently reported registry investigating newly initiated therapies in patients with PAH (COMPERA) appears to support the use of anticoagulation, at least in patients with IPAH [24]. Patients who were anticoagulated had better survival than those who had never received anticoagulation. Benefit was not seen in patients with other forms of PAH.

Disease-targeted therapies

In the last 10 years, drug trials have demonstrated favourable outcomes in PAH with disease-targeted therapies. Treatments available act in one of three ways:

1. prostanoids potentiate the prostacyclin pathway;
2. endothelin receptor antagonists (ERAs) inhibit the endothelin pathway;
3. phosphodiesterase-5 inhibitors enhance the nitric oxide pathway.

Previously there has been limited evidence of drugs improving survival [26] but new evidence to continues to emerge providing more options for treatment of this challenging condition. Because of the nature of patient selection for trials, these drugs are only licensed for patients with group I disease (IPAH, heritable, drug-associated, and associated PAH), and the European Society of Cardiology guidelines restrict treatment to patients with WHO class II or IV symptoms.

As patients deteriorate on monotherapy, a combination of different agents (mostly two oral agents, ERA, and sildenafil) is usually the next step. A meta-analysis showed a small benefit of combination therapy over standard monotherapy, but results should be taken with caution, as the studies sampled were heterogeneous in their choices of drugs used as well as their routes of administration [27]. Two trials (PACES [28] and BREATHE-2 [16]) showed encouraging results but only looked at oral therapy combined with IV epoprostenol, rather than dual oral therapy. More recently the AMBITION trial (see Evidence base, p. 212) [29] was published showing significant benefits from combination therapy (ambrisentan and tadalafil) compared to ambrisentan or tadalafil monotherapy.

Prostanoids are analogues of prostacyclin and can be administered in different pharmacological forms: IV (epoprostenol), subcutaneously (treprostenil), or by inhalation (iloprost). Even tablet formulations are under investigation. IV and subcutaneous prostanoids need to be given by continuous infusion due to their short half-life of <2 minutes. Achieving the right balance between symptomatic improvement and troublesome side effects (jaw pain, flushing, nausea, diarrhoea) can be tricky. All of them are a proven treatment strategy in PAH, but IV epoprostenol remains the only one proven to improve survival [26]. Because of their complexity of administration and side effects, they tend to be reserved for patients with severe haemodynamic compromise—either as third-line treatment or first-line for patients in WHO functional class III or IV.

ERAs, such as bosentan (dual-selective ET_A/ET_B receptor antagonist) can be taken orally and have been shown to improve exercise capacity, haemodynamics, and time to worsening in five RCTs (Pilot [30], BREATHE-1 [15], BREATHE-2 [16], BREATHE-5 [31], and EARLY [17]). The SERAPHIN trial provided evidence for the use of macitentan, a dual endothelial receptor antagonist (see Evidence base, p. 213) developed from altering the structure of bosentan. The reduction in the primary end point mainly came from a reduction in the rates of worsening of PAH. The side effects included headaches, nasopharyngitis and anaemia [37].

Phosphodiesterase-5 inhibitors are the newest class of drug available, with two non-randomized studies in 2004 and two RCTs in 2005 (SERAPH [33], SUPER-1 [14]). Sildenafil and tadalafil are both licensed in the UK for the treatment of PAH and have been shown to improve exercise capacity, symptoms, haemodynamics, and time to worsening. They cause enhanced pulmonary vasodilatation via the nitric oxide

Evidence base

AMBITION, 2015: multicentre, randomized, double-blind, phase 3-4 study comparing ambrisentan and tadalafil (combination-therapy group), ambrisentan plus placebo (ambrisentan-monotherapy group) and tadalafil plus placebo (tadalafil-monotherapy group). 605 participants 18 to 75 years old with (WHO) functional class II or III with a diagnosis of PAH over a mean duration of 609 days. The primary end point was the first event of clinical failure.

In the combination-therapy group a primary end point occurred in 18% compared with 34% and 28% in the ambrisentan-monotherapy and tadalafil-monotheray groups respectively.

At 24 weeks the combination-therapy group versus the pooled monotherapy group had:

Greater reductions in N-terminal pro-brain natriuretic peptide levels;

Increased percentage of patients with a satisfactory clinical response;

Greater improvement in 6MWT (48.98m vs. 23.80m; $P<0.001$) [29].

Evidence base

Barst *et al.*, 1996: randomized, unblinded study comparing IV epoprostenol versus supportive therapies over 12 weeks in 81 patients with functional classes III/IV IPAH. Showed statistically significant survival benefit in the epoprostenol group and statistically significant improvement in quality of life and symptom scores [26].

pathway by inhibiting the breakdown of cyclic GMP. They also have an antiproliferative effect of the pulmonary vascular smooth muscle. Side effects reported are mild to moderate and include headaches, flushing, and epistaxis.

Atrial septostomy

Patients with PH and a patent foramen ovale are known to have improved survival. This is because the right-to-left shunt helps to reduce the right ventricular preload which relieves the failing right ventricle and can help to improve cardiac output and systemic oxygen delivery despite reducing the arterial oxygen saturation. Atrial septostomy is performed by percutaneous balloon dilatation and is generally viewed as a palliative procedure or a bridge to transplantation in those patients failing on maximal medical therapy.

Pulmonary endarterectomy

Surgical pulmonary endarterectomy is the treatment of choice in CTEPH and remains the only curative treatment for PH.

Transplantation

With the development of disease-targeted therapies, the need for lung or heart–lung transplant in PH has reduced. Overall survival for patients with PAH, according to the American REVEAL registry [34], is 85% at 1 year, 68% at 3 years, 27% at 5 years, and 49% at 5 years. These figures are considerably better than survival figures prior to the modern treatment era, but PH remains a serious, and often fatal, condition.

It has been suggested that one-quarter of patients with IPAH fail to improve on medical therapies, and the prognosis for these patients with WHO functional classes III and IV remains very bleak. In particular, patients with pulmonary veno-occlusive disease and pulmonary capillary haemangiomatosis have a particularly poor response to medical therapies and should be referred early for transplantation. Patients with systemic sclerosis-associated PH also have a worse prognosis.

Patients presenting with WHO functional class IV should be referred for transplantation immediately. Patients with poor prognostic features should be referred if they fail to respond after 3 months of targeted medical therapy. The overall 5-year survival after transplantation is 45–50% [35].

> **Evidence base**
>
> **SERAPHIN, 2013**: multicentre, double-blind, randomized, placebo-controlled, event-driven, phase 3 trial comparing macitentan 3 mg or 10 mg with placebo. 250 participants over the age of 12-years-old with (WHO) functional class II, III or IV over a mean of 96 weeks. The primary end point was the time from the initiation of treatment to the first occurrence of a composite end point of death, atrial septostomy, lung transplantation, initiation of treatment with intravenous or subcutaneous prostanoids, or worsening of pulmonary arterial hypertension.
>
> In the 10-mg macitentan group the primary end point occurred in 31.4% compared with 38% in 3-mg macitentan group and 46.4% in the placebo group (statistically significant in each treatment group vs. placebo) [32].

A final word from the expert

This case study highlights the difficulties in diagnosis and management of patients with PAH. Despite the discovery of key pathways involved in endothelial dysfunction, observed in patients with PAH, and the consequent design and use of pulmonary vasodilator drugs, morbidity and mortality remain unacceptably high. It is also true that, despite advances in our understanding of the molecular biology and genetics of PAH, patients are not being diagnosed any earlier than they were 10 years ago; the majority of patients are still diagnosed 18 months after symptoms start, in NYHA functional class III, i.e. with significant limitations. This is important, as several studies have shown that patients do better if they present in a better functional class and with longer 6MWT distances. Having said that, the EARLY study, mentioned in this chapter, has demonstrated that patients in functional class II still have significantly impaired haemodynamics and evidence of disease progression if left untreated. Therefore, one significant challenge for the future is to identify patients earlier in their disease process. It is likely that this will only be done with improved education, for instance with circulation of articles like this one.

It is also an exciting time to be involved in the management of patients with PAH. There are several new therapies that have been, or are about to be, licensed for use in patients. Related to the medications previously mentioned are riociguat, a new class of drug called a soluble guanylate activator, and macitentan, a new dual endothelin receptor antagonist. Riociguat works by enhancing intracellular levels of cyclic guanosine monophosphate (GMP) (resulting in vasodilation) in both a nitric oxide-dependent and independent fashion. It has recently been shown to be beneficial in terms of 6MWT and haemodynamics in patients with IPAH (PATENT) and CTEPH (CHEST), in well-designed double-blind, placebo-controlled studies [36, 37]. The recently reported SERAPHIN study demonstrated that macitentan was superior to placebo in patients with PAH, in terms of a combined morbidity and mortality outcome [32]. This study was a landmark study in that it used such an outcome, rather than the traditional 6MWT change over 12 weeks. As such, it has probably set the bar for future studies in this field.

Finally, the race is on to develop new drugs that target the basic pathological entity—the remodelled pulmonary vessel. These drugs are likely to target both proliferation and apoptosis. Vascular cells from patients with PAH proliferate more to stimuli in vitro and are more resistant to apoptosis. Herein lies the analogy with human cancer. In fact, trials using agents used in patients with cancer have been performed. Imatinib, a tyrosine kinase inhibitor, did demonstrate haemodynamic benefits in patients with severe PAH but unfortunately had intolerable side effects, include intracranial haemorrhage [38]. However, it is possible that related tyrosine kinase inhibitors may be of benefit in the future. There is also evidence that epigenetic control of key genes involved in vascular cell turnover is abnormal in patients with PAH. By targeting these abnormalities, it has been possible to reverse pulmonary vascular remodelling in animal models.

References

1. Mesquita SM, Castro CR, Ikari NM, Oliveira SA, Lopes AA. Likelihood of left main coronary artery compression based on pulmonary trunk diameter in patients with pulmonary hypertension. *Am J Med* 2004;**116**:369–74.
2. Abenhaim L, Moride Y, Brenot F *et al*. Appetite-suppressant drugs and the risk of primary pulmonary hypertension. *N Engl J Med* 1996;**335**:609–16.
3. Galiè N, Hoeper MM, Humbert M *et al*.; ESC Committee for Practice Guidelines (CPG). Guidelines for the diagnosis and treatment of pulmonary hypertension: the Task Force for the Diagnosis and Treatment of Pulmonary Hypertension of the European Society of Cardiology (ESC) and the European Respiratory Society (ERS), endorsed by the International Society of Heart and Lung Transplantation (ISHLT). *Eur Heart J* 2009;**30**:2493–537.
4. Simonneau G, Gatzoulis MA, Adatia I *et al*. Updated clinical classification of pulmonary hypertension. *J Am Coll Cardiol* 2013;**62**(25 Suppl):D34–41.
5. Morrell N (2009). Pulmonary hypertension. In: Maskell N, Miller A (eds.) *Oxford Desk Reference Respiratory Medicine*. Oxford: Oxford University Press, pp.264–L 71.
6. Mauritz GJ, Rizopoulos D, Groepenhoff H *et al*. Usefulness of serial N-terminal pro-B-type natriuretic peptide measurements for determining prognosis in patients with pulmonary arterial hypertension. *Am J Cardiol* 2011;**108**:1645–50.
7. British Cardiac Society Guidelines and Medical Practice Committee. Recommendations on the management of pulmonary hypertension in clinical practice. *Heart* 2001;**86**(Suppl I):i1–13.

8. National Pulmonary Hypertension Centres of the UK and Ireland. Consensus statement on the management of pulmonary hypertension in clinical practice in the UK and Ireland. *Thorax* 2008;**63**(Suppl II):ii1–41.
9. Janda S, Shahidi N, Gin K, Swiston J. Diagnostic accuracy of echocardiography for pulmonary hypertension: a systematic review and meta-analysis. *Heart* 2011;**97**:612–22.
10. American Thoracic Society. Guidelines for the six-minute walk test. *Am J Respir Crit Care Med* 2002;**166**:111–17.
11. Miyamoto S, Nagaya N, Satoh T *et al*. Clinical correlates and prognostic significance of six-minute walk test in patients with primary pulmonary hypertension. Comparison with cardiopulmonary exercise testing. *Am J Respir Crit Care Med* 2000;**161**(2 Pt 1):487–92.
12. Rich S, Dantzker DR, Ayres SM *et al*. Primary pulmonary hypertension. A national prospective study. *Ann Intern Med* 1987;**107**:216–23.
13. Sitbon O, Humbert M, Jais X *et al*. Long-term response to calcium channel blockers in idiopathic pulmonary arterial hypertension. *Circulation* 2005;**111**:3105–11.
14. Galiè N, Ghofrani HA, Torbicki A *et al*. (2005). Sildenafil citrate therapy for pulmonary arterial hypertension. *N Engl J Med* 2005;**353**:2148–57.
15. Rubin LJ, Badesch DB, Barst RJ *et al*. Bosentan therapy for pulmonary arterial hypertension. *N Engl J Med* 2002;**346**:896–903.
16. Humbert M, Barst RJ, Robbins IM *et al*. Combination of bosentan with epoprostenol in pulmonary arterial hypertension: BREATHE-2. *Eur Resp J* 2004;**24**:353–9.
17. Galiè N, Rubin Lj, Hoeper M *et al*. Treatment of patients with mildly symptomatic pulmonary arterial hypertension with bosentan (EARLY study): a double-blind, randomised controlled trial. *Lancet* 2008;**371**:2093–100.
18. Shah AA, Wigley FM, Hummers LK. Telangiectases in scleroderma: a potential clinical marker of pulmonary arterial hypertension. *J Rheumatol* 2010;**37**:98–104.
19. Behr J, Ryu JH. Pulmonary hypertension in interstitial lung disease. *Eur Respir J* 2008;**31**:1357–67.
20. White B. Interstitial lung disease in scleroderma. *Rheum Dis Clin North Am* 2003;**29**:371–90.
21. Fuster V, Steele PM, Edwards WD, Gersh BJ, McGoon MD, Frye RL. Primary pulmonary hypertension: natural history and the importance of thrombosis. *Circulation* 1984;**70**:580–7.
22. Kawut SM, Horn EM, Berekashvili KK *et al*. New predictors of outcome in idiopathic pulmonary arterial hypertension. *Am J Cardiol* 2005;**95**:199–203.
23. Rich S, Kaufmann E, Levy PS. The effect of high doses of calcium-channel blockers on survival in primary pulmonary hypertension. *N Engl J Med* 1992;**327**:76–81.
24. Olsson KM, Delcroix M, Ghofrani HA *et al*. Anticoagulation and survival in pulmonary arterial hypertension: results from the Comparative, Prospective Registry of Newly Initiated Therapies for Pulmonary Hypertension (COMPERA). *Circulation* 2014;**129**:57–65.
25. British Thoracic Society Working Group on Home Oxygen Services (2006). *Clinical component for the home oxygen service in England and Wales*. Available at: <https://www.brit-thoracic.org.uk/document-library/clinical-information/oxygen/home-oxygen-guideline-(adults)/bts-home-oxygen-in-adults-clinical-component/>.
26. Barst RJ, Rubin LJ, Long WA *et al*.; Primary Pulmonary Hypertension Study Group. A comparison of continuous intravenous epoprostenol (prostacyclin) with conventional therapy for primary pulmonary hypertension. *N Engl J Med* 1996;**334**:296–302.
27. Fox BD, Shimony A, Langleben D. Meta-analysis of monotherapy versus combination therapy for pulmonary arterial hypertension. *Am J Cardiol* 2011;**108**:1177–82.
28. Simonneau G, Rubin LJ, Galiè N *et al*.; PACES Study Group. Addition of sildenafil to long-term intravenous epoprostenol therapy in patients with pulmonary arterial hypertension: a randomized trial. *Ann Intern Med* 2008;**149**:521–30.
29. Galiè N, Barberà JA, Frost A *et al*. Initial Use of Ambrisentan plus Tadalafil in Pulmonary Arterial Hypertension. *N Engl J Med* 2015;**373**:834–844.

30. Ibrahim R, Granton JT, Mehta S. An open-label, multicentre pilot study of bosentan in pulmonary arterial hypertension related to congenital heart disease. *Can Respir J* 2006 Nov-Dec;**13**:415–20.
31. Galiè N, Beghetti M, Gatzoulis MA *et al.* Bosentan therapy in patients with Eisenmenger syndrome: a multicenter, double-blind, randomized, placebo-controlled study. *Circulation* 2006;**114**:48–54.
32. Pulido T, Adzerikho I, Channick RN *et al.*; SERAPHIN Investigators. Macitentan and morbidity and mortality in pulmonary arterial hypertension. *N Engl J Med* 2013;**369**:809–18.
33. Wilkins MR, Paul GA, Strange JW, *et al.* Sildenafil versus Endothelin Receptor Antagonist for Pulmonary Hypertension (SERAPH) study. *Am J Respir Crit Care Med* 2005;**171**:1292–7.
34. McGoon MD, Miller DP. A contemporary US pulmonary arterial hypertension register. *Eur Respir Rev* 2012;**21**:8–18.
35. Trulock EP, Edwards LB, Taylor DO *et al.* Registry of the International Society for Heart and Lung Transplantation: twenty-third official adult lung and heart-lung transplantation report—2006. *J Heart Lung Transplant* 2006;**25**:880–92.
36. Ghofrani HA, Galiè N, Grimminger F *et al.*; PATENT-1 Study Group. Riociguat for the treatment of pulmonary arterial hypertension. *N Engl J Med* 2013;**369**:330–40.
37. Ghofrani HA, D'Armini AM, Grimminger F *et al.*; CHEST-1 Study Group. Riociguat for the treatment of chronic thromboembolic pulmonary hypertension. *N Engl J Med* 2013;**369**:319–29.
38. Hoeper MM, Barst RJ, Bourge RC *et al.* Imatinib mesylate as add-on therapy for pulmonary arterial hypertension: results of the randomized IMPRES study. *Circulation* 2013;**127**:1128–38.

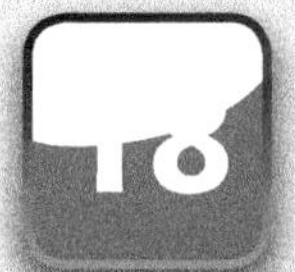

Sleep-disordered breathing in the obese

Swapna Mandal

Expert commentary Joerg Steier

Case history

A 48-year-old female in acute respiratory distress was brought by ambulance to the A&E department. The family informed the medical team that she has been increasingly unwell over the past 4 days; she has become more breathless and could no longer get up from her chair due to her breathlessness. She has been confused and increasingly sleepy. On the day of admission, her family were having difficulty waking her and therefore called an ambulance.

On examination, she was morbidly obese with a BMI of >50 kg/m^2; the family informed the medical team she was 1.62 m (5 ft 4 inches) and weighed approximately 150 kg. She was confused, with a GCS score of 11/15 (eyes: opening to pain; voice: her speech was confused and disoriented; movement: she localized to painful stimuli; E2 V4 M5). Auscultation of her heart sounds was difficult, but she had bilateral crepitations to the mid zones; her JVP was elevated at 4 cm (normal <3 cm above the sternal angle)l and she has peripheral oedema up to her abdomen.

An ECG was performed and demonstrated right ventricular hypertrophy with a strain pattern (Figure 18.1). Her ABG showed decompensated hypercapnic respiratory failure (Table 18.1).

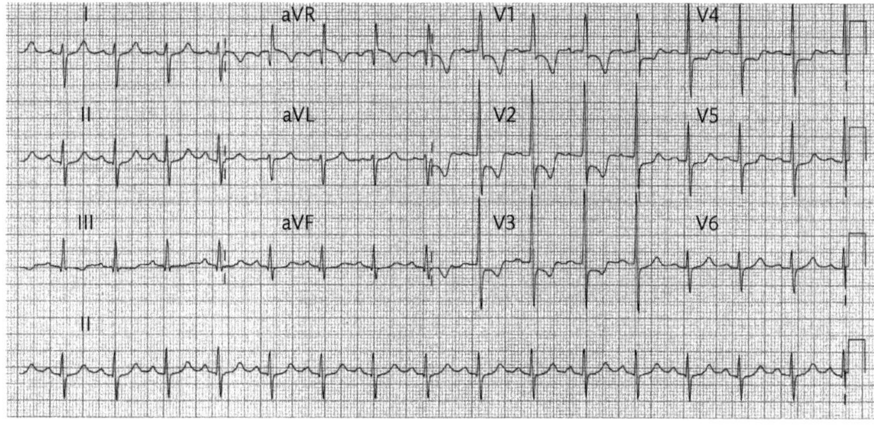

Figure 18.1 The patient's ECG demonstrating right ventricular hypertrophy with a strain pattern. Diagnostic criteria for right ventricular hypertrophy on ECG include: right axis deviation, dominant R wave in V1, and dominant S wave in V5 or V6. Supporting characteristics include: right ventricular strain pattern (ST depression or T wave inversion in V1–V4 and II, III, and aVF) and deep S waves in I and aVL.

Source: Reproduced with permission from Dr Mike Cadogan, *www.lifeinthefastlane.com*.

Table 18.1 Arterial blood gas taken on room air demonstrating acidotic type 2 respiratory failure (low pO_2 and high pCO_2)

Parameter (normal values)	Patient value (unit)
pH (7.35–7.45)	7.28
pO_2 (11–13)	6.87 kPa
pCO_2 (4.5–6.0)	10.81 kPa
HCO_3 (22–26)	32.3 mEq/L

Learning point Definitions of obesity

There are various ways to define obesity, but most commonly obesity is defined by the body mass index (BMI). The BMI is derived from an individual's body weight (in kilograms), compared to their height (in metres) squared. To calculate the BMI, the following equation is used [1]:

$$\text{BMI} = \text{Weight (kg)} / \text{height (m)}^2$$

The classification of obesity by the WHO is shown below (Table 18.2).

Table 18.2 Classification of body mass index

BMI (kg/m^2)	Classification
<18.5	Underweight
18.5–24.9	Normal
25–29.9	Overweight
30–34.9	Class I obesity
35–39.9	Class II obesity
>40	Class III obesity

Further definitions have been added by the surgical literature, which classifies a BMI of >40 kg/m^2 as severe obesity and >50 kg/m^2 as super obese.

It must be mentioned that these thresholds are valid for the Caucasian population but may be different in other populations.

Further history from her family revealed that she has had a 6-month history of increasing daytime somnolence and often fell asleep during meal times; her weight had been steadily increasing, whilst her mobility had been decreasing. She has been housebound for the last 4 months; she could no longer walk to her bedroom and therefore slept in a chair in the lounge. Her family have also noted that she has episodes of choking, whilst asleep, and sometimes stops breathing. Her past medical history includes type 2 diabetes mellitus and hypertension; she takes metformin 1 g tds, furosemide 40 mg od, and ramipril 5 mg od.

Based on the history and following the clinical assessment, a diagnosis of acute decompensated hypercapnic respiratory failure secondary to likely combined obstructive sleep apnoea hypopnoea syndrome (OSAHS) and obesity hypoventilation syndrome (OHS) with concomitant right heart failure was made.

Learning point Definitions of sleep-disordered breathing

Obesity has become more prevalent, with a quarter of the UK population estimated to have a BMI of >30 kg/m^2 [2]. Sleep-disordered breathing, which includes OSAHS and OHS, is common in the obese population, with up to 50% of patients with a BMI of >40 kg/m^2 having OSA [3]. The prevalence of OHS is more difficult to estimate; however, it is suggested that 0.37% of the general population in the US have OHS (i.e. one in 270 adults) [4].

The AASM has established standard definitions for sleep-disordered breathing [5].

Obstructive sleep apnoea hypopnoea syndrome is defined as:

- excessive daytime somnolence not explained by other factors, or
- two of the following:
  - recurrent wakening from sleep;
  - episodes of choking or gasping during sleep;
  - daytime fatigue;
  - impaired concentration;
  - unrefreshing sleep.

And

- overnight sleep study demonstrating >5 obstructive respiratory (apnoeas, hypopnoeas) events per hour.

Obesity hypoventilation syndrome is defined as:

- one or more of the following:
  - excessive daytime somnolence;
  - cor pulmonale;
  - raised haematocrit;
  - evidence of PH;
  - daytime hypercapnia ($PaCO_2$ >6 kPa or >45 mmHg).

And

- one of the following:
  - oxygen desaturations during overnight monitoring not explained by obstructive apnoeic or hypopnoeic events;
  - an increase in $PaCO_2$ of >1.3 kPa or 10 mmHg during sleep, compared to baseline awake values.

Expert comment

Sleep-disordered breathing is common in the general population. Frequently, it is not recognized for years, and we know from surveys of hospital services that it is rarely screened for systematically. The commonest diagnoses of sleep-disordered breathing are OSA and OHS. However, different forms of sleep-disordered breathing may present as CSA, Cheyne–Stokes respiration due to a medical or neurological condition, medication, or altitude. Similarly, alveolar hypoventilation syndrome may be caused by numerous conditions of central origin or different neuromuscular or medical co-morbidities [6]. Less well-known upper airway resistance syndrome has been described to cause sleep disturbance as well [7]. Most sleep-disordered breathing can be successfully treated, and early diagnosis is therefore important to avoid social, occupational, or medical complications.

Treatment

The patient was given 80 mg of IV furosemide and started on bilevel non-invasive ventilation (NIV) via a full face mask, with an IPAP of 18 cmH_2O and an EPAP of 4 cmH_2O. An FiO_2 of 0.40 was delivered via NIV, and the machine set to a backup rate of 18 breaths/minute (four breaths below their respiratory rate when the patient was off NIV),

Table 18.3 Arterial blood gas after 1 hour of treatment with NIV, revealing progression of the patients' respiratory acidosis

Parameter (normal values)	Patient value (unit)
pH (7.35–7.45)	7.16
pO_2 (11–13)	7.8 kPa
pCO_2 (4.5–6.0)	12.2 kPa
HCO_3 (22–26)	31.8 mEq/L

with an inspiratory time (Ti) of 1.2 s. Over the course of an hour, the pressures were increased to an IPAP of 22 cmH_2O and an EPAP of 6 cmH_2O, and an ABG was repeated (Table 18.3).

The patient was noted to be fatiguing. Furthermore, blood tests revealed a deteriorating renal function, with a urea of 22.4 mmol/L (1.7–8.3 mmol/L) and a creatinine of 305 micromoles/L (45–84 micromoles/L). The intensive care team was called to review the patient. It was elicited from the family that furosemide had only been started a week prior to admission, and, since the patient had been so drowsy over the past 4 days, she had not been eating or drinking as she would normally, thus explaining her renal failure. At this time, since the patient had two organ failure (respiratory and renal) and her condition was deteriorating, a decision was made to intubate the patient and take her to the ICU.

Learning point Pulmonary mechanics in the obese

The mechanisms underlying ventilatory failure in obese patients are complex and multifactorial. Pulmonary mechanics in the obese are different, compared to lean individuals, with an increased work of breathing and load on the respiratory system which is further exacerbated when the supine position is adopted.

The BMI is known to correlate positively with airways resistance and the work of breathing, with studies demonstrating smaller peripheral airways in the obese. Obesity frequently causes a restrictive defect, with these individuals breathing at a low functional residual capacity (FRC) [8, 9]. It has been demonstrated that, compared to normal individuals, those with obesity have reduced respiratory compliance, and this reduction in compliance is more marked in those with OHS [10].

Breathing at low lung volumes causes expiratory flow limitation, due to early airway closure, and increases the intrinsic PEEP [11]; this results in an increased work of breathing [12, 13] and high neural respiratory drive [11].

In uncomplicated obesity, subjects tend to breathe more rapidly at lower tidal volumes to overcome the hypoxia and hypercapnia imposed by these physiological changes [14]; however, this response does not occur in OHS, suggesting that the changes in pulmonary mechanics alone cannot explain the diurnal hypercapnia. It is thought that the development of hypercapnia in OHS may be due to an interaction between various factors, including sleep-disordered breathing, altered pulmonary mechanics, and ventilatory drive.

Studies have demonstrated high neural respiratory drive in uncomplicated obesity, compared to non-obese subjects; however, hypercapnic and hypoxic ventilatory challenges in OHS have demonstrated a blunted response [11, 15-17], suggesting an imbalanced load-to-capacity ratio in obesity.

Furthermore, OHS causes sleep fragmentation, which may further blunt the hypercapnic and hypoxic response, and prolonged repetitive oxygen desaturations experienced during sleep may further contribute to daytime hypercapnia [18].

Evidence base

To study the load imposed upon the respiratory system by obesity, Steier *et al.* recorded the neural respiratory drive, as measured by the diaphragm electromyography (EMGdi), and the work of breathing, as measured by the oesophageal, gastric, and transdiaphragmatic pressures, in 30 obese and 30 normal-weight subjects.

Those subjects with obesity had an increased ventilatory load and neural respiratory drive, as measured by EMGdi (21.9 (9.0) versus 8.4 (4.0) % max; $p < 0.001$). Furthermore, in the supine posture, the efficacy of ventilation deteriorated only in obese subjects. This was, in part, explained by an intrinsic PEEP (PEEPi) of 5.3 (3.6) cmH_2O that developed in the obese subjects with a supine posture; applying CPAP in a subset of this group abolished the PEEPi.

This study demonstrated that obese subjects have an increased neural respiratory drive, comparable to patients with moderate to severe COPD, which further increases with a supine posture [11].

Clinical tip The use of NIV in obese patients

The underlying pathophysiology of hypercapnic respiratory failure in OSA/OHS is different to that of COPD, and a different approach to NIV management should therefore be adopted.

When starting patients with isolated OHS or combined OSA/OHS on NIV, consideration of the following points may be useful:

- initial EPAP should be set to ≥4 cmH_2O for those with isolated OHS;
- initial EPAP should be set to ≥8 cmH_2O for those with combined OSA/OHS;
- pressure support (pressure support = IPAP – EPAP) should be set to ≥10 cmH_2O;
- backup rate should be set to four breaths lower than the respiratory rate off NIV;
- Ti should be set at 1.2 s.

Monitor the patient, and, if they remain hypercapnic, consider increasing the IPAP. Increasing the IPAP by 2 cmH_2O will increase the pressure support and improve alveolar ventilation. In the case of acutely unwell patients, the aim should be to decrease the $PaCO_2$ by 1 kPa each hour, until they become eucapnic. In stable patients who are starting domiciliary NIV, the aim should be to decrease the $PaCO_2$ by 0.5–1 kPa overnight or to a $PaCO_2$ of ≤6.5 kPa. Most individuals with OSA/OHS and isolated OHS will require an IPAP of at least 18 cmH_2O.

The EPAP reduces the work of breathing by overcoming the intrinsic PEEP but also prevents upper airway obstruction, and it is therefore comparable to the effect of CPAP, with respect to upper airway collapsibility. The patient should be monitored for ongoing apnoeas and desaturations; if these are noted, mask fitting and leak should be checked, and, if these are satisfactory, the EPAP should be increased by 2 cmH_2O. Patients with OSA/OHS will frequently require EPAP levels of 8–10 cmH_2O to abolish upper airway obstruction. However, adequate pressure support is also needed; therefore, the IPAP should be appropriately adjusted [19].

Over the course of 5 days on the ICU, the patient's ABGs improved. She was invasively ventilated with synchronized intermittent mandatory ventilation, with a PEEP of 10 cmH_2O, a pressure support of 15 cmH_2O above the PEEP, and a respiratory rate of 15 breaths/minute, with the aim of keeping the pCO_2 below 8 kPa. She was gradually weaned and extubated on day 5; she was then placed on to NIV and transferred to the respiratory ward to be established on long-term domiciliary NIV. She also underwent an echocardiogram which demonstrated evidence of moderate tricuspid regurgitation and PH with right ventricular dilatation and a reduced LVEF of 33% (echocardiogram report shown in Table 18.4). Her cardiac medications were optimized; her diuretic (furosemide) dose was increased to 80 mg bd, and she

Table 18.4 Echocardiogram report suggesting moderate PH with left and right ventricular dysfunction

Echocardiogram parameter	Measurement	Normal range
LVEF (%)	33%	>55%
LV diameter (diastolic)	6.2 cm	3.9-5.3 cm
RA	15 mmHg	<10 mmHg
RV systolic function TAPSE (cm−2)	1.7 cm	>2 cm
S^1	9 cm/s	>12 cm/s
RVSP	58 mmHg	<25 mmHg
IVC	IVC mildly dilated (2.4 cm) with some <50% collapse	Fully collapsible, <2 cm in diameter

IVC, inferior vena cava; LV, left ventricle; LVEF, left ventricular ejection fraction; RA, right atrium; RV, right ventricle; RVSP, right ventricular systolic pressure; TAPSE, tricuspid annular plane systolic excursion; TR, tricuspid regurgitation.

was started on a low dose of a beta-blocker (bisoprolol 2.5 mg od). The patient was reviewed by the dietician and given weight loss advice. After further discussion with the medical team, the patient was referred for consideration of bariatric surgery.

Learning point Weaning from invasive ventilation

Weaning obese patients from invasive mechanical ventilation can be particularly challenging. Obese patients with OSA and OHS are particularly at risk of respiratory failure, since the sedative effects of drugs given to intubate these individuals may exacerbate their underlying condition.

Obese patients often develop basal atelectasis, promoted by high intra-abdominal pressures (intra-abdominal hypertension) and posture rendering them hypoxaemic, thus making extubation difficult. Therefore, weaning patients with OHS from ventilation often takes longer due to altered pulmonary mechanics and neural respiratory drive. Furthermore, when extubating sedated patients, thought needs to be given to upper airway patency [20].

The use of NIV in the post-extubation period in the obese decreases ICU length of stay, reduces the risk of respiratory failure, and confers a survival benefit in those who are hypercapnic [21].

Learning point NICE guidance for bariatric surgery

Bariatric surgery for obesity can be considered:

- in those with a BMI ≥40 kg/m^2;
- or a BMI >35 kg/m^2 if they have another significant co-morbid illness, e.g. diabetes mellitus, hypertension, that could be improved with weight loss:
    - providing that other non-surgical interventions have been tried for at least 6 months without success;
    - the patient will be managed by a specialist obesity service;
    - the patient is fit for anaesthesia and surgery;
    - the patient is committed to long-term follow-up.
- as first-line treatment in those with a BMI >50 kg/m^2.

The patient in this case had a BMI of >40 kg/m^2 and had tried other weight loss methods, but had failed and could therefore be considered for bariatric surgery.

Expert comment

Bariatric surgery summarizes the interventions to modify the stomach in order to achieve weight loss. There are different procedures that have been developed, predominantly classified into restrictive (e.g. gastric banding) or malabsorptive (e.g. bypass) interventions; different methods can be combined. The amount of achievable weight loss and side effects are dependent on the procedure selected.

However, patients undergoing bariatric surgery need to adjust their lifestyle if they want to avoid a 'yo-yo' effect of their weight. It has been shown that the weight increases again following the first year post-bariatric surgery [22]. The effect of surgery is less likely to be maintained over time if no other intervention is in place to support the patient in their effort to maintain weight loss. It is therefore crucial to have a multidisciplinary approach towards the morbidly obese patient undergoing bariatric surgery, including medical and respiratory management, psychological, dietician, and motivational support, including exercise training.

Evidence base

A meta-analysis of 136 studies of bariatric surgery, involving a total of 22,094 patients, demonstrated that, in 85.7% of those patients with OSA who underwent bariatric surgery, OSA improved or resolved following significant weight loss [24].

Evidence base

An observational study examining the effects of weight loss in 38 patients with OSA or OHS following bariatric surgery demonstrated significant improvements in respiratory function (FEV_1, FVC, expiratory reserve volume (ERV), FRC, and TLC). Similarly, PaO_2 and $PaCO_2$ significantly improved ($p < 0.01$; see below) over time. There was also an improvement in secondary polycythaemia in some patients (n = 12); the mean haemoglobin content decreased from 16.9 g/dL prior to surgery to 14.9 g/dL post-procedure. The percentage of patients with evidence of OSA decreased from 44% to 8% following surgery [23].

Parameter	Pre-surgery	Post-surgery (3–12 months)
ERV (% predicted)	37 ± 8	76 ± 14
PaO_2 (kPa)	53 ± 9	68 ± 11
$PaCO_2$ (kPa)	51 ± 7	41 ± 4

Discussion

This case discusses an increasingly common presentation to A&E departments; with the increasing prevalence of obesity, so will the prevalence of obesity-related sleep-disordered breathing rise. Current estimates suggest the prevalence of OSA to be 2–24% [25-27] and that of obesity hypoventilation to be up to 30% in hospitalized obese patients [28].

OSAHS is characterized by recurrent complete or partial upper airway obstruction during sleep, in spite of ongoing respiratory effort. The respiratory events cause intermittent oxygen desaturations, sleep fragmentation, and daytime symptoms such as excessive daytime somnolence.

The diagnosis of OSAHS is made through eliciting a careful history of symptoms associated with OSAHS and respiratory polygraphy (Figure 18.2).

An obstructive apnoea is defined as a complete cessation of airflow, demonstrated by a reduction in amplitude in nasal airflow lasting longer than 10 s with ongoing respiratory effort (thoraco-abdominal movement); this is usually followed by a >3% oxygen desaturation or an arousal (sometimes a 4% oxygen desaturation is used).

An obstructive hypopnoea is defined as a reduction in nasal airflow (>50% from baseline) that is associated with a 3% oxygen desaturation or arousal which lasts 10 s or longer, or a reduction of ≥30% in nasal airflow with a ≥4% desaturation.

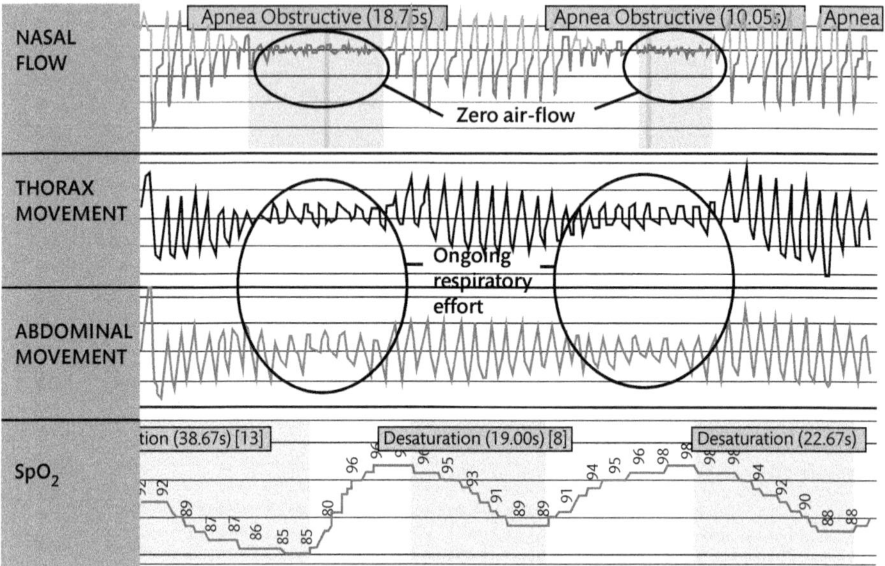

Figure 18.2 Obstructive apnoea with cessation in nasal airflow and ongoing inspiratory effort (measured by thoraco-abdominal movement), followed by oxygen desaturation (SpO_2).

Table 18.5 Severity classification of OSAHS

AHI (h^{-1})	Severity of OSAHS
<5	None (within normal limits)
5–15	Mild
15–30	Moderate
>30	Severe

The severity of OSAHS is determined by the AHI, the number of apnoeas or hypopnoeas per hour of sleep (Table 18.5).

Expert comment

The standard descriptive index to quantify sleep-disordered breathing is the apnoea–hypopnoea index (AHI), counting the number of apnoeas and hypopnoeas per hour of sleep. However, it has become more obvious that sometimes this index does not accurately reflect sleep disturbance from respiratory effort. Some patients arouse from sleep due to RERAs that do not fulfil any of the criteria used to describe apnoeas or hypopnoeas. The number of RERAs plus the number of apnoeas and hypopnoeas per hour of sleep are commonly summarized in the respiratory disturbance index (RDI).

Excessive daytime somnolence can be measured using the MSLT (Table 18.6) or subjectively by asking the patient to complete the validated ESS. This is an 8-item scale in which patients score the likelihood of falling asleep in certain situations (0–3 points for each item, with a score of 0 indicating no likelihood and 3 indicating a high likelihood). A total score of >10 out of a possible 24 points is considered to be indicative of excessive daytime somnolence. However, in the sleep clinic population, lower cut-offs, e.g. 8/24, may be used as well [29].

Table 18.6 Severity of excessive daytime somnolence measured by the MSLT. This test involves asking patients to sleep for four or five 20-minute periods across a day, whilst measuring their EEG activity and the time taken to fall asleep, with a shorter time to sleep indicating more severe sleepiness

Minutes to onset of sleep	Sleepiness
<5	Severe
<10	Moderate
<15	Mild

More recently, other tools have been developed to screen for the likelihood of OSAHS such as the STOP-BANG questionnaire. This questionnaire is currently used as a preoperative screening tool in patients awaiting surgery [30].

Learning point STOP-BANG questionnaire

This questionnaire asks four questions (STOP) and performs four simple measurements (BANG) for completion:

STOP

S—Do you **S**nore loudly?
T—Do you feel **T**ired?
O—Has anybody **O**bserved you stop breathing during your sleep?
P—Do you have high blood **P**ressure?

BANG

B—**B**ody mass index >35 kg/m^2
A—**A**ge >50 (years)
N—**N**eck circumference >40 cm
G—Male **G**ender?

For each question that is answered with a yes, a score of 1 point is given.

The risk of OSA is considered high if a score of 3 or greater is achieved.

The standard management of patients with moderate to severe OSAHS is CPAP. Mandibular advancement devices are an alternative to CPAP in mild OSAHS and can be used in individuals with simple snoring, mild OSAHS patients without daytime somnolence, or those unable to tolerate CPAP. However, these devices are less effective than CPAP in controlling apnoeas and hypopnoeas [31, 32].

CPAP has been shown to restore normal upper airway respiratory control at night and improve daytime symptoms, mood, cognitive function, and HRQoL, including cardiovascular and metabolic risk factors. CPAP acts as a 'pneumatic splint' and maintains upper airway patency during sleep. Ideally, patients should be titrated to an individual pressure level, and this can be achieved by manual titration overnight or by using an autoset CPAP [33, 34]. These devices determine the pressure required to maintain the upper airway patency. The usage data can be stored and interrogated to find the minimum pressure required to maintain upper airway patency. Eventually, patients are given a fixed-pressure CPAP machine. CPAP should be used for a minimum of 4 hours per night, but longer use achieves greater effects [35, 36].

Evidence base

The first landmark trial evaluating the use of CPAP in OSA was published in 1981 in *The Lancet*. Sullivan *et al.* generated CPAP for five patients with severe OSA by connecting a vacuum cleaner blower motor to soft plastic tubes which were inserted into the nostrils. At that time, the patients would have been offered tracheostomies to treat their OSA due to a lack of alternative treatment options.

Application of 7.5 cmH_2O of CPAP abolished the obstructive events in these five patients when asleep. It was also demonstrated that CPAP could be worn for consecutive nights without adverse effects, thus heralding the beginning of a new era of treatment for OSA [37].

Patients with enlarged tonsils or other anatomical abnormalities, e.g. polyps, should be referred to an ENT surgeon for consideration of removal in order to improve symptoms. Uvulopalatopharyngoplasty (UPPP) is no longer recommended as treatment for patients with OSA. Patients should also be advised of general sleep hygiene measures (see Learning point, p. 226). Weight loss through medical or surgical methods can contribute significantly to reducing the AHI and, in some cases, can be curative [38, 39].

Expert comment

Currently, the best treatments for sleep-disordered breathing are the use of CPAP or NIV therapy, as indicated. However, it has to be mentioned that CPAP requires individual pressure adjustment, and NIV requires further patient–ventilator synchronization, which complicates the initial set-up.

For CPAP treatment, it is possible to have pressures titrated manually using feedback via a monitoring device (e.g. sleep study) or to use an automated (autoset) pressure titration; both options are similarly effective [33, 40].

For NIV, it is difficult to generate correct settings automatically. NIV requires more specific adjustment of several pressure levels for different conditions, and, due to the complexity of inspiratory and expiratory pressures, timing, and trigger sensitivities, it is more accurately guided by experienced clinicians. However, self-titrating semi-automated devices to adjust several features (e.g. EPAP) are currently developed, and future advances in technology and understanding of pathophysiological conditions may allow easier and more successful automated NIV set-up.

Learning point Sleep hygiene

All patients attending sleep disorder clinics should be advised of the following to improve their sleep quality.

- Have a fixed sleep and wake time.
- Avoid sleeping during the day.
- Avoid alcohol 4 hours prior to sleep.
- Avoid caffeine 4 hours prior to sleep.
- Avoid nicotine 4 hours prior to sleep.
- Avoid distractions in the bedroom, e.g. televisions; do not use the bedroom as workspace.
- Ensure the bedroom is dark and quiet and is at an optimal temperature.
- Regular exercise is good for sleep; however, refrain from doing this 4 hours prior to sleep.

OHS is defined as the development of daytime hypercapnia ($PaCO_2$ >45 mmHg or >6 kPa) in individuals with a BMI of >30 kg/m^2, in association with features of PH and demonstration of episodes of prolonged severe desaturation without repetitive

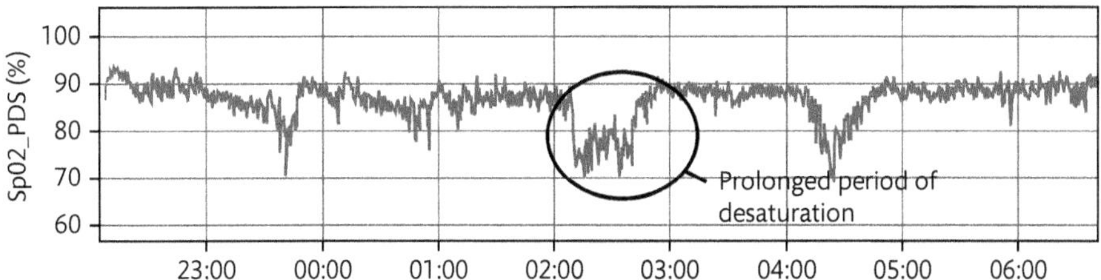

Figure 18.3 Overnight oximetry demonstrating several periods of prolonged desaturation, with the oxygen saturations dropping to approximately 70%; the 4% oxygen desaturation index (a marker of AHI) for this oximetry was 9 events/hour.

apnoeic/hypopnoeic episodes on sleep studies, no signs of neuromuscular weakness, or concomitant pulmonary disease (Figure 18.3) [5].

Hypoventilation syndrome in obesity can exist as isolated OHS and OHS with OSA, with studies demonstrating that up to 30% of obese patients with OSA may have an element of OHS [41].

Treatment of OHS requires a multidisciplinary approach. Most importantly, steps should be taken to encourage weight loss. Significant weight loss through either conventional or surgical methods can result in significant improvement in pulmonary mechanics and ventilation and sometimes even provide a cure. Bariatric surgery has been more successful than medical methods in achieving significant weight loss; but without lifestyle adjustment, there is a certain degree of fluctuation in weight following gastric banding or gastric bypass surgery. Timely institution of positive airway pressure treatment is essential, but it has not been established whether CPAP or bilevel positive airway pressure (NIV) is the most effective mode of treatment, with studies demonstrating some efficacy in both [42, 43]. Bilevel positive airway pressure may be seen as the more advantageous mode of treatment, as it is a mode of ventilation which maintains upper airway patency, but also reduces respiratory muscle loading and improves gas exchange. This treatment has been shown to improve symptoms, quality of life, ventilatory parameters, and outcomes both in the short and long term [44]. A reasonable approach is to start patients on bilevel positive airway pressure ventilation and repeat an ABG at 3 months; if the patient has become eucapnic, they can be changed to CPAP, and those who remain hypercapnic should continue with bilevel positive airway pressure ventilation [45] (Figure 18.4).

Evidence base

Murphy *et al.* compared an autotitrated NIV mode (average volume-assured pressure support, AVAPS) with fixed-level pressure support in OHS, to determine if this hybrid mode of ventilation was advantageous, compared to a manual titrated NIV set-up.

A total of 50 patients were randomized, and, at 3 months, significant improvements in $PaCO_2$ were noted (AVAPS $PaCO_2\Delta$ −0.6 kPa; $p < 0.01$ versus manual pressure support mode (PS) $PaCO_2\Delta$ −0.6 kPa; $p = 0.02$); however, no significant differences were noted between the manual and automated set-ups.

There were also significant improvements in severe respiratory insufficiency questionnaire scores and daytime physical activity, with no group differences, suggesting that both modes of ventilation were similarly effective in the management of OHS [19].

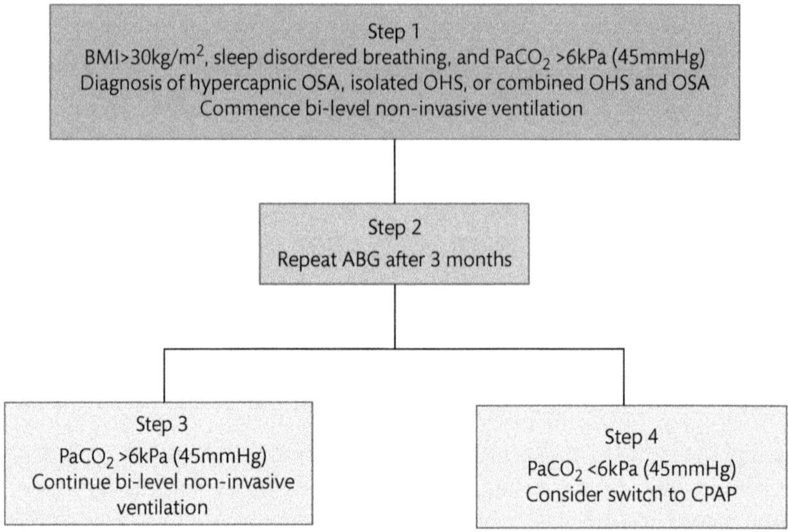

Figure 18.4 Management strategy for patients with obesity-related respiratory failure.

Source: Mandal & Hart, Clinical Medicine 2012. Modified and reproduced with permission from Clinical Medicine [45].

Obesity can also complicate other chronic respiratory conditions such as asthma and COPD.

Patients with COPD may develop hypoxia and hypercapnia due to the severity of their underlying disease. These physiological changes may worsen during sleep and, when combined with OSA, result in a failure to restore normal ventilation following apnoeic events. This combination of OSA and COPD, termed the **overlap syndrome**, is seen more commonly in COPD patients who tend to be more obese than those with isolated COPD. This syndrome should be considered in patients in whom the severity of COPD would not fully explain their respiratory failure or symptoms. Diagnosis of overlap syndrome requires a sleep study with oximetry and transcutaneous capnography. The treatment is complicated by the fact that some treatments given to treat COPD may worsen OSA. LTOT may worsen nocturnal hypercapnia; oral steroids may be required for exacerbation periods but contribute not only to weight gain, but also to muscle weakness, and, in some cases, patients will have been prescribed anxiolytics which will interfere with their ventilatory response and neural respiratory drive. Studies investigating the optimum treatment for this group of patients are similarly difficult to design. In those with predominant OSA without significant type 2 respiratory failure, CPAP can be the treatment of choice. In patients with significant type 2 respiratory failure, bilevel positive airway pressure ventilation (NIV) should be considered. In the past, studies have been focussed on patients with isolated COPD but have demonstrated improvements in symptoms and HRQoL [46].

Epidemiological studies have suggested a relationship between obesity and asthma. However, there have been conflicting data regarding the underlying pathophysiological mechanisms. It is known that obesity is associated with systemic inflammation, and this may contribute to an inflammatory response in asthma. There is evidence to suggest that increased bronchial hyper-reactivity correlates with the BMI. Obesity is associated with diminished lung volumes, early airway closure, and a reduction in the diameter of the peripheral airways, and this may mimic airway obstruction, similar to asthma. Furthermore, the relationship between obesity and sleep-disordered breathing and obesity and gastro-oesophageal reflux is well established, and these co-morbidities are known to contribute to poor asthma control [47-50]. Coexisting obesity results in increased symptoms, hospital attendances, and medication use in asthma. Weight loss in these individuals improves airflow limitation and symptom control, increases the FRC, and reduces the diurnal PEF variability, exacerbation rates, and medication use [51-54].

With an increase in the prevalence of obesity, physicians are likely to see a rise in patients with the respiratory complications of obesity. Obese patients deserve careful consideration when managing or preventing respiratory failure. Invasive ventilation during emergencies can be technically difficult but can also result in a prolonged, difficult weaning period. Patients with stable hypercapnic respiratory failure should be managed with non-invasive positive airway pressure treatment at the earliest opportunity to achieve good clinical and physiological outcomes [43]. However, ultimately, the underlying problem of excess weight needs to be targeted to prevent patients from developing acute or chronic respiratory complications.

A final word from the expert

Sleep-disordered breathing affects large parts of the population. If present, it significantly impairs social functioning, causes excessive daytime sleepiness, and increases cardiovascular and metabolic risks. It also puts the patient at risk of developing hypercapnic respiratory failure and may only be recognized when it causes acute problems (e.g. in the perioperative period). Treatment of sleep-disordered breathing is highly effective and well established, but, as the patient is often unaware of the condition, it is important that health-care professionals ask for specific symptoms and screen systematically.

Sleep-disordered breathing has a positive correlation with obesity. It is therefore likely that health-care professionals will be confronted with more severe and untreated cases in the future. In morbidly obese subjects, it will be important to consider an MDT approach, including exercise programmes, to improve success in the management of such patients.

References

1. World Health Organization. *BMI classification*. Available at: <http://apps.who.int/bmi/index.jsp?introPage=intro_3.html>.
2. Craig R, Mindell J, Hirani V (2008). *Health Survey for England 2008. Volume 1: Physical Activity and Fitness*. Leeds: NHS Information Centre.
3. Resta O, Foschino-Barbaro MP, Legari G *et al*. Sleep-related breathing disorders, loud snoring and excessive daytime sleepiness in obese subjects. *Int J Obes Relat Metab Disord* 2001;**25**:669–75.
4. Mokhlesi B, Saager L, Kaw R. Should we routinely screen for hypercapnia in sleep apnea patients before elective noncardiac surgery? *Cleve Clin J Med* 2010;**77**:60–1.
5. The Report of an American Academy of Sleep Medicine Task Force. Sleep-related breathing disorders in adults: recommendations for syndrome definition and measurement techniques in clinical research. *Sleep* 1999;**22**:667–89.

6. American Academy of Sleep Medicine (2001). *The International Classification of Sleep Disorders, Revised (Diagnostic and Coding Manual)*. Westchester, IL: American Academy of Sleep Medicine.
7. Guilleminault C, Stoohs R, Clerk A, Cetel M, Maistros P. A cause of excessive daytime sleepiness. The upper airway resistance syndrome. *Chest* 1993;**104**:781–87.
8. Zerah F, Harf A, Perlemuter L, Lorino H, Lorino AM, Atlan G. Effects of obesity on respiratory resistance. *Chest* 1993;**103**:1470–6.
9. King GG, Brown NJ, Diba C *et al*. The effects of body weight on airway calibre. *Eur Respir J* 2005;**25**:896–901.
10. Naimark A, Cherniack RM. Compliance of the respiratory system and its components in health and obesity. *J Appl Physiol* 1960;**15**:377–82.
11. Steier J, Jolley CJ, Seymour J, Roughton M, Polkey MI, Moxham J. Neural respiratory drive in obesity. *Thorax* 2009;**64**:719–25.
12. Sharp JT, Henry JP, Sweany SK, Meadows WR, Pietras RJ. The total work of breathing in normal and obese men.*J Clin Invest* 1964;**43**:728–39.
13. Pelosi P, Croci M, Ravagnan I *et al*. The effects of body mass on lung volumes, respiratory mechanics, and gas exchange during general anesthesia. *Anesth Analg* 1998;**87**:654–60.
14. Luce JM. Respiratory complications of obesity. *Chest* 1980;**78**:626–31.
15. Lopata M, Onal E. Mass loading, sleep apnea, and the pathogenesis of obesity hypoventilation. *Am Rev Respir Dis* 1982;**126**:640–5.
16. Javaheri S, Colangelo G, Lacey W, Gartside PS. Chronic hypercapnia in obstructive sleep apnea-hypopnea syndrome. *Sleep* 1994;**17**:416–23.
17. Sampson MG, Grassino K. Neuromechanical properties in obese patients during carbon dioxide rebreathing. *Am J Med* 1983;**75**:81–90.
18. White DP, Douglas NJ, Pickett CK, Zwillich CW, Weil JV. Sleep deprivation and the control of ventilation. *Am Rev Respir Dis* 1983;**128**:984–6.
19. Murphy PB, Davidson C, Hind MD *et al*. Volume targeted versus pressure support non-invasive ventilation in patients with super obesity and chronic respiratory failure: a randomised controlled trial.*Thorax*, 2012;**67**:727–34.
20. Miehsler W. Mortality, morbidity and special issues of obese ICU patients. *Wien Med Wochenschr* 2010;**160**(5–6):124–8.
21. El-Solh AA, Aquilina A, Pineda L, Dhanvantri V, Grant B, Bouquin P. Noninvasive ventilation for prevention of post-extubation respiratory failure in obese patients. *Eur Respir J* 2006;**28**:588–95.
22. Christiansen T, Bruun JM, Madsen EL, Richelsen B. Weight loss maintenance in severely obese adults after an intensive lifestyle intervention: 2- to 4-year follow-up. *Obesity (Silver Spring)* 2007;**15**:413–20.
23. Sugerman HJ, Fairman RP, Baron PL, Kwentus JA. Gastric surgery for respiratory insufficiency of obesity. *Chest* 1986;**90**:81–6.
24. Buchwald H, Avidor Y, Braunwald E *et al*. Bariatric surgery: a systematic review and meta-analysis. *JAMA* 2004;**292**:1724–37.
25. Young T, Palta M, Dempsey J, Skatrud J, Weber S, Badr S. The occurrence of sleep-disordered breathing among middle-aged adults. *N Engl J Med* 1993;**328**:1230–5.
26. Young T, Peppard PE, Taheri S. Excess weight and sleep-disordered breathing. *J Appl Physiol* 2005;**99**:1592–9.
27. Young T, Shahar E, Nieto FJ *et al*. Predictors of sleep-disordered breathing in community-dwelling adults: the Sleep Heart Health Study. *Arch Intern Med* 2002;**162**:893–900.
28. Nowbar S, Burkart KM, Gonzales R *et al*. Obesity-associated hypoventilation in hospitalized patients: prevalence, effects, and outcome. *Am J Med* 2004;**116**:1–7.
29. Rosenthal LD, Dolan DC. The Epworth sleepiness scale in the identification of obstructive sleep apnea. *J Nerv Ment Dis* 2008;**196**:429–31.

30. Chung F, Yegneswaran B, Liao P *et al.* STOP questionnaire: a tool to screen patients for obstructive sleep apnea. *Anesthesiology* 2008;**108**:812–21.
31. Engleman HM, Martin SE, Deary IJ, Douglas NJ. Effect of continuous positive airway pressure treatment on daytime function in sleep apnoea/hypopnoea syndrome. *Lancet* 1994;**343**:572–5.
32. Giles TL, Lasserson TJ, Smith BH, White J, Wright J, Cates CJ. Continuous positive airways pressure for obstructive sleep apnoea in adults. *Cochrane Database Syst Rev* 2006;**3**:CD001106.
33. Teschler H, Berthon-Jones M, Thompson AB, Henkel A, Henry J, Konietzko N. Automated continuous positive airway pressure titration for obstructive sleep apnea syndrome. *Am J Respir Crit Care Med* 1996;**154**(3 Pt 1):734–40.
34. Brown LK. Autotitrating CPAP: how shall we judge safety and efficacy of a 'black box'? *Chest* 2006;**130**:312–14.
35. Montserrat JM, Ferrer M, Hernandez L *et al.* Effectiveness of CPAP treatment in daytime function in sleep apnea syndrome: a randomized controlled study with an optimized placebo. *Am J Respir Crit Care Med*, 2001;**164**:608–13.
36. Monasterio C, Vidal S, Duran J *et al.* Effectiveness of continuous positive airway pressure in mild sleep apnea-hypopnea syndrome. *Am J Respir Crit Care Med* 2001;**164**:939–43.
37. Sullivan CE, Issa FG, Berthon-Jones M, Eves L. Reversal of obstructive sleep apnoea by continuous positive airway pressure applied through the nares. *Lancet* 1981;**1**:862–5.
38. Barvaux VA, Aubert G, Rodenstein DO. Weight loss as a treatment for obstructive sleep apnoea. *Sleep Med Rev* 2000;**4**:435–52.
39. Rao A, Tey BH, Ramalingam G, Poh AG. Obstructive sleep apnoea (OSA) patterns in bariatric surgical practice and response of OSA to weight loss after laparoscopic adjustable gastric banding (LAGB). *Ann Acad Med Singapore* 2009;**38**:587–93.
40. Meurice JC, Marc I, Sériès F. Efficacy of auto-CPAP in the treatment of obstructive sleep apnea/hypopnea syndrome. *Am J Respir Crit Care Med* 1996;**153**:794–8.
41. Mokhlesi B, Tulaimat A, Faibussowitsch I, Wang Y, Evans AT. Obesity hypoventilation syndrome: prevalence and predictors in patients with obstructive sleep apnea. *Sleep Breath* 2007;**11**:117–24.
42. Piper AJ, Wang D, Yee BJ, Barnes DJ, Grunstein RR. Randomised trial of CPAP vs bilevel support in the treatment of obesity hypoventilation syndrome without severe nocturnal desaturation. *Thorax* 2008;**63**:395–401.
43. Masa JF. The Obesity Hypoventilation Syndrome Can Be Treated With Noninvasive Mechanical Ventilation. *Chest* 2001;**119**:1102–7.
44. de Llano LAP. Short-term and long-term effects of nasal intermittent positive pressure ventilation in patients with obesity-hypoventilation syndrome. *Chest* 2005;**128**:587–94.
45. Mandal S, Hart N. Respiratory complications of obesity. *Clin Med* 2012;**12**:75–8.
46. Clini E, Sturani C, Rossi A. The Italian multicentre study on noninvasive ventilation in chronic obstructive pulmonary disease patients. *Eur Respir J* 2002;**20**:529–38.
47. Beuther DA, Sutherland ER. Overweight, obesity, and incident asthma: a meta-analysis of prospective epidemiologic studies. *Am J Respir Crit Care Med* 2007;**175**:661–6.
48. Greenberg AS, Obin MS. Obesity and the role of adipose tissue in inflammation and metabolism. *Am J Clin Nutr* 2006;**83**:461S–5S.
49. Chinn S, Jarvis D, Burney P. Relation of bronchial responsiveness to body mass index in the ECRHS. European Community Respiratory Health Survey. *Thorax* 2002;**57**:1028–33.
50. Sabaté JM, Jouët P, Merrouche M *et al.* Gastroesophageal reflux in patients with morbid obesity: a role of obstructive sleep apnea syndrome? *Obes Surg* 2008;**18**:1479–84.

51. Rodrigo GJ, Plaza V. Body mass index and response to emergency department treatment in adults with severe asthma exacerbations: a prospective cohort study. *Chest* 2007;**132**:1513–19.
52. Eneli IU, Skybo T, Camargo CA Jr. Weight loss and asthma: a systematic review. *Thorax* 2008;**63**:671–6.
53. Hakala K, Stenius-Aarniala B, Sovijarvi A. Effects of weight loss on peak flow variability, airways obstruction, and lung volumes in obese patients with asthma. *Chest* 2000;**118**:1315–21.
54. Stenius-Aarniala B, Poussa T, Kvarnström J, Grönlund EL, Ylikahri M, Mustajoki P. Immediate and long term effects of weight reduction in obese people with asthma: randomised controlled study. *BMJ* 2000;**320**:827–32.

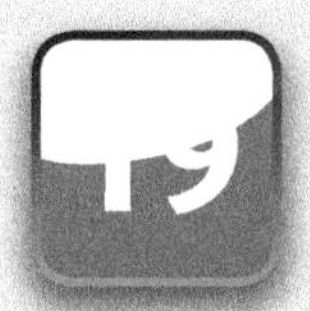

Pulmonary sarcoidosis

Chloe Bloom

Expert commentary Seamus Donnelly

Case history

A 25-year-old female was referred to the respiratory clinic after a diagnosis of intermediate uveitis. She had initially presented with painless, dry eyes, with visual impairment and floaters. She had felt otherwise well in herself. She had a treated vitamin B12 deficiency in the past and did not take any regular medications. She was born in Kenya and moved to the UK 15 years ago. Her parents were originally from India. She was married, with a 1-year-old daughter, smoked about five cigarettes a day and did not drink alcohol. Her mother and aunt had both been diagnosed with sarcoidosis in the past. Her father had treated hypertension.

In the respiratory clinic, her eye symptoms were improving with corticosteroid eye drops. She had no respiratory symptoms, including no complaints of cough, chest pain, or breathlessness. Her CXR showed bilateral hilar lymph node enlargement, with no focal lung lesions (Figure 19.1). She had a number of blood tests requested, including full blood count, angiotensin-converting enzyme (ACE), immunoglobulins, and interferon-gamma release assay (IGRA). She also had a tuberculin skin test (TST), lung function tests, and an HRCT requested. She was booked for a bronchoscopy and transbronchial biopsy (TBBx).

Clinical tip Familial sarcoidosis

There is a significant risk of sarcoidosis in first- and second-degree relatives of patients with sarcoidosis. This risk is highest in siblings and higher in white Americans than African-Americans [1]. This tendency towards familial clustering provides strong evidence for a genetic susceptibility in sarcoidosis.

Expert comment

Familial sarcoidosis is well recognized and a significant concern to sarcoidosis patients. An analysis of US patients in the ACCESS study found an enhanced risk in children of sarcoidosis patients, with an overall odds ratio of 5.8. However, Caucasian patients had a significantly enhanced risk, with an odds ratio of 18.0 [1].

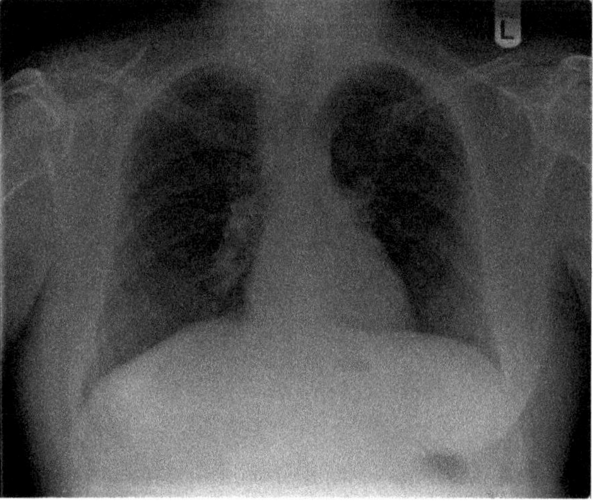

Figure 19.1 CXR demonstrating bilateral hilar lymph node enlargement.

Table 19.1 **Scadding's criteria describing the radiological grading for sarcoidosis**

CXR stage	Radiological findings	Spontaneous resolution
Stage 1	BHL	75%
Stage 2	BHL and lung opacities	60%
Stage 3	Shrinking BHL and lung opacities	<30%
Stage 4	Lung fibrosis	None

*BHL, bilateral hilar lymphadenopathy.

Learning point Diagnosis of pulmonary sarcoidosis

Patients often present with a heterogeneous clinical picture, with pulmonary involvement occurring in over 90%. The skin is involved in at least 30% of patients and the eye in about 25%. When assessing patients with suspected sarcoidosis, no single test is specific enough or sensitive enough for diagnosis. The ATS, ERS, and World Association for Sarcoidosis and Other Granulomatous Disorders (WASOG) consensus statement asserts that a diagnosis should only be made by those with a specialist interest in sarcoidosis, using compatible histological, radiological, and clinical findings, with the exclusion of other granulomatous disorders [2]. This remains the most acknowledged and recognized diagnostic pathway of pulmonary sarcoidosis.

- Non-caseating granulomas and exclusion of alternative cause (e.g. TB, histoplasmosis, beryllium).
- TBBx is the recommended procedure in most cases.
- Endobronchial ultrasound (EBUS)-guided biopsies of mediastinal adenopathy is being utilized much more.
- In patients with Löfgren's syndrome (see Clinical tip, p. 235), a biopsy is not required.
- CXR is graded according to the Scadding's criteria (Table 19.1).
- HRCT may be useful in selected patients with stage I or III disease to discriminate alveolitis from fibrosis [3].
- As sarcoidosis is a multi-organ disorder, patients can present with a plethora of manifestations.
- Findings relating specifically to the lungs include dyspnoea, dry cough, and chest pain, which occur in up to half of all patients.

In the past, a standard diagnostic test was the reaction to an intradermal injection of homogenates of human sarcoid tissue called the Kveim–Siltzback reagent. However, due to concerns of transmission of infections, the reagent was discontinued in the UK in 1996.

Clinical tip Difficulties in diagnosis

On average, symptomatic sarcoidosis patients have symptoms for >3 months prior to diagnosis and require three or more encounters with health-care providers prior to a specific diagnosis [4]. Sarcoidosis patients presenting with pulmonary symptoms often have a further relative delay in the diagnosis of sarcoidosis, as their symptoms are non-specific, and alternative diagnoses are therefore often considered.

Expert comment

It is extremely important to chase a tissue diagnosis, particularly in the non-erythema nodosum (EN) patient with mediastinal adenopathy. A significant percentage of patients with non-EN mediastinal adenopathy referred with possible sarcoidosis have an alternative diagnosis, principally lymphoma and TB.

Her investigations showed a normal full blood count, normal immunoglobulins, but a slightly raised serum ACE at 77 IU/L. Her IGRA and TST were negative, and her lung function tests were all within normal ranges. Her HRCT showed extensive superior mediastinal and hilar lymphadenopathy, but the lungs were clear. On bronchoscopy, there were no abnormal endobronchial findings. Histology of her TBBx reported non-necrotizing epithelioid granulomas of varying sizes, with multinucleate giant cells in some of the granulomas. Ziehl–Neelsen stain for AFB was negative.

Expert comment

Serum ACE is raised in only up to 60% of patients at acute presentation. If it is initially raised, then it can be helpful in monitoring systemic disease. The level is believed to reflect the total systemic granulomatous burden in the body, and not specifically lung disease.

Clinical tip Testing for *Mycobacterium tuberculosis* exposure in suspected sarcoidosis patients

- A negative TST is highly sensitive for sarcoidosis, even in TB-endemic areas, and, as such, can be used to help distinguish between TB and sarcoidosis.
- A positive TST in 141 patients with biopsy-proven sarcoidosis was shown to have a high specificity for TB in a cohort residing in India, suggesting any patient with a positive TST should be investigated for TB [5].
- Two studies have shown IGRA tests for latent TB screening show good predictive values in sarcoidosis patients, which is of benefit when considering TNF-alpha inhibitors.

The patient was reviewed in clinic and informed of her diagnosis. As she was clinically well and had evidence of stage I disease, with normal lung function, she was advised to stop smoking, as this may make her sarcoidosis worse, and to return for clinical review and repeat blood tests in 3 months' time.

Evidence base

The ACCESS study remains the largest study of sarcoidosis patients and was carried out in the US across ten different sarcoidosis centres, recruiting over 700 patients and their relatives, between 1997 and 1999 [6]. The objective of this study was to generate hypotheses about the aetiology of sarcoidosis. Although it did not identify a single cause of sarcoidosis, the data collected represent the best clinical description of sarcoidosis patients at new presentation. This and other epidemiological studies clearly delineate the heterogeneity of sarcoidosis.

Expert comment

Indeed, the ACCESS study was an impressive landmark study of sarcoidosis patients. Unfortunately, patients were only studied at one time point and were not followed prospectively, which would have added additional significant scientific and clinical value to the work.

Learning point Evaluating a sarcoidosis patient

The natural history and prognosis of sarcoidosis are protean. Patients should be assessed for disease activity and prognosis to help guide treatment management. Currently, the Scadding's criteria, devised in 1961, are the only accepted and widely used classification system. Although it is insufficient for clinical decision-making, the correlation between the CXR stage and the likelihood of spontaneous resolution can be helpful. Disease activity assessment should reflect persistent inflammation with evolving granuloma formation [7]. Many clinical findings are thought to correlate with disease activity, including:

- symptoms;
- elevated serum ACE;
- serum hypergammaglobulinaemia;
- serum lymphopenia;
- raised BAL lymphocyte count—lymphocytosis of $>2 \times 10^5$ cells/mL or 16% or above and CD4:CD8 ratio of >3.5;
- change in thoracic radiographic disease;
- presence of pulmonary nodules on CT scan;
- gallium scan activity;
- activity on PET scans
- change in lung function test (10–15% decrease in DLCO).

However, none of these markers of disease activity are specific for sarcoidosis.

Expert comment

BAL lymphocytosis is characteristically seen in sarcoidosis, TB, and HP. A predominance of CD4 cells favours sarcoidosis. A ratio of CD4/CD8 of >3.5 is reported to have a sensitivity, with respect to sarcoidosis, of 94%. The most practical use for BAL analysis is in patients who have had sarcoidosis and are worried about recurrence. A normal BAL lymphocyte count and a CD4/CD8 ratio approaching 1.0 help to exclude active pulmonary disease.

Clinical tip Categorizing a sarcoidosis patient

A commonly used categorization system is based on a patient's outcome: acute, chronic, or refractory.

- Acute disease resolves within 2 years (regardless of treatment). An example of acute disease is Löfgren's syndrome—bilateral hilar lymphadenopathy, EN, and ankle arthritis—typically associated with a good prognosis and spontaneous remission.
- Chronic disease continues for over 2 years.
- Refractory patients require continuous aggressive treatment. Patients with lupus pernio or bronchial stenosis often have refractory disease.

Expert comment

Whilst it is well recognized that an EN presentation in the context of sarcoidosis is associated with a good prognosis, i.e. an 85% expectation of spontaneous remission over 2–3 years, it is important to remember that 15% persist and progress. It is important to follow patients with EN over a 2- to 3-year time period to ensure identifying early patients where the disease is progressing.

On return to clinic, the patient had developed intermittent chest pain and a dry cough since the previous visit. Her blood tests showed no change from previously. The patient was concerned about receiving steroids, particularly in regards to putting on weight, and she also mentioned she was keen for another pregnancy in due course. It was agreed to review her again in 3 months' time, with repeat lung function tests and blood tests.

Clinical tip Does treatment help?

- Whilst spontaneous resolution occurs in two-thirds of patients within 5 years, approximately one-quarter of cases will go on to develop progressive lung disease.
- The challenge remains for many cases in deciding whether systemic treatment is appropriate, in view of the known side effects. This difficulty is perhaps reflected by the wide range of patients (20–70% across different studies) physicians start on systemic treatment [8].
- Oral glucocorticoids are the first line of therapy.
- Bisphosphonates should be added to prevent steroid-induced osteoporosis in men and post-menopausal women, and considered in females of childbearing age.
- Gastric protection should be considered.
- In asymptomatic patients with stage 0 or I radiological disease, there is strong evidence that no treatment is required.
- Ninety-five per cent of patients with stage I disease will have a normal CXR within 10 years.
- In symptomatic patients with stage I disease, other causes of the symptoms should also be sought, e.g. proximal bronchial stenosis which will not be detected by a CXR.
- For asymptomatic patients with stage II–IV disease, the current recommendation is observation only.

Evidence base

2002—Finnish RCT

- Patients with normal lung function were treated with oral glucocorticoids for 3 months, followed by 15 months of inhaled glucocorticoids and a 5-year clinical follow-up.
- The treatment group were less likely to have remaining radiographic changes, and stage II patients had a small improvement in FVC and DLCO.
- Sixty-one per cent of stage II–III disease patients had spontaneous resolution to stage I or 0.

2009 Cochrane review of oral and inhaled glucocorticoids

- Five RCTs of oral glucocorticoids [9].
- At 3–24 months, there was an overall improvement in radiological disease in the treated patients.
- BUT RCTs included patients with stage I through to stage III radiological disease.
- A subgroup analysis performed on four trials showed the improvement was only in patients with stage II–III disease at 6 and 24 months [10].
- Patients with stage II–III disease were 2.5 times more likely to show radiological improvement, if commenced on oral corticosteroid therapy for at least 6 months. Also importantly, untreated patients were more likely to show deterioration in chest radiology.
- Overall the subgroup analysis determined a small, but statistically significant, difference in FVC (4.2% predicted) and diffusing capacity (5.7% predicted).

After her 3-month review, the patient's symptoms had progressed. She continued to have intermittent chest pain; her cough was becoming more intrusive, and she was more fatigued. Her lung function tests showed a 10% drop in her diffusion capacity, and she had developed small pulmonary nodules on a repeat CXR. She was started on oral prednisolone 20 mg per day, which she was to continue for 1 month, then to taper the dose down to reach 5 mg on alternate days by 3 months. A further review was planned in 4 months' time.

Learning point Oral corticosteroid dosing regimen

- Steroid dosing typically involves:
  - initial high doses to control inflammation;
  - tapering to a maintenance dose to lessen the risk of side effects (during this time, steroid-sparing drugs may be started);

(Continued)

  - continuing the maintenance dose;
  - tapering the dose for complete steroid withdrawal.
- The British guidelines (2008 BTS in collaboration with the Thoracic Society of Australia and New Zealand and the Irish Thoracic Society ILD guidelines) differ slightly from international guidelines (1999 ATS/ERS/WASOG consensus statement).
- The BTS guidelines recommend initiation of prednisolone (or equivalent) at 0.5 mg/kg/day for 4 weeks. Maintenance dose should be reduced to a level that will control symptoms and disease progression, for a period of 6–24 months. Typically, this is about 5–15 mg/day and is continued for several months before further tapering.
- The international guidelines recommend an initial dose of 20–40 mg/day, tapering after 1–3 months in those who respond by 5–10 mg/day, and treating for a total of at least 12 months.
- A Delphi consensus study carried out in the US between 2008 and 2009 documented the typical clinical practice of experts treating pulmonary sarcoidosis [11]. Oral corticosteroid therapy was usually initiated at 0.3–0.6 mg/kg/day (20–40 mg/day) and continued for 4–6 weeks. If the response was stable or improved, the dose was tapered by 5–10 mg every 4–8 weeks. Once reaching a dose of 0.2–0.4 mg/kg/day or about 10–20 mg/day, if there was no improvement, the same dose was continued for a further 4–6 weeks.
- Oral glucocorticoids may also be given on alternate days at twice the dose; however, it is noteworthy there are little data to support a reduction in side effects.
- There are no optimal tools for measuring a patient's response, but a selection of compatible parameters, such as symptoms (pulmonary and systemic), thoracic radiological features, lung function tests (FVC, TLC, TLCO), blood biomarkers (ACE, full blood count, calcium, erythrocyte sedimentation rate (ESR), CRP), and ambulatory oximetry readings are often assessed.

Data on long-term benefits of continuing oral glucocorticoids for longer than 2 years remain unclear. Many sarcoidosis specialists suggest that, in some patients, treatment should be continued to prevent relapses [12]. This is apparent, as over half of those started on systemic treatment continue treatment for >2 years. However, most chronic patients are managed on relatively low-dose treatment regimens.

Clinical tip Relapsed disease during maintenance dose

- Recurrence of symptoms, such as cough and chest pain, often occurs during tapering, so many physicians will initiate a brief course of higher doses, e.g. 10–20 mg above the maintenance dose for 2–4 weeks. One study has shown benefit, after relapse during maintenance therapy, from 20 mg daily prednisolone, with a significant improvement in lung function after just 3 days [13].
- Some patients relapse during steroid withdrawal and develop an acute respiratory or extrathoracic exacerbation. In the past, studies from the 1970s and 1990s suggested the dose for acute respiratory exacerbations should be between 20 and 40 mg, or even up to 1 mg/kg, daily. However, a more recent study has shown that a short course (2–4 weeks) of 20 mg daily prednisolone significantly improves lung function within 3 days of initiation [13].

She was seen again in clinic and was at that time taking 5 mg of prednisolone on alternate days. However, her cough had worsened since she started tapering her dose, and she felt in the last few weeks it was worse than before she started the treatment. She also noticed pains in her left ankle. After a long discussion with the patient, her prednisolone dose was increased to 20 mg daily, and she was commenced on azathioprine as a steroid-sparing agent. She tolerated the azathioprine well and had a good symptomatic response.

Learning point Treatment guidelines—alternative regimens

Alternative immunosuppressive regimens are commenced to reduce the long-term effects of oral glucocorticoids in patients who are unable to tolerate glucocorticoids and in patients with progression of disease despite adequate corticosteroid therapy.

- Evidence to support alternative therapies is limited, but the largest body of literature is available for methotrexate.
- One RCT demonstrated that methotrexate had steroid-sparing effects, but results took up to 12 months to be seen. Several small case series have also supported the use of methotrexate as a steroid-sparing agent, with an average of 40–60% response rate. Methotrexate was the most commonly used second-line agent, after glucocorticoids, in the Delphi consensus on the treatment of sarcoidosis.
- The BTS guidelines say alternative immunosuppressives have a limited role but should be considered when oral glucocorticoids are unable to control the disease or in patients intolerant of steroid-induced side effects. They recommend methotrexate as the primary alternative drug.
- Other alternative drugs that are used include azathioprine, cyclophosphamide, chloroquine, hydroxychloroquine, pentoxyfilline, ciclosporin, thalidomide, leflunomide, and chlorambucil. Although case series report benefits for each of these drugs, there are no RCTs. The BTS recommends, in view of their side effects, that they should only be used with caution where disease is progressing and no other alternatives are available.
- Azathioprine is frequently used to replace methotrexate, due to its lower hepatotoxic effects, but there are few trials published on its efficacy.
- TNF-alpha is thought to play a role in maintaining granuloma formation. Over the past decade, several monoclonal antibodies to TNF-alpha have become available and have been used to treat sarcoidosis. A phase 2 RCT comparing infliximab to placebo for chronic pulmonary sarcoidosis showed a significant improvement in lung function and supports further evaluation of anti-TNF-alpha therapy [14].
- In end-stage lung disease, transplantation should be considered; although granulomas can occur in the transplanted lung, they appear to have little clinical consequence.

Clinical tip Immunosuppression in patients of childbearing age

Sarcoidosis typically affects young adults; therefore, many female patients are of childbearing age. Hence, this should be considered when deciding on a treatment plan and in discussion with the patient. For example, methotrexate and leflunomide are contraindicated during pregnancy, as they are teratogenic, whereas azathioprine and antimalarial drugs are considered as safe options. In patients with rheumatic disease, it is advised patients should not take methotrexate at least 3 months before trying for a planned pregnancy. It is unclear whether it is safe for male patients to take methotrexate before conception. During pregnancy itself, sarcoidosis symptoms may improve, possibly due to a higher level of maternal free cortisol.

Expert comment

Biologic therapies, in particular those targeting the pro-inflammatory cytokine TNF, are being increasingly used therapeutically in sarcoidosis. There is an increasing body of evidence of their clinical effectiveness in refractory disease, particularly aggressive uveitis and skin and central nervous system (CNS) disease.

Discussion

This clinical case undoubtedly alludes to the many difficulties and challenges both in diagnosing pulmonary sarcoidosis and in the clinical decisions surrounding treatment. These difficulties are exacerbated by the lack of well-conducted RCTs and the reliance on only expert-driven evidence-based guidelines. What is required are large international sarcoidosis clinical networks with well-defined and stratified sarcoidosis patient groups in which to investigate novel biological therapies in well-designed RCTs.

The natural history and prognosis of sarcoidosis are protean. Pulmonary involvement occurs in about 90%, but the presentation is heterogeneous. A typical pulmonary sarcoidosis patient will endure a prolonged diagnostic pathway, similar to the patient in this clinical case, to confirm the diagnosis. The level of evidence for the recommendations made in the diagnosis of sarcoidosis in the ATS/ERS/WASOG statement was mostly derived from expert opinion developed by a consensus. In this case, the patient initially presented with Scadding stage I radiological disease, with no respiratory symptoms and a normal respiratory examination; however, her pulmonary sarcoidosis progressed over a period of months.

Once the diagnosis is established, decisions must be made regarding management. Oral glucocorticoids have been widely used since the 1960s to treat sarcoidosis. There are both international (ATS/ERS/WASOG 1999) and British (BTS 2008) guidelines on the management of sarcoidosis patients. These guidelines focus much of their recommendations on the presence or absence of symptoms. Although there is a general consensus that symptomatic patients respond favourably to oral glucocorticoids, the evidence for the decision to treat for symptom control should perhaps be considered further, as it is based predominantly only on two non-RCTs (the BTS and Finnish studies mentioned earlier). Furthermore, due to the paucity of acceptable RCTs, our understanding of the benefits of oral glucocorticoids on radiological disease or lung function parameters is based on RCTs with non-comparable outcomes and confounding variables. Of the 150 studies examined for the *JAMA* systematic review of glucocorticoid therapy in pulmonary sarcoidosis, only eight met the criteria for inclusion, of which only six examined oral therapy alone. However, the RCTs included in the Cochrane 2006 review and the *JAMA* systematic review still had many potential confounding factors such as a study with no placebo received by the control group, a study with patients with respiratory disease whilst the other studies had patients with multisystem disease, variable doses of prednisolone, some given methylprednisolone, treatment course length varying between 3 and 24 months, and heterogeneity in the ethnicity of the study populations not taken into consideration. In addition, there is no consensus on the outcome variables that should be measured, such that treatment studies have used a variety of different scoring systems (combinations of radiological/lung function/symptom scores). For example, the BTS 1996 study did not use the commonly applied Scadding criteria, but an alternative radiological system developed specifically for that study. In this regard, not only do we need more well-conducted RCTs, but we should also be considering a standardized scoring system from which we can compare studies.

A final word from the expert

Sarcoidosis, whilst uncommon, has higher prevalence amongst individuals of Irish, Scottish, and Scandinavian descent. A recent Irish prevalence study found 85 cases/100,000. A US study suggested a lifetime risk for African-Americans of 2.4% and amongst Caucasians of 0.85%. It is not as rare as one thinks.

The non-specific nature of presenting symptoms of sarcoidosis often leads to a delay in diagnosis. Studies have shown significant delay, particularly with pulmonary involvement. A US study showed the presentation of cough was associated with >4 physician visits until the diagnosis of sarcoidosis was established. In addition, whilst the age profile of disease presentation is classically 20–40 years, there is a significant later peak at 60+ years, particularly in females. In the ACCESS study of over 700 sarcoidosis patients, over 25% of patients were diagnosed at 60+ years of age. So in elderly patients with a cough—although not common—sarcoidosis should be part of your differential.

Unfortunately, it is not unusual for delayed referrals to the chest clinic of patients with an initial EN/bihilar lymphadenopathy presentation of sarcoidosis and patients being discharged at diagnosis with no follow-up, then presenting later with progressive disease. It is important to remember that, even in this 'good prognostic group', up to 20% of patients will progress.

It is important to chase a tissue diagnosis, particularly in a non-EN presentation, as up to 15% of patients with mediastinal adenopathy and no EN will have an alternative diagnosis to sarcoidosis.

References

1. Rybicki BA, Iannuzzi MC, Frederick MM *et al.* Familial aggregation of sarcoidosis. A case-control etiologic study of sarcoidosis (ACCESS). *Am J Respir Crit Care Med* 2001;**164**:2085–91.
2. Costabel U, Hunninghake GW. ATS/ERS/WASOG statement on sarcoidosis. Sarcoidosis Statement Committee. American Thoracic Society. European Respiratory Society. World Association for Sarcoidosis and Other Granulomatous Disorders. *Eur Respir J* 1999;**14**:735–7.
3. Nunes H, Brillet PY, Valeyre D, Brauner MW, Wells AU. Imaging in sarcoidosis. *Semin Respir Crit Care Med* 2007;**28**:102–20.
4. Judson MA, Thompson BW, Rabin DL *et al.* The diagnostic pathway to sarcoidosis. *Chest* 2003;**123**:406–12.
5. Smith-Rohrberg D, Sharma SK. Tuberculin skin test among pulmonary sarcoidosis patients with and without tuberculosis: its utility for the screening of the two conditions in tuberculosis-endemic regions. *Sarcoidosis Vasc Diffuse Lung Dis* 2006; 23: 130–134.
6. Baughman RP, Teirstein AS, Judson MA *et al.* Clinical characteristics of patients in a case control study of sarcoidosis. *Am J Respir Crit Care Med* 2001;**164**:1885–9.
7. [No authors listed]. Consensus conference: activity of sarcoidosis. Third WASOG meeting, Los Angeles, USA, September 8–11, 1993. *Eur Respir J* 1994;**7**:624–7.
8. Baughman RP, Nunes H. Therapy for sarcoidosis: evidence-based recommendations. *Expert Rev Clin Immunol* 2012;**8**:95–103.
9. Paramothayan NS, Lasserson TJ, Jones PW. Corticosteroids for pulmonary sarcoidosis. *Cochrane Database Syst Rev* 2005;**2**:CD001114.
10. Paramothayan S, Jones PW. Corticosteroid therapy in pulmonary sarcoidosis: a systematic review. *JAMA* 2002;**287**:1301–7.
11. Schutt AC, Bullington WM, Judson MA. Pharmacotherapy for pulmonary sarcoidosis: a Delphi consensus study. *Respir Med* 2010;**104**:717–23.
12. Coker RK. Guidelines for the use of corticosteroids in the treatment of pulmonary sarcoidosis. *Drugs* 2007;**67**:1139–47.
13. McKinzie BP, Bullington WM, Mazur JE, Judson MA. Efficacy of short-course, low-dose corticosteroid therapy for acute pulmonary sarcoidosis exacerbations. *Am J Med Sci* 2010;**339**:1–4.
14. Baughman RP, Drent M, Kavuru M *et al.* Infliximab therapy in patients with chronic sarcoidosis and pulmonary involvement. *Am J Respir Crit Care Med* 2006;**174**:795–802.

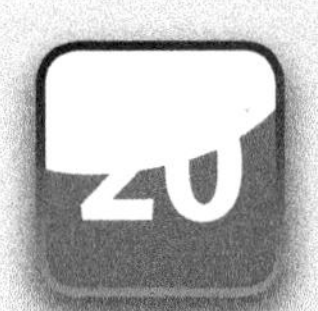

Swine 'flu' in pregnancy

Mark H Almond

Expert commentary Mark J Griffiths

Case history

A 26-year-old pregnant female referred herself to the labour ward, reporting reduced fetal movements and a 3-day history of an influenza-like illness comprising coryzal symptoms, hot and cold sweats, headaches, fevers, and myalgia. Examination revealed that she was febrile (>38°C), resulting in her admission for observation and cardiotocography (CTG), which was reportedly normal.

Her medical history included recurrent urinary tract infections, childhood asthma, hypertension, whilst taking the oral contraceptive pill, and an episode of numbness of the right hand that had previously been investigated for demyelination by MRI. She was a non-smoker, took no regular medications, and had no known drug allergies.

Learning point Pulmonary physiology and pathology during pregnancy

As serum progesterone concentrations increase throughout pregnancy, hyperventilation (with an associated respiratory alkalosis) may occur due to increased stimulation of the respiratory centres within the brain. The gravid uterus results in decreases in both the RV and FRC, whilst the TLC decreases slightly in the third trimester. The FEV_1, FVC, and peak expiratory flow rate (PEFR) do not change significantly [1].

Pregnancy results in a state of relative immunosuppression, and the following pulmonary complications should be borne in mind (Table 20.1, derived from [1]).

Table 20.1 Pulmonary complications of pregnancy

Deterioration of pre-existing	Respiratory disease	Asthma (worsens in one-third) Lymphangioleiomyomatosis (LAM)
	Cardiac disease	Peripartum cardiomyopathy Structural heart disease, e.g. mitral stenosis
	Autoimmune disease	SLE Wegener's granulomatosis
Pulmonary infection	Bacterial	*S. pneumoniae*, commonest pathogen *M. pneumoniae*, commonest atypical
	Viral	Influenza A Varicella Measles
	Other	TB Pneumocystis Fungal
ARDS	Secondary to	Emboli Pneumonia Sepsis Aspiration
PE	Thrombotic Air Amniotic fluid Trophoblastic	

Data from Pereira A, Krieger BP. Pulmonary complications of pregnancy. *Clinics in chest medicine*. 2004;**25**:299–310.

Following her admission, she remained febrile, despite paracetamol, and, by day 3, had developed a cough productive of clear sputum. Her chest was noted to be clear on auscultation; however, as her pyrexia remained at >38°C, she was commenced on IV co-amoxiclav and clarithromycin for CAP.

Expert comment

During an influenza pandemic, the patient who was at risk, in the case of A/H1N1 2009 influenza, owing to the history of asthma and current pregnancy, ideally should have been treated with antiviral agents on presentation. In the review of maternal deaths in the UK related to A/H1N1 2009 influenza from April 2009 to January 2010, seven out of eight deaths reported were associated with an avoidable delay in the administration of antiviral agents, and none of the women had been vaccinated.

The following day, fetal tachycardia was noted, resulting in a subsequent emergency lower segment Caesarean section (LSCS) under spinal anaesthesia. Intraoperatively, the patient's oxygen saturations were 92% on 10 L of oxygen, subsequently dropping post-operatively to 90% on 15 L via a non-rebreathe mask. A boy was delivered and subsequently transferred to the special care baby unit (SCBU).

She was reviewed by the medical registrar on the labour ward who noted diminished breath sounds and crepitations at the left base, with a subsequent chest radiograph revealing extensive left-sided consolidation. An ABG showed a PaO_2 of 8.5 kPa on 15 L/minute of oxygen, and she was transferred to the HDU for CPAP and arterial line insertion. Concurrently, an H1N1 throat swab was sent for reverse transcriptase polymerase chain reaction (rt-PCR), in addition to *Legionella* and pneumococcal urinary antigens.

Clinical tip Clinical diagnostic criteria for pandemic influenza (pH1N1)

- Fever (>38°C) or a history of fever; AND
- Influenza-like illness (two or more of the following symptoms: cough, sore throat, rhinorrhoea, limb or joint pain, headache, vomiting, or diarrhoea); OR
- Severe and/or life-threatening illness suggestive of an infectious process.

Notably, gastrointestinal symptoms (diarrhoea, vomiting, and abdominal pain) are more prominent in pH1N1, relative to seasonal influenza (<10%), and up to one-third of patients may be afebrile at presentation [2]. Most adults with pH1N1 experience mild symptoms, with 50% recovering within 7 days of symptom onset and a further 25% within 10 days.

Clinical tip Diagnostic criteria for ARDS

Following the initial description of ARDS in 1967, it took a further 27 years before it was formally defined in 1994 by the AECC; however, issues regarding reliability and validity of the definition emerged. The 2012 Berlin definition eliminates the term 'acute lung injury' (Table 20.2) [3].

Table 20.2 2012 Berlin definition of ARDS

Timing	Within 1 week of a known clinical insult or new or worsening respiratory symptoms
Chest imaging	Bilateral opacities—not fully explained by effusions, lobar/lung collapse, or nodules
Origin of oedema	Respiratory failure not fully explained by cardiac failure or fluid overload Need objective assessment (e.g. echocardiography) to exclude hydrostatic oedema if no risk factor present
Oxygenation	Mild: 200 mmHg < PaO_2/FiO_2 < 300 mmHg, with PEEP/CPAP >5 cmH_2O Moderate: 100 mmHg < PaO_2/FiO_2 < 200 mmHg, with PEEP >5 cmH_2O Severe: PaO_2/FiO_2 < 100 mmHg, with PEEP >5 cmH_2O

Learning point Complications of pandemic H1N1 influenza A

Influenza viruses are a significant cause of morbidity and mortality globally, resulting in severe illness in 3–5 million people and death in up to 500,000 during epidemic years. These viruses are members of the *Orthomyxoviridae* family and subclassified into influenza A, B, and C, of which only influenza A has pandemic potential. Influenza pandemics occur when a virus expressing a novel haemagglutinin (HA) or neuraminidase (NA) surface glycoprotein infects a population with no prior immunity. The devastating effects of this were demonstrated by the 1918 H1N1 pandemic in which approximately 20–50 million people died worldwide.

Over the past century, four pandemics have taken place:

- 1918: Spanish influenza (H1N1);
- 1957: Asian influenza (H2N2);
- 1968: Hong Kong influenza (H3N2);
- 2009: Mexican influenza (H1N1).

Although it is now generally considered that the 2009 H1N1 pandemic resulted in mild disease in most individuals, serious complications still occurred, as listed in Table 20.3, both pulmonary and extrapulmonary [4].

Table 20.3 Pulmonary and extrapulmonary complications of 2009 H1N1 pandemic

Pulmonary	Primary influenza pneumonia Secondary bacterial pneumonia Pulmonary superinfection with atypical pathogens Exacerbations of chronic lung disease (asthma and COPD) Respiratory failure and ARDS
Extrapulmonary	Cardiac: pericarditis and myocarditis Muscular: myositis and rhabdomyolysis Neurologic: encephalopathy, encephalomyelitis, transverse myelitis, aseptic meningitis, Guillain–Barré syndrome Gastrointestinal: acute pancreatitis

Rothberg MB, Haessler SD. Complications of seasonal and pandemic influenza. Crit. Care Med. 2010 Apr;38(4 Suppl):e91–7.

Expert comment

Following cellular endocytosis of the influenza virus, pathogen-associated molecular patterns (PAMPs), such as single- or double-stranded RNA, are detected by endosomal (toll-like receptors (TLRs)) or cytoplasmic (retinoic inducible gene 1 (RIG-1)) pathogen recognition receptors (PRRs) that, in turn, induce the expression of type I and III interferons. Interferons act in an autocrine and paracrine fashion to induce an antiviral state through the upregulation of interferon-stimulated genes (ISGs) such as the myxovirus resistance gene A (MxA) and interferon-induced transmembrane protein 3 (IFITM3) [5]. Peripheral blood mononuclear cells (PBMCs) isolated from healthy pregnant women have been shown to produce significantly less type I and III interferon when stimulated with pH1N1/09, compared with PBMCs from non-pregnant women, potentially contributing to their increased susceptibility to adverse outcomes [6].

Despite a PEEP of 10 cmH_2O and an FiO_2 of 1.0, she remained in type 1 respiratory failure, with a PaO_2 of 6.8 kPa, resulting in her transfer to the adult intensive care unit (AICU) for intubation. By this point, her chest radiograph had deteriorated, demonstrating bilateral patchy changes, consistent with ARDS, and dense left lower lobe collapse and consolidation (Figure 20.1).

Her throat swab tested positive on rt-PCR for pH1N1, and she was commenced on oseltamivir, a NA inhibitor. After she was placed in the prone, rather than supine,

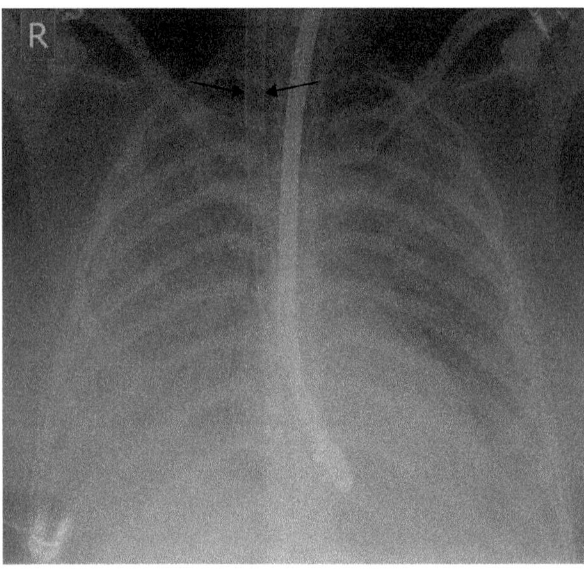

Figure 20.1 Frontal portable chest radiograph shortly after placement of a right internal jugular catheter for extracorporeal membrane oxygenation (ECMO: arrow heads). In the midline, an endoscope has been placed to carry out a transoesophageal echocardiogram. This was used to determine the cardiac structure and function, to exclude intracardiac shunts, and to optimize the placement of the ECMO cannula.

position, her PaO_2 improved to 9.23 kPa; however, with no significant progress made, the decision was made to transfer her to a tertiary centre for ECMO.

Expert comment

Management of an antenatal patient on the ICU necessitates special consideration. Failed intubation is significantly commoner in the obstetric population, relative to other anaesthetic intubations, with diminished FRC and increased oxygen consumption, resulting in rapid desaturation upon hypoventilation [7]. These factors should predispose to intubations being carried out electively and by the most experienced operators available. Haemodynamic instability may result from compression of the vena cava by the gravid uterus in the supine position. This can be mitigated by positioning patients on their left side or with the right hip elevated, in preference to repeated fluid challenges which will increase the formation of pulmonary oedema. Mechanical hyperventilation should be avoided, as this may adversely affect uterine blood flow. Neither prone positioning nor ECMO are absolutely contraindicated by pregnancy, although both present particular challenges to the intensive care team.

Clinical tip Referral criteria to secondary care and critical care

Hospital:

- signs of respiratory distress;
- hypoxia (oxygen saturations <94% on air);
- dehydration or shock;
- any signs of sepsis;
- altered conscious level.

(Continued)

Critical care:

- severe dyspnoea;
- hypoxaemia with PaO_2 <8 kPa despite maximal oxygen therapy;
- refractory hypotension;
- septic shock;
- GCS <10 or deteriorating conscious level;
- severe acidosis (pH <7.26);
- influenza-related pneumonia and CURB-65* ≥4 or bilateral primary viral pneumonia.

* CURB-65 score: confusion, urea >7 mmol/L, respiratory rate ≥30/minute, low systolic (<90 mmHg) or diastolic (≤60 mmHg), blood pressure, age ≥65 years.

Source: from reference [2].

On arrival at the tertiary ECMO centre, her oxygen saturations ranged from 70% to 82% on 100% oxygen. Veno-venous ECMO was instituted, following which her systolic blood pressure dropped to 40 mmHg, recovering with vasopressor support. On arrival in the ICU, she had a sinus tachycardia, maintaining a mean arterial pressure (MAP) of 86 mmHg supported by high levels of noradrenaline. Transthoracic echocardiography revealed a markedly impaired global systolic function and a pericardial effusion, presumed to be secondary to influenza-induced myocarditis and pericarditis that was not causing a tamponade. Her antibiotics were changed at this point to include piperacillin with tazobactam, in addition to clarithromycin and oseltamivir.

Evidence base Referral to an ECMO centre and mortality amongst patients with severe 2009 influenza A (H1N1)

Background

- ECMO was used to treat H1N1/09-related ARDS during the 2009 pandemic [8].

Participants

- Patients with H1N1-related ARDS.

Design

- Retrospective cohort study.
- ECMO-referred versus matched non-ECMO-referred patients.
- (ECMO-referred patients defined as all patients with H1N1-related ARDS who were referred, accepted, and transferred to one of four adult ECMO centres in the UK during winter 2009–2010).

Primary outcome

- Survival to hospital discharge analysed according to intention-to-treat.

Results

- Mortality in ECMO-referred patients versus non-ECMO-referred patients:
  - 23.7% versus 52.5% (when individual matching used);
  - 24.0% versus 46.7% (when propensity matching used);
  - 24.0% versus 50.7% (when GenMatch matching used).

Conclusions

- For patients with H1N1-related ARDS, referral and transfer to an ECMO centre was associated with lower hospital mortality, compared with matched non-ECMO-referred patients.

Clinical tip Distinguishing between primary viral pneumonia and secondary bacterial pneumonia

During the 2009 H1N1 pandemic, influenza-related pneumonia was found in 40% of hospitalized patients in the US, and, in Australasia, 49% of the critically ill patients were diagnosed with viral pneumonia and 20% had secondary bacterial pneumonia [2].

Signs suggestive of the development of influenza-related pneumonia include dyspnoea, recrudescent fever, tachypnoea, cyanosis, and bilateral crepitations. Distinguishing between a primary viral pneumonia and a secondary bacterial pneumonia can be difficult in the clinical setting. The clinical parameters listed in Table 20.4 may aid differentiation [9,10].

Table 20.4 Clinical parameters that help distinguish between a primary viral pneumonia and a secondary bacterial pneumonia

	Primary viral pneumonia	Secondary bacterial pneumonia
Onset of respiratory compromise	1–2 days after initial symptoms	4–7 days after initial symptoms
Antibiotic response	Slow or non-responsive	Rapid
WCC	Normal to low	Increased
Biomarkers	CRP <20 mg/L Procalcitonin <0.5 micrograms/L	CRP >20 mg/L Procalcitonin >0.5 micrograms/L
Lower respiratory tract diagnostic specimen	Normal flora	Gram stain/culture shows predominant organism
Fever	Primary fever	Secondary fever after period of defervescence

Over the following 3 days, the patient's inflammatory markers deteriorated, with her WCC reaching 20.2 × 10^9/L and her CRP increasing from 149 to 443 mg/L. A CT thorax revealed dense consolidation, bilateral pleural effusions, and anteriorly a predominantly ground glass appearance with few patchy areas of normal lung parenchyma. To aid recruitment and ventilation, a right-sided intercostal chest drain was inserted under ultrasound guidance, subsequently draining 1.7 L. Despite the positive H1N1 throat swab rt-PCR, BAL fluid was negative for influenza A and B, herpes simplex virus, and *Pneumocystis jirovecii*; additionally, *Legionella* and pneumococcal urinary antigens were negative. In light of the deteriorating inflammatory markers, IV zanamivir was commenced after successful application for its use on a compassionate basis.

By day 20, intravascular haemolysis had developed, complicating her ECMO, and a large right-sided pleural collection had developed (Figure 20.2), necessitating a right anterolateral thoracotomy for evacuation of the haematoma, whilst on ECMO. Two litres of blood were drained, and two surgical chest drains subsequently placed. When the patient returned to the AICU, the drains became blocked by a blood clot, necessitating an immediate drain replacement.

The following day, N-acetylcysteine (NAC) was commenced, as her LFTs unexpectedly deteriorated, with the alkaline phosphatase (ALP) rising to 947 from 115 IU/L, gamma-glutamyl transpeptidase (GGT) to 1543 from 102, and aspartate transaminase (AST) to 143 from 21 IU/L. Her bilirubin remained normal, and a liver ultrasound failed to demonstrate any architectural abnormalities, thrombosis, or biliary tract obstruction. Furthermore, a widespread erythematous, blanching, papular rash developed predominantly on her limbs, associated with an elevated eosinophil

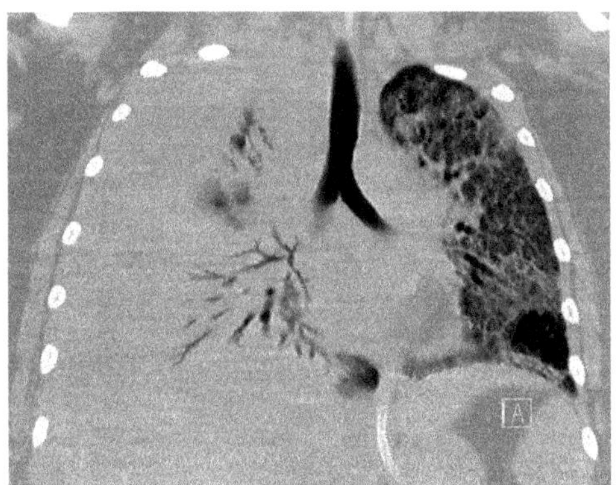

Figure 20.2 CT thorax revealing a large right-sided haemothorax with compression of the consolidated right lung.

count of 12.3 × 10^9/L, which may have been a manifestation of DRESS (drug reaction, eosinophilia, systemic symptoms), possibly secondary to piperacillin/tazobactam. Due to the reduced cardiac output, her renal function also deteriorated, with a rise in her creatinine from a baseline of 62–253 micromoles/L; continuous veno-venous haemodiafiltration (CVVHDF) was subsequently commenced.

A significant left-sided pneumothorax developed on day 23, requiring insertion of a third chest drain. A subsequent CT thorax revealed the progression of ARDS, with diffuse ground glass shadowing, superimposed on reticular changes and traction dilatation of the bronchioles, consistent with fibrotic change, in addition to a further right-sided pneumothorax, for which a fourth chest drain was inserted (Figure 20.3).

By day 31, despite the presence of four chest drains on suction, her ventilatory requirements had improved to such a degree that she could be weaned from ECMO to an arteriovenous extracorporeal carbon dioxide removal (ECCOR) device, which

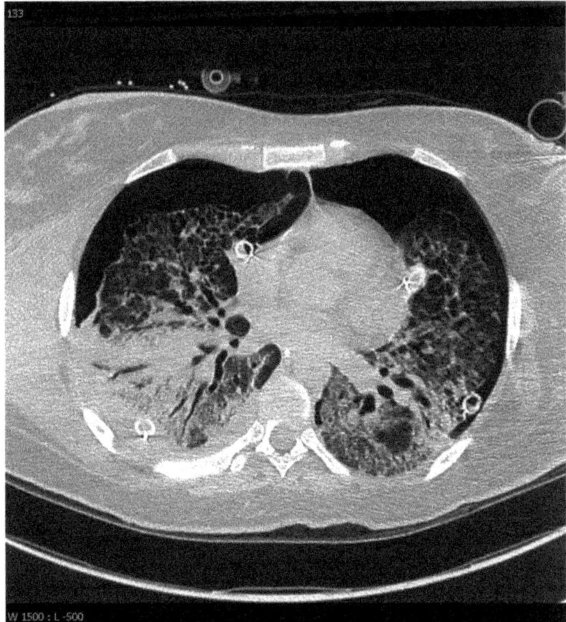

Figure 20.3 Late in the clinical course, the lung parenchyma is distorted, contracted, and riddled with cystic airspaces. There are large bilateral pneumothoraces, four intercostal chest drains visible, and a small right-sided haemothorax.

is associated with a lower risk of haemorrhagic complications. Unfortunately, she developed gross icterus, as her liver function continued to deteriorate, the bilirubin rising to 390 micromoles/L. Consequently, her case was discussed with the local tertiary liver unit who felt that it was likely to be sepsis-related liver dysfunction, with a prognosis of survival of only 5–10%.

By day 33, the patient's list of diagnoses was extensive, and ultimately overwhelming, including ARDS with increasing ventilatory requirements whilst on ECCOR, renal failure necessitating haemofiltration, liver failure (on NAC), ongoing sepsis, and increasing vasopressor and inotrope requirements in the context of myocarditis-induced biventricular cardiac failure. The possibility of restarting ECMO was discussed with the family; however, it was decided that it would not change the ultimate outcome. The patient died on day 36, after spending >800 hours on ECMO.

Discussion

Following the emergence of the first cases of pH1N1 in Mexico in March 2009, the virus spread rapidly, achieving pandemic status within 3 months. The pH1N1 virus resulted from the combination of two genes from a Eurasian swine virus with six genes from a 'triple-reassortant' North American swine virus lineage (see Learning point, p. 249). In the US alone, the pandemic accounted for an estimated 59 million illnesses, 265,000 hospitalizations, and 12,000 deaths by mid-February 2010 [11].

The pandemic virus differed from seasonal influenza in its propensity to affect young and middle-aged adults (aged 20–65), rather than the elderly. In the UK, 474 deaths were reported in the pandemic phase, of whom one-third had minimal or no underlying health problems. Risk factors for severe disease included asthma, cardiac disease, immunosuppression, pregnancy and post-partum states, diabetes mellitus, and obesity. Fewer than 1% of patients in the UK were admitted to hospital; however, of these, 12–15% required critical care, placing a huge burden on services [2].

Learning point Origins of the 2009 H1N1 influenza A pandemic

Epidemic influenza viruses are derived from pandemic viruses by antigenic drift, i.e. gradual minor antigenic changes caused by point mutations in HA and NA molecules, whereas reassortment and interspecies transmission result in the introduction of viruses with new HA and NA subtypes into human populations, thus resulting in pandemics. Epidemics are caused by influenza A and B viruses, whereas only influenza A viruses have pandemic potential [12].

The 1918 'Spanish' influenza pandemic was most probably caused by the transmission of an avian H1N1 virus to humans. Following 1918, H1N1 from that outbreak continued to circulate in humans, causing annual epidemics. Due to the segmented nature of the genome in influenza viruses, they are especially prone to reassortment events if one host is co-infected by two different viruses. This allows genetic material from viruses that usually circulate in birds to be introduced to human adapted viruses. The 1957 Asian pandemic was caused by a novel H2N2 virus that retained five genome segments from the 1918 H1N1 virus but obtained three new segments from an avian H2N2 virus. Similarly, in 1968, the circulating human H2N2 recombined with the HA from an avian H3 virus, resulting in the H3N2 'Hong Kong' pandemic. The H3N2 and H1N1 subtypes have continued to co-circulate and to cause human seasonal influenza outbreaks into the twentieth-first century [13].

The 2009 H1N1 pandemic was unexpected (an H5N1 pandemic was predicted) and challenged the concept that the introduction of a new HA subtype is necessary to result in a pandemic [12]. In fact,

(Continued)

the eight gene segments for the 2009 pandemic virus originate from at least four different sources and three different hosts. In the late 1990s, a 'triple reassortant' virus emerged in pigs, comprising the PA and PB2 genes from an avian reservoir, the PB1 and NA of a human H3N2, and the four other genes, including the HA, from the 'classical' swine virus that had been circulating since 1918. This 'triple reassortant' virus subsequently recombined with a Eurasian avian-like H1N1 virus that had been circulating in pigs since the 1970s (receiving the NA and M genes), resulting in the 2009 H1N1 pandemic virus.

The 2009 H1N1 virus is not the same as the H1N1 virus that has been circulating in humans, causing seasonal epidemics, since the 1918 pandemic. Although both viruses have HA proteins derived from the 1918 pandemic, the 2009 virus contained the HA from the 'classical' swine influenza virus, which, unlike the seasonal human H1, had been under relatively little antigenic pressure, thus introducing a novel antigen into the human population [13].

The diagnosis in this case was based upon both the clinical presentation and the positive rt-PCR throat swab. Laboratory diagnosis of pH1N1/09 is best achieved through real-time rt-PCR analysis of both combined nasopharyngeal and throat swabs and nasopharyngeal aspirates plus tracheobronchial aspirates in ventilated patients [14]. There is a high incidence of false-negative results, so repeated testing of both upper respiratory swabs and tracheobronchial aspirates is required to exclude a viral infection with confidence. If there is a high index of suspicion, antiviral therapy should be continued until repeated samples are negative [15]. Although rt-PCR is the most sensitive and specific method of diagnosis, it has limited availability, and nasopharyngeal aspiration can be both unpleasant and negative in the presence of influenza-related pneumonia. Rapid influenza antigen and immunofluorescent antibody tests are available that can distinguish influenza A and B; however, they are not able to distinguish seasonal and pandemic influenza A, nor are they as sensitive and specific as rt-PCR [16]. Confirmation of pH1N1/09 infection can only be made by rt-PCR or viral culture.

With regard to management, the Department of Health issued recommendations in October 2009, outlining the treatment of pH1N1 in both the primary and secondary care settings, updating previous BTS guidelines [2]. The recommendation for clinically diagnosed uncomplicated influenza infection is prompt commencement of antiviral therapy plus symptomatic management (antipyretics, good fluid intake, smoking avoidance, rest, and topical decongestants). Hospitalized patients should be administered antibiotics within 4 hours of admission. For severe influenza-related pneumonia, 10 days of parenteral co-amoxiclav plus a macrolide (e.g. clarithromycin) should be given (for penicillin-allergic patients, second-generation cephalosporins may be used as an alternative), extending to 14–21 days where *Staphylococcus aureus* or Gram-negative enteric bacilli pneumonia is suspected or confirmed. The routine use of corticosteroids in influenza-associated pneumonia is not recommended, and their use may increase mortality.

The NA inhibitor oseltamivir (75 mg orally bd for 5 days) is the drug of choice for most patients because it achieves higher systemic levels than inhaled zanamivir. Early administration of antiviral agents is associated with a better prognosis and limits progression to pulmonary infiltrates, but they still confer benefit if started >48 hours and up to 7 days after symptom onset. H1N1 is resistant to the adamantanes (e.g. amantadine), but oseltamivir-resistant strains have remained relatively rare, with only 45 cases recognized in the UK from 6,379 influenza-positive samples tested [17]. Zanamivir (10 mg inhaled bd for 5 days) is the antiviral of choice in renal failure and for pregnant women—unless they have asthma, COPD, or difficulty using inhaled preparations, in which case oseltamivir should be used. IV zanamivir is not licensed in the UK but has been used, as in this instance, as part of a compassionate-use programme for critically ill patients.

In contrast to seasonal H1N1 influenza, oseltamivir resistance remained relatively low throughout the 2009 pandemic. In the 2 years prior to April 2011, 27,000 pH1N1/09 viruses were tested for NA resistance by the WHO, and only 447 oseltamivir-resistant viruses were identified [18]. The majority of resistant organisms were detected in patients undergoing oseltamivir treatment; however, 14% were isolated from patients with no previous history of oseltamivir treatment, suggesting either spontaneous mutation conferring resistance or transmission of resistant strains from patients who received treatment.

Unsurprisingly, immunocompromised patients, especially those with haematological malignancies or haematopoietic stem cell transplantation (HSCT), were at greatest risk of developing oseltamivir-resistant influenza. Almost half (49%) of the oseltamivir-resistant cases were isolated from immunosuppressed patients, and, of these, half had no prior exposure to antiviral drugs [18]. The majority of resistant cases were associated with a histidine-to-tyrosine mutation (H275Y) in the NA of the virus (alternatively called the H274Y mutation, depending on the NA numbering system used), although other mutations have been identified.

Infection control is of paramount importance during an influenza pandemic, and nosocomial outbreaks were identified during the 2009 H1N1 pandemic, emphasizing the need for adherence to infection control standards in hospitals. Naturally, hand hygiene is a critical element of infection control precautions and, in order to inactivate influenza A, should be carried out for 20–30 s with alcohol hand gel and 40–60 s with handwashing (including thorough drying). Good respiratory hygiene measures ('catch it, bin it, kill it') should also be adhered to, not only in the ward environment, but also in communal waiting areas and during patient transport. Respiratory droplets typically travel only 1 m, but ideally patients should be isolated, rather than cohorted, and fluid-repellent surgical masks worn when working in close contact with symptomatic patients. Aerosol-generating procedures, including the use of NIV, should be carried out in well-ventilated single rooms, with the doors closed, wearing a gown, gloves, eye protection, and a filtering face piece 3 (FFP3) face mask. Notably, the administration of nebulized medications and pressured humidified oxygen is not considered to represent a significant infection risk [19].

Vaccination is safe and effective and offers the best means of decreasing the number of individuals infected with influenza. In a study involving over 95,000 children and young adults in Beijing, a monovalent vaccine was 87.3% effective in preventing pH1N1, and there was no association with Guillain–Barré syndrome [20]. During the winter of 2010, a trivalent vaccine that included protection against pH1N1 was available, but uptake was poor in at-risk groups and amongst health-care workers (25% in the National Health Service (NHS)). Health-care workers in the UK accept that vaccination against hepatitis B is required to perform their role, but this is not yet the case for influenza.

Learning point Influenza vaccination

The WHO monitors the epidemiology of influenza viruses throughout the world. Each year, it makes recommendations about the three strains to be included in vaccines for the forthcoming winter. The majority of current inactivated influenza vaccines are trivalent, containing two subtypes of influenza A and one type B virus. Trivalent vaccines give around 60–70% protection against infection when

(Continued)

influenza virus strains in the vaccine are well matched with those in circulation. Quadrivalent vaccines, with an additional strain of influenza B virus, were first authorized for use in the UK in 2013. Following immunization, antibody levels may take up to 10–14 days to reach protective levels. In 2012, the Joint Committee on Vaccination and Immunization (JCVI) recommended that the influenza vaccination programme be extended to all children aged 2 to <17 years old.

Goals of immunization:

- protection of those who are most at risk of serious illness/death;
- reducing transmission of infection.

Trivalent influenza vaccine should be offered, ideally before the virus starts to circulate, to:

- all those aged 65 years or older;
- all those aged 6 months or older in clinical risk groups:
  - chronic respiratory disease: asthma, COPD, cystic fibrosis, bronchiectasis, ILD;
  - chronic heart disease: chronic heart failure, congenital heart disease;
  - chronic kidney disease: chronic kidney disease 3, 4, and 5, nephrotic syndrome, transplant;
  - chronic liver disease: cirrhosis, chronic hepatitis, biliary atresia;
  - chronic neurological disease: stroke, transient ischaemic attack, compromised respiratory function;
  - diabetes mellitus;
  - immunosuppression;
  - pregnant women: at any stage of pregnancy;
  - morbid obesity (class III): adults with a BMI of ≥40 kg/m^2 [21].

A final word from the expert

The clinical issues presented by this case illustrate the need for intensivists to liaise closely with other specialties. The organisms which cause pneumonia, their treatment, and identification change quite markedly from year to year, requiring input from clinical microbiologists and public health physicians. Similarly, obstetricians and midwives, where appropriate, should be constantly available to support the intensive care team to optimize care for the mother and baby. After the A/H1N1 2009 influenza pandemics of 2009–2010, a national ECMO service was commissioned to provide retrieval to one of five specialist centres and advanced organ support for the patients most severely affected by ARDS.

References

1. Pereira A, Krieger BP. Pulmonary complications of pregnancy. *Clin Chest Med* 2004;**25**:299–310.
2. Department of Health (2009). *Pandemic H1N1 2009 influenza: clinical management guidelines for adults and children*. Available at: <http://www.rcpch.ac.uk/sites/default/files/asset_library/Research/Clinical%20Effectiveness/Practice%20Statements/DH%20Clinical%20Management%20Guideline.pdf>.
3. ARDS Definition Task Force, Ranieri VM, Rubenfeld GD, Thompson BT *et al*. Acute respiratory distress syndrome: the Berlin Definition. *JAMA* 2012;**307**:2526–33.
4. Rothberg MB, Haessler SD. Complications of seasonal and pandemic influenza. *Crit Care Med* 2010;**38**(4 Suppl):e91–7.
5. García-Sastre A. Induction and evasion of type I interferon responses by influenza viruses. *Virus Res* 2011;**162**:12–18.

6. Forbes RL, Wark PA, Murphy VE, Gibson PG. Pregnant women have attenuated innate interferon responses to 2009 pandemic influenza A virus subtype H1N1. *J Infect Dis* 2012;**206**:646–53.
7. Lapinsky SE, Pasadas-Calleja JG, McCullagh I. Clinical Review: Ventilatory strategies for obstetric, brain-injured and obese patients. *Crit Care* 2009;**13**:206.
8. Noah MA, Peek GJ, Finney SJ *et al.* Referral to an extracorporeal membrane oxygenation center and mortality among patients with severe 2009 influenza A(H1N1). *JAMA* 2011;**306**:1659–68.
9. Ruuskanen O, Lahti E, Jennings LC, Murdoch DR. Viral pneumonia. *Lancet* 2011;**377**:1264–75.
10. Wright PF, Kirkland KB, Modlin JF. When to consider the use of antibiotics in the treatment of 2009 H1N1 influenza-associated pneumonia. *N Engl J Med* 2009;**361**:e112.
11. Writing Committee of the WHO Consultation on Clinical Aspects of Pandemic (H1N1) 2009 Influenza, Bautista E, Chotpitayasunondh T, Gao Z *et al.* Clinical aspects of pandemic 2009 influenza A (H1N1) virus infection. *N Engl J Med* 2010;**362**:1708–19.
12. Klenk HD, Garten W, Matrosovich M. Molecular mechanisms of interspecies transmission and pathogenicity of influenza viruses: Lessons from the 2009 pandemic. *Bioessays* 2011;**33**:180–8.
13. Elderfield R, Barclay W. Influenza pandemics. *Adv Exp Med Biol* 2011;**719**:81–103.
14. de la Tabla VO, Masiá M, Antequera P *et al.* Comparison of combined nose-throat swabs with nasopharyngeal aspirates for detection of pandemic influenza A/H1N1 2009 virus by real-time reverse transcriptase PCR. *J Clin Microbiol* 2010;**48**:3492–5.
15. Health Protection Agency (2009). *Pandemic (H1N1) 2009 influenza testing in the critical care setting.* Available at: <http://webarchive.nationalarchives.gov.uk/20140714084352/http://hpa.org.uk/web/hpawebfile/hpaweb_c/1259152349491>.
16. Almond MH, McAuley DF, Wise MP, Griffiths MJD. Influenza-related pneumonia. *Clin Med* 2012;**12**:67–70.
17. Health Protection Agency (2011). *HPA weekly national influenza report: Summary of UK surveillance of influenza and other seasonal respiratory illnesses 6 October 2011–Week 40.* Available at: <http://webarchive.nationalarchives.gov.uk/20140714084352/http://www.hpa.org.uk/webc/HPAwebFile/HPAweb_C/1317130965576>.
18. Hurt AC, Chotpitayasunondh T, Cox NJ, *et al.*; WHO Consultation on Pandemic Influenza A (H1N1) 2009 Virus Resistance to Antivirals. Antiviral resistance during the 2009 influenza A H1N1 pandemic: public health, laboratory, and clinical perspectives. *Lancet Infect Dis* 2012;**12**:240–8.
19. Department of Health (2009). *Pandemic (H1N1) 2009 influenza: a summary of guidance for infection control in healthcare settings.* Available at: <http://webarchive.nationalarchives.gov.uk/20130107105354/http://www.dh.gov.uk/prod_consum_dh/groups/dh_digitalassets/@dh/@en/@ps/documents/digitalasset/dh_110899.pdf>.
20. Wu J, Xu F, Lu L *et al.* Safety and effectiveness of a 2009 H1N1 vaccine in Beijing. *N Engl J Med* 2010;**363**:2416–23.
21. Public Health England (2013). *Influenza: the green book, chapter 19.* Available at: <https://www.gov.uk/government/publications/influenza-the-green-book-chapter-19>.

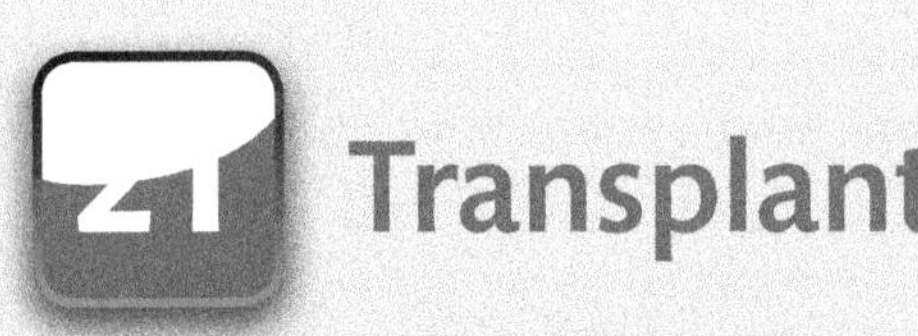

Transplant

Jessica Barrett

Expert Commentary Martin Carby

Case history

A 58-year-old man presented to his local hospital with difficulty breathing. Over the past fortnight, he had become increasingly breathless and was now symptomatic, even when walking round his house. In A&E, his clinical examination was unremarkable, aside from a faint monophonic wheeze, and his oxygen saturations were normal. His other observations and initial blood tests were also normal. His CXR showed some slight volume loss in the right lower lobe, and he was admitted for further assessment.

As a child, he had a severe episode of whooping cough, resulting in bilateral bronchiectasis which progressed over the next 50 years. He worked full-time as a security officer until he took early retirement from ill health, aged 52. Over the years, he had frequent exacerbations, but following his retirement his health deteriorated, with weight loss and frequent episodes of haemoptysis. His FVC had dropped from 62% to 33% predicted, and his FEV_1 from 40% to 30% predicted. He was placed on the transplant register and received a double-lung transplant, aged 57.

Expert comment

Early referral of patients with end-stage lung disease to the transplant team allows timely preparation and listing for organ transplantation, allowing both the best chance of being matched with an organ donor in time and maximizing the potential for good post-operative recovery and long-term survival. It also allows the patient time to come to terms with the need for organ transplantation which is a psychologically, as well as physically, stressful time.

Clinical tip When to refer

Consider referral for patients with end-stage lung disease with declining function despite optimal therapy. Candidates are usually NYHA III or IV, with an expected survival of 2–3 years.

Absolute contraindications include severe hepatic or renal dysfunction, smoking, drug and alcohol misuse, progressive neuromuscular disease, and most malignancies [1].

The transplant centre will require information about the primary diagnosis, co-morbidities and medications, smoking status, bacterial colonization, current exercise capacity, social support, compliance with medications, and psychological state. Also supply results of recent imaging, echocardiogram, ABG, angiography, and bone densitometry, if available.

Learning point Indications for lung transplant (ISHLT 1995–2010)

Group A—obstructive lung disease: COPD (34.6%), alpha-1-antitrypsin deficiency (6.4%), bronchiectasis (2.8%), sarcoidosis (2.6%), lymphangioleiomyomatosis (1.0%).
Group B—pulmonary vascular disease: primary PH (3.2%), congenital heart disease (0.9%).
Group C: cystic fibrosis (16.8%).
Group D—restrictive lung disease: idiopathic pulmonary fibrosis (22.6%), OB (1% non-retransplant, 0.9% retransplant), connective tissue-associated pulmonary fibrosis (1.2%) [2].

The transplant was complicated by severe ischaemic airway injury in the immediate post-transplant period, but he recovered and had remained well for 8 months, until this episode of dyspnoea.

Learning point Early complications

1. Surgical complications: bleeding, air leak, anastomotic complications, and diaphragmatic weakness.
2. Anastomotic complications: anastomotic dehiscence can be partial or complete and presents with dyspnoea, pneumothorax, or collapse. Complete dehiscence is rare and often fatal; partial

(Continued)

Expert comment

Airway stents may have to cross the origin of the upper lobe bronchus in order to cross the narrowed anastomosis or segment of bronchomalacia in the main bronchi. Complications of stent insertion can be bleeding, movement of the stent, and cough, and the stent can become a focus for infection and blocked by secretions. Careful thought is required before stent placement, as the stent quickly (4 weeks) becomes incorporated into the airway wall and is problematic to remove.

Clinical tip

Hyperammonaemia can cause agitation, seizures, and cerebral oedema in the immediate post-operative period due to impaired handling of nitrogenous waste products. Early recognition is vital, and haemodialysis may be required.

Expert comment

Treatment of an acute rejection episode with augmented immunosuppression should be followed by adjustment of the maintenance immunosuppression regimen to try to prevent recurrent rejection—a major risk factor for chronic allograft dysfunction. Recurrent acute rejection can be treated with increasing pharmacological and non-pharmacological immunosuppression, but patient adherence to treatment should also be examined if there is failure of a usually potent immunosuppressive regimen.

Learning point Classification of graft rejection

A, acute rejection: perivascular and interstitial cell infiltrates (grade 0–4).
B, airway inflammation: lymphocytic bronchiolitis.
C, chronic airway rejection: OB—dense fibrous scarring, often eosinophilic.
D, chronic vascular rejection: fibrointimal thickening of pulmonary arteries and veins [10].

dehiscence may be treated conservatively with chest drains or may require placement of a temporary metal stent to promote granulation tissue formation. Anastomotic necrosis and infection may also occur in the first month.

3. Infections: either donor- or recipient-derived organisms.
4. Acute rejection: commonest in the first 6 months but is treatable.
5. PE: common in the immediate post-operative period [3], and the risk is increased by the use of central venous catheterization and underlying CTDs. Be aware of the risk of haemothorax when initiating anticoagulation.
6. Primary graft dysfunction (PGD):
   - occurs in 10–25% of patients due to endothelial damage from ischaemia and reperfusion during the operative period;
   - develops in the first few days following transplant and is commoner in recipients with a BMI >25 kg/m^2, elevated PAPs pre-transplant, and idiopathic or secondary pulmonary fibrosis. Donor risk factors include age, head trauma, and increased ischaemic time [4];
   - patients present with hypoxaemia and diffuse parenchymal infiltrates on CXR;
   - the International Society for Heart and Lung Transplantation (ISHLT) classifies the severity of PGD based on the PaO_2/FiO_2 at 0, 24, 48, and 72 hours, with mortality of over 50% in severe episodes [2];
   - treatment is supportive, with low tidal volume ventilation, progressing to ECMO, if necessary, and careful avoidance of fluid overload. Inhaled nitrous oxide does not improve morbidity and mortality [5].
7. Pleural effusion: during removal of the native lung, the pulmonary lymphatics are severed. Rarely, the thoracic duct may also be cut (particularly if there are mediastinal adhesions), and the resultant chyle leak can cause a persistent pleural effusion. Although mostly non-infectious, an empyema must be excluded, as there is a high associated mortality [6].
8. Ischaemia of bronchial artery circulation in the first month before collateral vessels develop.
9. Bronchomalacia: dynamic collapse of the airways. Occurs in the first 4 months and presents as cough, shortness of breath, and an obstructive spirometry pattern. Diagnosis is made with expiratory CT scanning and bronchoscopy, and the lesion can be stented, if necessary.

Learning point Acute rejection

Acute cellular rejection (ACR) usually occurs within the first 3 months, but occasionally after the first year. Some patients are asymptomatic; others have fever, malaise, cough, and dyspnoea. A drop in spirometry of >10% is a sensitive indicator, but not specific. Radiological findings are similarly wnon-specific. A CXR may show infiltrates, and a CT scan may show GGOs, septal thickening, or pleural effusions. The diagnosis is confirmed with TBBx findings of perivascular lymphocytic infiltrates. It is advisable to take a number of alveolated biopsies, as the pathology may be patchy. Many transplant centres will take surveillance biopsies during the first year to diagnose asymptomatic rejection; however, as the bronchoscopy complication rate varies, there is no universal consensus as to whether the risk outweighs the benefits [7, 8]. Treatment is with high-dose methylprednisolone for 3 days, then tapering doses of oral glucocorticoids [9]. Careful follow-up is essential to ensure adequate response.

On the ward, he was reviewed by the respiratory team. Spirometry was performed, and, although his FEV_1 and FVC were unchanged from recent readings, a terminal phase plateau was noted on the flow–volume loop.

He was transferred to his transplant centre and underwent bronchoscopy. A significant stenosis was found distal to the right main bronchus, with an estimated 50% of the lumen obstructed. A stent was placed using a rigid bronchoscope, and he made a good recovery.

Learning point Bronchial stenoses

Anastomotic complications tend to occur late, with an increase in bronchial stenosis from the second month onwards. The majority of stenoses affect the anastomosis, blocking the lumen with granulation or scar tissue, but some affect the distal airways, causing a 'vanishing airway syndrome'. Initially, the obstruction may be asymptomatic but will progress, causing dyspnoea, cough, or post-obstruction pneumonia.

Fernández-Bussy *et al.* [11] advise attempting bronchoscopic balloon dilatation at least three or four times before considering stent insertion, as this is often complicated by mucus plugging, further granulation tissue formation, and stent migration.

He remained well for a year, over which time he was able to walk his dog a couple of miles a day. His daily spirometry readings remained stable, and his immunosuppressive regime of ciclosporin 100 mg and 75 mg, mycophenolate 500 mg bd, and prednisolone 20 mg od was well tolerated.

During winter, he became unwell, with increasing daytime somnolence, and was drowsy and confused when woken. He developed a productive cough, with increasing shortness of breath, leaving him housebound. In A&E, he was found to be hypoxic, and an initial ABG on 2 L of oxygen showed an acute-on-chronic type 2 respiratory failure (pH 7.30, PaO_2 8.9, $PaCO_2$ 10, HCO_3 42). A CXR showed a right lower lobe consolidation. He was started on NIV and broad-spectrum antibiotics. Over the next 2 days, he began to improve, and, after discussion with his transplant team, another bronchoscopy was performed. Pus was found in his right bronchus intermedius and lower lobe. Two hours after the procedure, he desaturated and became unresponsive. His ABG deteriorated (pH 7.05, PaO_2 7, $PaCO_2$ 22). He had a respiratory arrest, was intubated, and was started on tazobactam–piperacillin. After 5 days of mechanical ventilation and 4 days of NIV, he was sufficiently recovered for discharge planning.

He went home with a NIPPY machine and 0.5 L/minute of oxygen. Over the next 18 months, he had multiple chest infections and two further respiratory arrests, with high CO_2 levels measured each time. His sputum grew a variety of pathogens, including *Candida* spp., *Haemophilus influenza*, atypical *Mycobacterium chelonae* and *Pseudomonas aeruginosa*, which he was known to be colonized with prior to his transplant.

He required a course of antibiotics every 8 weeks so was started on regular azithromycin. The antibiotic choice was tailored according to sputum culture results. Bronchiectasis was detected in both transplanted lungs, probably secondary to the episode of ischaemic airway injury following the operation. In addition to the frequent infections, he had also developed complications from his immunosuppressive regime. He was found to have osteoporosis from the prednisolone and, following an episode of shingles, had persistent, burning neuropathic pain across his upper abdomen.

Expert comment

Although the starting point for an immunosuppressive regimen is according to a standard perioperative protocol, it can thereafter be tailored to the needs of the individual. There is often a misconception that measuring the level of immunosuppressant in blood gives a precise guide to the requirements of the drug. Rather, measuring levels helps to avoid toxicity and gives some surety regarding efficacy; thereafter, target drug levels are determined in an individual according to the history of rejection episodes, also taking into account the frequency and diversity of infective episodes and drug toxicities.

Learning point ICU outcomes for lung transplant patients

Of 51 lung transplant patients admitted to a Canadian ICU, 37% died during that admission [12]. Predictors of mortality were high APACHE III score, the need for mechanical ventilation, and a lower FEV_1 to best FEV_1 ratio. Whilst the authors acknowledge the high mortality in this group, they also stress the good medium-term outcomes for survivors, particularly those with reversible causes for ICU admission.

Expert comment

Whilst common pathogens also remain common in lung transplant recipients, there is a pressing need to try to make a microbiological diagnosis, rather than give empirical antibacterial treatment. Community-acquired viral infections and fungi can both cause LRTIs and require urgent treatment with potentially toxic medications with potential interactions with immunosuppressive drugs. Close liaison with, or transfer to, the transplant centre is advised.

Clinical tip Preventing infections

- Pre-transplant: influenza, tetanus, hepatitis B, and *Pneumococcus* vaccinations.
- Post-transplant: avoid live vaccines.
- Cultures from donor and recipient lungs, broad-spectrum post-transplant, and tailor to culture results, if necessary.
- CMV prophylaxis (with serum CMV monitoring).
- *Pneumocystis* prophylaxis.
- *Aspergillus* prophylaxis.

Clinical tip Consider the possibility of recurrence of primary disease in. ..

- Sarcoidosis (granulomas recur in two-thirds, rarely symptomatic).
- Diffuse panbronchiolitis.
- Giant cell interstitial pneumonia.
- Langerhans cell histiocytosis.
- Lymphangioleiomyomatosis.
- Bronchoalveolar cell carcinoma.

Learning point Non-infective complications of immunosuppressants

Osteoporosis is a common finding both pre- and post-transplant. Approximately 61% of patients on the transplant list have osteoporosis [13], as most will have been prescribed steroids for their underlying lung disease and will continue to take them as post-transplant immunosuppression. Previous smoking history and low BMI also contribute, and patients with cystic fibrosis are particularly vulnerable due to pancreatic insufficiency and malabsorption. Over the first year following transplantation, bone mineral density falls by around 5%, even in patients treated with calcium and vitamin D supplementation [14]. Patients awaiting transplant should have a dual-energy X-ray absorptiometry (DEXA) scan to assess bone mineral density and receive calcium and vitamin D supplementation. If osteoporosis is diagnosed, they should also receive bisphosphonates, and, following transplant, annual follow-up is advised [13].

Calcineurin inhibitors have acute and long-term effects on renal function. There is an immediate fall in the glomerular filtration rate (GFR), secondary to afferent arteriole vasoconstriction which is reversible with dose adjustment. Over a longer period, renal function may deteriorate due to tubular atrophy and glomerulosclerosis, with around 7% of lung and heart-lung transplant patients progressing to end-stage renal disease [15]. Excellent blood pressure control and preferential use of tacrolimus may slow progression in these patients.

Neurological complications are also relatively frequent post-transplant, with reported rates of serious complications as high as 50% at 10 years [16].

Expert comment

Calcineurin inhibitors cause hypertension (further exacerbating renal impairment), diabetes, and hyperlipidaemia. In the longer term, they predispose patients to lymphoproliferative disorders (sometimes related to Ebstein-Barr virus (EBV) infection) and skin cancer, particularly in those with a history of high sun exposure. There is a large potential for drug interactions, and recently generic formulations of calcineurin inhibitors are available. These are not bioequivalent at the same doses, and swapping between formulations should be done in expert hands, with appropriate drug and patient monitoring.

Three years following his initial transplant, his condition stabilized. The infections had become less frequent, and his immunosuppression was at a safe minimum. His last respiratory infection was 6 months ago, and he did not require intubation during his stay in hospital. He uses NIPPY at home for 8 hours a day and is making good progress.

Discussion

This case highlights several of the common complications following lung transplantation, most prominently the high risk of post-transplant infections.

Bacterial infections

Transplanted lungs are at a greater risk of infection than other solid organ transplants. The graft is constantly exposed to environmental pathogens and requires greater immunosuppression, as pulmonary tissue is highly immunogenic. The transplant process affects the intrinsic protective mechanisms by reducing lymphatic drainage and causing ciliary dysfunction from ischaemia. Denervation of the graft lung during transplantation and post-operative pain may both result in blunting of the cough reflex [17].

Bacterial infections are common immediately post-operatively, so transplant centres routinely start broad-spectrum antibiotics to cover this period. Washings of the donor lung are cultured, as transplanted bacteria can cause serious infections. These results, and pre-transplant sputum cultures for patients with cystic fibrosis, can be used to refine antibiotic choice [18].

Expert comment

Another clinically useful way to consider infections is with different pathogens common in early post-operative care, compared to during later follow-up. In the perioperative period, infections are commonly either donor- or recipient-derived organisms, hence the importance of a microbiological history, whilst a patient is on the waiting list, and material for culture from the organ donor. Infection with latent CMV can occur but is much less common with effective valganciclovir prophylaxis. Later on, chronic colonization with Gram-negative organisms is common, as are community-acquired viruses and fungal pathogens and occasionally infections with NTM.

Clinical tip Useful investigations in pneumonia

Imaging

- CXR.
- Blood cultures.
- Serum CMV PCR.
- *Legionella* and pneumococcal urinary antigen.
- *Mycoplasma* serology.

BAL

- Microscopy and Gram stain: bacteria, fungi, *Pneumocystis jirovecii*, mycobacteria.
- Aerobic and anaerobic culture, fungal and mycobacterial culture.
- Galactomannan antigen.
- CMV, herpes simplex virus, varicella-zoster virus, influenza, respiratory syncytial virus, adenovirus PCR/direct fluorescent antibody.

The majority of infections are caused by Gram-negative bacteria, most commonly *Pseudomonas* and *Enterobacteriaceae*. *Burkholderia cepacia* can cause devastating post-operative infection and is a much greater risk for severe pneumonia than *Pseudomonas* colonization in patients with cystic fibrosis [19]. Patients with cystic fibrosis also retain an increased risk of pneumonia, as the upper airway chloride channel defect remains despite native lung removal. In these patients, a CT scan of the sinuses is advisable pre-transplant to allow eradication of sinus infections [18].

Clinical tip

The presentation of respiratory tract infections (pneumonia is rare) in the transplant patient group may be atypical due to heavy immunosuppression. The signs and symptoms may also closely mimic those of rejection, or there may be concurrent pathology, so TBBx are often taken, in addition to the usual spectrum of investigations.

Mycobacterial infections

Clinically significant mycobacterial infections are relatively rare following a lung transplant, and they may represent reactivation [20]. Both tuberculous and NTM infections are treated with standard therapy in this patient group.

Fungal infections

Aspergillus and *Candida* are the commonest fungal infections, and the risk is increased in the first 6 months [21]. *Candida* infections are perioperative and rarely seen after the first month, whilst *Aspergillus* infection has a peak incidence at 3.2 months [22]. Around 25% of patients will be colonized with *Aspergillus*, with higher rates amongst those transplanted for cystic fibrosis [22]. Colonization is a risk factor for invasive disease, along with CMV infection [18], ischaemic injury, and OB.

Aspergillosis can present as tracheobronchitis, subacute infections with low-grade fever, pulmonary nodules or tree-in-bud shadowing on CT scan, or disseminated disease [23]. Fungal endocarditis and endophthalmitis can also occur. Tracheobronchitis usually presents with a cough or fever but may progress to haemoptysis, with severe infections even eroding the pulmonary artery [24]. The diagnosis is made on bronchoscopy which may show mucosal oedema, ulceration, or pseudomembranes, particularly at the anastomosis site. BAL can be tested for galactomannan antigen and stained and cultured for fungi. If necessary, the diagnosis is confirmed with histopathology.

Patients with pulmonary invasion present in a similar way, but usually later, and with signs of an LRTI. A CXR may show consolidation or cavitations and nodules. The classical finding on a CT scan is the ‘halo sign’ which describes a rim of ground

Clinical tip

Voriconazole and itraconazole interact with immunosuppressives (tacrolimus, sirolimus, ciclosporin), causing elevated levels—check and reduce the dose, if necessary. It is also important to monitor trough voriconazole levels.

Expert comment

Voriconazole and posaconazole have potent interactions with tacrolimus, and even more so with sirolimus. Both these immunosuppressants should be adjusted prospectively on institution of antifungal treatment. Tacrolimus should be halved, sirolimus reduced to about 15% of the original dose, and close monitoring continued until blood levels of immunosuppressants are stable.

Trough voriconazole level measurement may help to improve the efficacy and avoid the side effects of this drug. Side effects include visual disturbance, hallucinations, photosensitivity, and abnormalities in LFTs.

glass attenuation surrounding a central nodule. Disseminated infection is less common and preferentially affects the sinus, CNS, and spine.

The mainstay of treatment for invasive aspergillosis is voriconazole. Patients with extensive necrosis from tracheobronchitis should also receive nebulized amphotericin and be considered for debridement.

Evidence base Voriconazole versus amphotericin

- Randomized, unblinded trial comparing the efficacy of voriconazole with amphotericin in treating invasive aspergillosis [25].
- A total of 144 patients were treated with IV voriconazole for at least 7 days, followed by oral voriconazole, and 133 patients were treated with IV amphotericin.
- At 12 weeks, there were significantly better outcomes in the voriconazole group, with 52.8% showing a response to treatment versus 31.6% in the amphotericin group. Survival rates were also significantly higher, and drug-related side effects lower in the voriconazole group [25].

Pneumocystis jirovecii can be detected in the vast majority of transplanted lungs if prophylaxis is not used. Transplant centres routinely prescribe co-trimoxazole which is extremely effective, both as treatment and prophylaxis, and also provides protection against *Listeria*, *Nocardia*, and *Toxoplasma* [26]. For those patients who experience side effects, nebulized or IV pentamidine may be used instead for prophylaxis. Pentamidine is ineffective as a treatment if nebulized and takes several days to reach a therapeutic level in the lungs when administered IV; therefore, overlap for this period with another treatment is important.

Viral infections

CMV is a relatively common pathogen in this patient group and is important not only for the immediate effects of the infection, but also for its contributory role in the development of OB. There is growing evidence that episodes of CMV pneumonia increase the risk of both acute and chronic rejection [27] and also increase the likelihood of invasive fungal infections occurring.

CMV may be present as either CMV infection, where there is evidence of active viral replication, or CMV disease where there are signs or symptoms resulting from the infection. CMV syndrome, commonly presenting with fever, leucopenia, and thrombocytopenia, and tissue invasive disease are both classified under the latter heading. Tissue invasive disease usually affects the lung parenchyma and can present very similarly to acute rejection. Other organs may also be affected, particularly within the gastrointestinal tract.

The diagnosis is most securely made via a biopsy; however, the presence of CMV in the serum and broncheoalveolar fluid, together with radiological changes, are helpful. CXR and CT findings are variable but often show patchy GGOs and small nodules. Histopathological evidence of viral cytopathic changes and inclusion bodies can help to distinguish acute rejection with CMV infection from invasive CMV pneumonitis.

Where possible, seronegative recipients should receive CMV-negative donor lungs; however, this lengthens waiting list times so may not be practical. Prophylaxis with oral valganciclovir is important, but there is currently no consensus on the optimal length of treatment. Less than 3 months of prophylaxis produces worse outcomes, and there is continued benefit to at least 12 months. A recent study argued indefinite prophylaxis as a practical strategy to delay or prevent the development of bronchiolitis obliterans syndrome (BOS) [28]. Treatment of mild disease is with oral valganciclovir, and severe disease with IV ganciclovir, adjusted for renal function. Foscarnet can be used if there is resistance to ganciclovir, although rates of resistance are only around 6% [29].

Expert comment

Although CMV prophylaxis is recommended in the UK, other centres may well take an approach of frequent monitoring, and, if either PCR or pp65 antigen becomes positive, pre-emptive therapy is provided before clinical disease is apparent. This approach does not seem to be inferior, in terms of patient outcomes, and may be relevant to consider, in light of increasing drug costs in the context of financial constraints.

Obliterative bronchiolitis

There has been a significant improvement in early morbidity and mortality in lung transplant recipients over the past 10 years; however, this trend is not seen after the first year. The cause of this is chronic rejection, which is still the main reason why survival for lung transplants lags behind that of other solid organ transplants. Reported prevalence varies between transplant centres; however, the largest volume of data are from the ISHLT. Their 2008 report stated 51% of recipients will have evidence of chronic rejection at 5.6 years [30]. Following diagnosis of chronic rejection, the median survival is only 3 years [31].

The histopathological presentation of chronic rejection is OB, but the diagnosis is frequently made clinically, due to the low sensitivity of TBBx, and is therefore referred to as bronchiolitis obliterans syndrome (BOS).

Initial presentation is usually after the first 6 months, and the incidence increases steadily, affecting almost 50% by 5 years. Symptoms are non-specific and varied—some patients have upper respiratory symptoms; others notice a slight decline in their exercise tolerance or a non-productive cough. As the syndrome progresses, the dyspnoea becomes much more significant, and the cough may become productive. *Pseudomonas* can often be found in sputum samples, and spirometry will deteriorate, showing a severely obstructive picture in the later stages. Clinical findings vary from a completely clear chest to crackles, pops, and squeaks, as the bronchiolitis progresses.

Risk factors and prevention

The usual inexorable decline following the onset of BOS makes prevention a vital consideration. The risk factors for BOS include immunological and non-immunological insults, which have led to some dispute about the underlying aetiology. As factors other than episodes of rejection clearly play a role in the onset of BOS, the picture is probably more complex than simply a manifestation of chronic rejection.

Learning point Risk factors for BOS

Probable	Potential
Acute rejection	*Aspergillus* colonization of the lower airways
CMV pneumonitis	Aspiration
HLA mismatching	CMV infection without pneumonitis
Lymphocytic bronchitis/bronchiolitis	Donor antigen-specific activity
Non-compliance with medications	EBV reactivation
PGD	Aetiology of native lung disease
	Gastro-oesophageal reflux
	Older donor age
	Pneumonia (Gram-negatives, Gram-positives, fungi)
	Prolonged allograft ischaemia
	Recurrent infection other than CMV

From reference [32].

A major risk factor is acute rejection, particularly severe or frequent episodes [33, 34]. Episodes of lymphocytic bronchiolitis are commoner in patients who go on to develop BOS. Other findings that suggest a strong immunological basis are an increased risk in recipients with a HLA mismatch with their donor [34] and that some patients improve with altered or increased immunosuppression.

Non-immunological factors are also important. The risk is increased by episodes of CMV pneumonitis, ischaemic injury from PGD, and gastro-oesophageal reflux. Invasive CMV pneumonitis has been found to significantly increase the risk of BOS development, with worse outcomes if the infection occurs within the first 6 months post-transplant [35].

Evidence base Davis *et al.* (2003)

- A retrospective study of 128 lung transplant patients who had an oesophageal pH assessment.
- Seventy-three per cent had abnormal studies, and 43 patients subsequently underwent fundoplication.
- Sixteen of 26 patients with BOS pre-procedure showed an improvement in the FEV_1.
- Overall survival was significantly better in patients who had fundoplication and those who had normal pH studies [36].

A subsequent retrospective study [37] found similarly improved survival and decreased rates of BOS in patients who had early surgical treatment of reflux disease following lung transplant [37].

Diagnosis

Diagnosis of BOS is one of exclusion. CXR and HRCT findings are non-specific but may show hyperinflation and expiratory air trapping. In advanced disease, there may also be evidence of bronchiectasis.

As long as the patient can tolerate the procedures, bronchoscopy and TBBx are useful to exclude other causes of the clinical presentation.

Early biopsy findings are submucosal lymphocytic infiltrates affecting the bronchioles and smaller airways. This progresses to epithelial cell necrosis and granulation tissue formation. Fibrosis then develops, gradually obliterating the airway. These findings are patchy and may be missed on TBBx; therefore, a diagnosis of BOS is made if the FEV_1 falls below 80% for >3 weeks, with no other obvious cause [38, 39]. There have been several attempts to find early or surrogate markers for BOS, including chemokine levels, exhaled nitrous oxide, and neutrophilic BAL washings, but so far none have been sufficiently specific or sensitive to be used for diagnosis.

Treatment

There is no established treatment for BOS, and strategies used vary between transplant centres. Broadly, the choices are amongst changing the immunosuppressive regime, aggressively treating any exacerbating factors such as infection, and some novel therapies that are discussed in later text. These strategies are often futile, and the only option left for many patients is retransplantation. It has previously been assumed that BOS occurs more quickly in patients following their second transplant; however, this is not borne out by data from long-term follow-up of 15 retransplanted patients [40].

Expert comment

Lung transplant recipients can successfully receive a second transplant but should fulfil all the same criteria as those being assessed for a transplant the first time. Sadly after surgery and medical treatment for BOS itself, this is rarely the case, and many patients with progressive BOS are supported with symptom control and terminal care.

A meta-analysis of three RCTs found tacrolimus reduced episodes of acute rejection, compared with ciclosporin, but had no impact on all-cause mortality or BOS occurrence [41]. Speich *et al.* found mycophenolate decreased graft loss from BOS but did not alter the incidence or overall mortality, compared with azathioprine [42]. Increasing the level of immunosuppression can slow the rate of progression but increases the mortality rate from other causes.

Strategies used in transplant centres across the world include total lymphoid irradiation, extracorporeal photophoresis, and inhaled ciclosporin. Inhaled corticosteroids have been found to have little effect. Some studies have demonstrated attenuation of lung function decline with montelukast or IV immunoglobulin, but more evidence for these approaches is needed.

Azithromycin may play a role in both treatment and prevention of BOS. Vos *et al.* found that 40% of patients with BOS showed a ≥10% improvement in FEV_1 after 3–6 months of treatment with azithromycin. This group of 'responders' had a higher BAL neutrophil count prior to treatment and, most importantly, had better long-term survival, compared to the group of 'non-responders' [43]. An RCT by the same group of researchers demonstrated both an improvement in FEV_1 and greater BOS-free survival in patients treated with prophylactic azithromycin post-transplant [44]. These studies used doses of 250 mg on alternate days. Although there are potential side effects associated with long-term use, including the development of resistance in colonizing bacteria and an increased risk of cardiac complications, many centres are starting to use this strategy.

Malignancies

Post-transplant lymphoproliferative disease

The incidence of post-transplant lymphoproliferative disease (PTLD) is highest in the first year post-transplant and usually occurs in the allograft. Early cases usually present as lung nodules, whereas late-onset cases present with disseminated pathology such as peripheral and intra-abdominal lymphadenopathy or intussusception. The source of EBV is usually the donor lung, and the highest risk for PTLD is in recipients who were EBV-negative pre-transplant; one paper describes an incidence of 33% in the EBV-negative group versus 2% in the EBV-positive group [45]. Cystic fibrosis, tacrolimus use, and the donor HLA A2 or DR7 status are also risk factors [46, 47]. Diagnosis is made with imaging and tissue sampling, preferably from a biopsy, rather than fine-needle aspiration. The histopathology usually shows B cell lymphoproliferation, and EBV infection of cells can be confirmed with *in situ* hybridization. Management is best undertaken at the transplant centre and involves reducing the level of immunosuppression to improve the cellular immune response to the virus. Ganciclovir and rituximab are also used, but chemotherapy can be problematic, as patients are already immunosuppressed.

Our patient's unstable course following lung transplantation is certainly not unusual, considering the high rate of short- and long-term complications in this group. The ongoing communication between his local hospital and the transplant centre has played a key role in providing him with optimal care during episodes of acute illness, and this link should be maintained by anyone caring for a patient post-lung transplant. With careful regulation of his immunosuppression and prompt treatment of infections, it is to be hoped his lung function will remain stable. However, 74% of lung transplant recipients have developed BOS 10 years post-operation, so he remains at high risk. With encouraging advances being made in the treatment of other complications, chronic rejection remains the critical problem to solve.

Clinical tip Be aware of the increased risk of other malignancies

Other than PTLD, the commonest malignancies found in lung transplant recipients are skin, vulval, and cervical tumours. Lung cancer has only been reported in patients transplanted for pulmonary fibrosis or COPD with a significant smoking history. In these patients, the tumour often progresses rapidly, possibly due to loss of tumour regulation caused by immunosuppression.

A final word from the expert

The case presented demonstrates several important principles concerning lung transplantation.

1. Whilst lung transplantation increases life expectancy and greatly improves the quality of life for many people with end-stage lung disease, it is not a cure, and ongoing medical follow-up, drug therapy, and frequent interventions are required.
2. Specific complications, such as in this case, anastomotic complications, and sudden deterioration during an infective exacerbation can occur.
3. Considering the lifelong immunosuppressive regimen following a lung transplantation, lung transplant recipients can be, in many ways, surprisingly robust, and good outcomes are expected from infective exacerbations with swift intervention and consideration of a range of infections requiring different treatments.
4. The major challenge in improving outcomes for lung transplant recipients remains prevention and treatment of OB. The identification of precipitants and early intervention with tailoring of appropriate treatments are having an impact, and survival is improving over time. The realization that OB is multifactorial in origin, and not just a manifestation of immune-mediated injury by the host immune system, is an important step towards further improvements.

References

1. Glanville AR, Estenne M. Indications, patient selection and timing of referral for lung transplantation. *Eur Respir J* 2003;**22**:845–52.
2. Christie JD, Carby M, Bag R, Corris P, Hertz M, Weill D; ISHLT Working Group on Primary Lung Graft Dysfunction. Report of the ISHLT Working Group on Primary Lung Graft Dysfunction part II: definition. A consensus statement of the International Society for Heart and Lung Transplantation. *J Heart Lung Transplant* 2005;**24**:1454–9.
3. Izbicki G, Bairey O, Shitrit D, Lahav J, Kramer MR. Increased thromboembolic events after lung transplantation. *Chest* 2006;**129**:412–16.
4. Kuntz CL, Hadjiliadis D, Ahya VN *et al*. Risk factors for early primary graft dysfunction after lung transplantation: a registry study. *Clin Transplant* 2009;**23**:819–30.
5. Tavare AN, Tsakok T. Does prophylactic inhaled nitric oxide reduce morbidity and mortality after lung transplantation? *Interact Cardiovasc Thorac Surg* 2011;**13**:516–20.
6. Nunley DR, Grgurich WF, Keenan RJ, Dauber JH. Empyema complicating successful lung transplantation. *Chest* 1999;**115**:1312–15.
7. McWilliams TJ, Williams TJ, Whitford HM, Snell GI. Surveillance bronchoscopy in lung transplant recipients: risk versus benefit. *J Heart Lung Transplant* 2008;**27**:1203–9.
8. Sandrini A, Glanville AR. The controversial role of surveillance bronchoscopy after lung transplantation. *Curr Opin Organ Transplant* 2009;**14**:494–98.
9. Levine SM; Transplant/Immunology Network of the American College of Chest Physicians. A survey of clinical practice of lung transplantation in North America. *Chest* 2004;**125**:1224–38.
10. Stewart S, Fishbein MC, Snell GI *et al*. Revision of the 1996 working formulation for the standardization of nomenclature in the diagnosis of lung rejection. *J Heart Lung Transplant* 2007;**26**:1229–42.
11. Fernández-Bussy S, Majid A, Caviedes I, Akindipe O, Baz M, Jantz M. Treatment of airway complications following lung transplantation. *Arch Bronconeumol* 2011;**47**:128–33.

12. Hadjiliadis D, Steele MP, Govert JA, Davis RD, Palmer SM. Outcome of lung transplant patients admitted to the medical ICU. *Chest* 2004;**125**:1040–5.
13. Ebeling PR. Approach to the patient with transplantation-related bone loss. *J Clin Endocrinol Metab* 2009;**94**:1483–90.
14. Spira A, Gutierrez C, Chaparro C, Hutcheon MA, Chan CK. Osteoporosis and lung transplantation: a prospective study. *Chest* 2000;**117**:476–81.
15. Ishani A, Erturk S, Hertz MI, Matas AJ, Savik K, Rosenberg ME. Predictors of renal function following lung or heart-lung transplantation. *Kidney Int* 2002;**61**:2228–34.
16. Mateen FJ, Dierkhising RA, Rabinstein AA, van de Beek D, Wijdicks EF. Neurological complications following adult lung transplantation. *Am J Transplant* 2010;**10**:908–14.
17. Kotloff RM, Ahya VN. Medical complications of lung transplantation. *Eur Respir J* 2004;**23**:334–42.
18. Speich R, van der Bij W. Epidemiology and management of infections after lung transplantation. *Clin Infect Dis* 2001;**33**(Suppl 1):S58–65.
19. Alexander BD, Petzold EW, Reller LB *et al.* Survival after lung transplantation of cystic fibrosis patients infected with *Burkholderia cepacia* complex. *Am J Transplant* 2008;**8**:1025–30.
20. Kesten S, Chaparro C. Mycobacterial infections in lung transplant recipients. *Chest* 1999;**115**:741–5.
21. Singh N, Husain S. *Aspergillus* infections after lung transplantation: clinical differences in type of transplant and implications for management. *J Heart Lung Transplant* 2003;**22**:258–66.
22. Singh N, Paterson DL. *Aspergillus* infections in transplant recipients. *Clin Microbiol Rev* 2005;**18**:44–69.
23. Mehrad B, Paciocco G, Martinez FJ, Ojo TC, Iannettoni MD, Lynch JP. Spectrum of *Aspergillus* infection in lung transplant recipients: case series and review of the literature. *Chest* 2001;**119**:169–75.
24. Kessler R, Massard G, Warter A *et al.* Bronchial-pulmonary artery fistula after unilateral lung transplantation: a case report. *J Heart Lung Transplant* 1997;**16**:674–7.
25. Herbrecht R, Denning DW, Patterson TF *et al.*; Invasive Fungal Infections Group of the European Organisation for Research and Treatment of Cancer and the Global Aspergillus Study Group. Voriconazole versus amphotericin B for primary therapy of invasive aspergillosis. *N Engl J Med* 2002;**347**:408–15.
26. Green H, Paul M, Vidal L, Leibovici L. Prophylaxis of *Pneumocystis* pneumonia in immunocompromised non-HIV-infected patients: systematic review and meta-analysis of randomized controlled trials. *Mayo Clin Proc* 2007;**82**:1052–9.
27. Snyder LD, Finlen-Copeland CA, Turbyfill WJ, Howell D, Willnaer DA, Palmer SM. Cytomegalovirus pneumonitis is a risk for bronchiolitis obliterans syndrome in lung transplantation. *Am J Respir Crit Care Med* 2010;**181**:1391–6.
28. Valentine VG, Weill D, Gupta MR *et al.* Ganciclovir for cytomegalovirus: a call for indefinite prophylaxis in lung transplantation. *J Heart Lung Transplant* 2008;**27**:875–81.
29. Bhorade SM, Lurain NS, Jordan A *et al.* Emergence of ganciclovir-resistant cytomegalovirus in lung transplant recipients. *J Heart Lung Transplant* 2002;**21**:1274–82.
30. Christie JD, Edwards LB, Aurora P *et al.* Registry of the International Society for Heart and Lung Transplantation: twenty-fifth official adult lung and heart/lung transplantation report—2008. *J Heart Lung Transplant* 2008;**27**:957–69.
31. Valentine VG, Robbins RC, Berry GJ *et al.* Actuarial survival of heart-lung and bilateral sequential lung transplant recipients with obliterative bronchiolitis. *J Heart Lung Transplant* 1996;**15**:371–83.
32. Hayes D. A review of bronchiolitis obliterans syndrome and therapeutic strategies. *J Cardiothorac Surg* 2011;**6**:92.
33. Bando K, Paradis IL, Similo S *et al.* Obliterative bronchiolitis after lung and heart-lung transplantation. An analysis of risk factors and management. *J Thorac Cardiovasc Surg* 1995;**110**:4–13.

34. Schulman LL, Weinberg AD, McGregor CC, Suciu-Foca NM, Itescu S. Influence of donor and recipient HLA locus mismatching on development of obliterative bronchiolitis after lung transplantation. *Am J Respir Crit Care Med* 2001;**163**:437–42.
35. Snyder LD, Finlen-Copeland CA, Turbyfill WJ, Howell D, Willnaer DA, Palmer SM. Cytomegalovirus pneumonitis is a risk for bronchiolitis obliterans syndrome in lung transplantation. *Am J Respir Crit Care Med* 2010;**181**:1391–6.
36. Davis RD Jr, Lau CL, Eubanks S *et al.* Improved lung allograft function after fundoplication in patients with gastroesophageal reflux disease undergoing lung transplantation. *J Thorac Cardiovasc Surg* 2003;**125**:533–42.
37. Cantu E 3rd, Appel JZ 3rd, Hartwig MG *et al.* J. Maxwell Chamberlain Memorial Paper. Early fundoplication prevents chronic allograft dysfunction in patients with gastroesophageal reflux disease. *Ann Thorac Surg* 2004;**78**:1142–51.
38. Boehler A, Kesten S, Weder W, Speich R. Bronchiolitis obliterans after lung transplantation: a review. *Chest* 1998;**114**:1411–26.
39. Cooper J, Billingham M, Egan T *et al.* A working formulation for the standardization of nomenclature and for clinical staging of chronic dysfunction in lung allografts: International Society for Heart and Lung Transplantation. *J Heart Lung Transplant* 1993;**12**:713–16.
40. Brugière O, Thabut G, Castier Y *et al.* Lung retransplantation for bronchiolitis obliterans syndrome: long-term follow-up in a series of 15 recipients. *Chest* 2003;**123**:1832–7.
41. Fan Y, Xiao YB, Weng YB, Weng YG. Tacrolimus versus cyclosporine for adult lung transplant recipients: a meta-analysis. *Transplant Proc* 2009;**41**:1821–4.
42. Speich R, Schneider S, Hofer M *et al.* Mycophenolate mofetil reduces alveolar inflammation, acute rejection and graft loss due to bronchiolitis obliterans syndrome after lung transplantation. *Pulm Pharmacol Ther* 2010;**23**:445–9.
43. Vos R, Vanaudenaerde BM, Ottevaere A *et al.* Long-term azithromycin therapy for bronchiolitis obliterans syndrome: divide and conquer? *J Heart Lung Transplant* 2010;**29**:1358–68.
44. Vos R, Vanaudenaerde BM, Verleden SE *et al.* A randomised controlled trial of azithromycin to prevent chronic rejection after lung transplantation. *Eur Respir J* 2011;**37**:164–72.
45. Aris RM, Maia DM, Neuringer IP *et al.* Post-transplantation lymphoproliferative disorder in the Epstein-Barr virus-naïve lung transplant recipient. *Am J Respir Crit Care Med* 1996;**154**(6 Pt 1):1712–17.
46. Parker A, Bowles K, Bradley JA *et al.*; Haemato-oncology Task Force of the British Committee for Standards in Haematology and British Transplantation Society. Diagnosis of post-transplant lymphoproliferative disorder in solid organ transplant recipients—BCSH and BTS Guidelines. *Br J Haematol* 2010;**149**:675–92.
47. Montone KT, Litzky LA, Wurster A *et al.* Analysis of Epstein-Barr virus-associated posttransplantation lymphoproliferative disorder after lung transplantation. *Surgery* 1996;**119**:544–51.

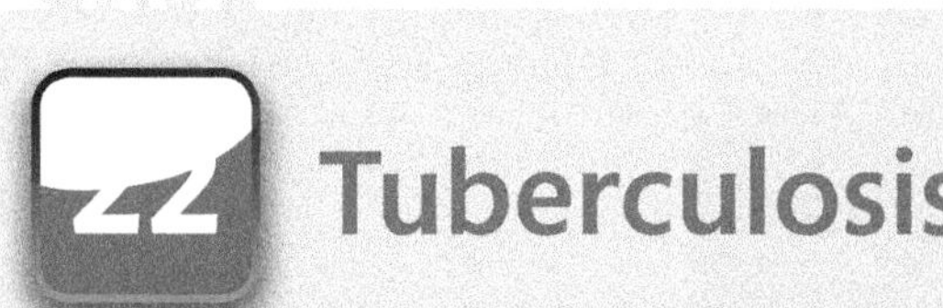

Tuberculosis

Georgina Russell

Expert commentary Onn Min Kon

Case history

A 34-year-old man was referred to the chest clinic with a 3-week history of cough productive of yellow sputum with streaks of fresh blood. He had lost 10 kg in weight and described sweating at night, such that he lay on a towel which he would have to change in the night. He had no documented fever and no chest pain and continued to work.

He had no past medical history, took no regular medication, and had no known allergies. He smoked five cigarettes a day and drank no alcohol.

He was born in northern Thailand and had been in the UK for the last 14 months. He worked full-time in a restaurant owned by his cousin and lived with his wife and their 3-year-old son in a house with his uncle and aunt. He played football twice a week, coaching a local youth team.

On examination, he was thin, with a BMI of 17.5. There were some small palpable cervical lymph nodes, but the remainder of his clinical examination was normal.

The patient was sent for a chest radiograph (Figure 22.1), and blood tests and sputum samples collected on 3 consecutive days were sent for analysis.

The blood tests showed a normal renal function, a low haemoglobin of 11.5 g/dL, an elevated WCC (12.4×10^9/L) with predominant neutrophilia, and a raised ALP (280 IU/L).

The patient returned to clinic a week later, his symptoms persisting, and he had now stopped work. He had submitted three sputum samples. Each underwent Gram staining and standard culture, as well as auramine staining and mycobacterial culture. The standard cultures did not grow any bacteria. The auramine stains were

Clinical tip Individuals at high risk of TB

- Homeless.
- Prisoners (or recent prisoners).
- HIV-positive individuals.
- Diabetics.
- People receiving immunosuppression (particularly anti-TNF-alpha).
- Young children.

Expert comment

In general, it is unusual to detect any clinical signs in the chest despite active TB, unless the disease is advanced or there is a significant pleural effusion, and hence signs should not be relied on in terms of ruling out TB.

Clinical tip Differential diagnoses

- Bacterial pneumonia.
- Viral pneumonia.
- NTM infection.
- Bronchiectasis exacerbation.
- Wegener's granulomatosis.
- Sarcoidosis.
- Lymphoma.

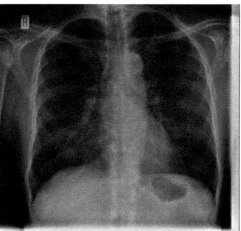

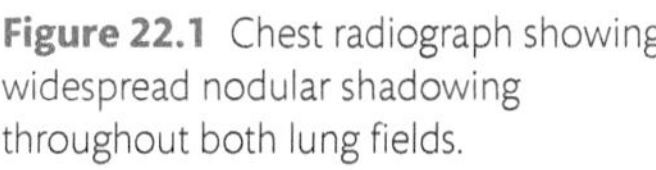

Figure 22.1 Chest radiograph showing widespread nodular shadowing throughout both lung fields.

Clinical tip How to read a Mantoux test

- 0.1 mL of 2 tuberculin units (TU) of tuberculin injected intradermally.
- Read at 48–72 hours from injection.
- Measure the area of induration (not erythema).
- Induration of ≥5 mm is considered positive in the absence of BCG vaccination.
- Induration of ≥14 mm is considered positive in the presence of BCG vaccination.

Expert comment

One should be cautious in over-reliance on a negative TST as a 'rule-out', or a positive result as a 'rule-in', test, as this can be negative in cases where there is advanced disease or the patient is immunocompromised. A positive test merely indicates that the individual has encountered the organism previously and may therefore merely represent latent infection, rather than prove active disease.

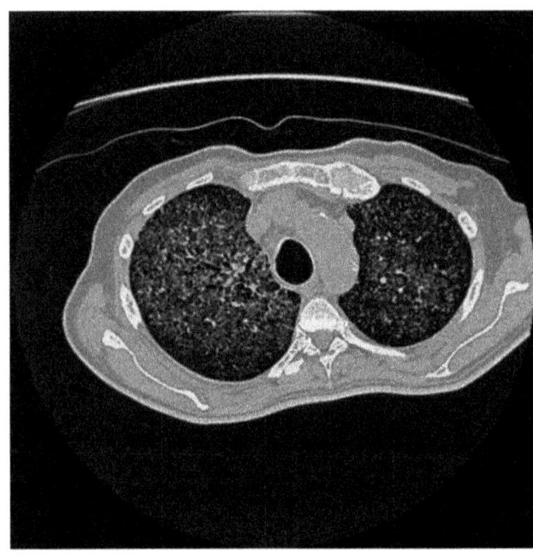

Figure 22.2 HRCT thorax showing widespread uniform small nodules with mediastinal lymph nodes (1.4 cm maximum diameter).

negative on all three samples. A HRCT of the thorax showed widespread small nodules and mediastinal lymphadenopathy (Figure 22.2), and a Mantoux test showed an induration of 18 mm at 72 hours. The nurses verified that the patient has had bacille Calmette–Guérin (BCG) vaccination as a child and documented the scar on his forearm. Direct questioning also revealed that the gentleman's uncle was treated for TB on a visit to Thailand a year ago.

The microbiology laboratory informed the clinician that the initial sputum sample was growing *Mycobacterium*.

Learning point TB diagnosis

A diagnosis of TB rests on positive microbiological confirmation of the TB bacillus from the infected individual. To see bacilli on initial inspection (or smear), there needs to be a minimum of 5000 bacilli/mL. This explains why the CSF and pleural fluid are so rarely 'smear'-positive. The highest yield is three sputum samples (ideally first thing in the morning). There is no increase in sensitivity beyond three samples. The sputum is stained either with Ziehl–Neelsen (using light microscopy) or with auramine (using immunofluorescence).

Sputum smear in the HIV-negative population has a sensitivity of between 34% and 80% from various studies, with highest rates in cavitatory disease and lowest in those with a weak cough.

If the individual is unable to produce sputum, but a diagnosis of pulmonary TB is suspected, then induced sputum (following inhalation of 3–7% hypertonic saline) can be performed. This aerosolizes *Mycobacterium*, so it must be carried out in line with infection control policies. In a study from Montreal of 500 patients unable to produce sputum or with smear-negative samples, an adequate sample was obtained in 99% of patients [1]. The yield from induced sputum has compared in some studies favourably to bronchoscopic sampling, particularly if repeat procedures are undertaken, and has significantly lower costs [2].

An alternative is bronchoscopy and washing taken from the affected lobe. If there is no radiograph abnormality, convention suggests it is sensible to wash both upper lobes. Studies have shown that a rapid diagnosis in the form of a positive smear ranges from 30% to 70% using fibreoptic bronchoscopy, and the yield of a positive culture varies according to the samples taken [3].

Most clinicians would advocate sending a bronchial washing and post-bronchoscopy sputum; some would also send bronchial brushings. A study of smear-negative miliary TB has shown that bronchoscopy provided a diagnosis in 83% of cases, from a variety of samples [4].

A diagnosis of miliary TB was made. The patient was closely questioned for the presence of any neurological symptoms, all of which he denied. However, given the risk of haematogenous spread to the meninges, a CT head and a lumbar puncture were performed which were normal.

Learning point

Miliary TB suggests haematogenous spread of bacilli, which raises the possibility of TB within the meninges. It is good practice therefore to consider whether a patient with miliary TB also has TB meningitis, because the length of treatment recommended for TB affecting the meninges or spine is 12 months, rather than the standard 6. Up to 20% of patients with miliary TB will also have TB meningitis. Any patient with neurological symptoms or headache should undergo a lumbar puncture. If there are no symptoms or signs of meningeal inflammation, a CT scan looking for meningeal enhancement may suffice.

TB meningitis can present asymptomatically or with headache, fever, confusion, and coma. Cranial nerve palsies are not uncommon. Mortality rates are reported to be between 20% and 30%, and permanent disability in 4–50% of survivors. Death is associated with late diagnosis.

Treatment with steroids significantly reduces the risk of death (risk ratio reduction of 22%) and disability (risk ratio reduction 17%) in all stages of TB meningitis [5]. A typical regime would be dexamethasone 0.4 mg/kg per 24 hours, with a reducing course over 6–8 weeks. Steroids are also universally accepted as beneficial in the treatment of pericardial TB.

In order to initiate treatment, the patient was weighed at 62 kg and eyesight-tested using a Snellen (for acuity) and Ishihara (for colour blindness) chart. He was started on ethambutol 1000 mg and Rifater® 6 tablets to be taken once a day. The side effects of the medication were explained, and he was assigned a TB specialist nurse to assist in adherence. He was then sent home with a prescription for 1 month, with a follow-up appointment in 2 weeks to check compliance and for side effects. The keyworker notified the Health Protection Agency of the new case of TB; this is a legal requirement.

Clinical tip Drug nomenclature

The standard TB regimen consists of four drugs, abbreviated using a single letter and a number indicating the length of time in months for the course of the drug. The standard regimen therefore is 6HRZE 4RH.

- H = isoniazid.
- R = rifampicin.
- Z = pyrazinamide.
- E = ethambutol.
- S = streptomycin.
- Rifater® contains rifampicin + isoniazid + pyrazinamide.
- Rifinah® contains rifampicin + isoniazid.

Ten days later, the patient presented to A&E with a 2-day history of vomiting and yellow sclerae. In A&E, he was jaundiced, dehydrated, febrile, and tachycardic. There were no chest findings to note, and his abdomen was soft, with active bowel sounds and some epigastric tenderness, but no organomegaly. He was given IV fluids and antiemetics, and blood tests were sent (Table 22.1).

Table 22.1 Results of blood tests on admission to A&E

Haematology	Result	Normal range	Biochemistry	Result	Normal range
Haemoglobin	12.0	13–18 g/dL	Sodium	140	135–145 mmol/L
MCV	84	83–105 fL	Urea	10	2.5–6.7 mmol/L
WCC	12	4–11 × 10^9/L	Creatinine	98	70–150 micromoles/L
Neutrophil	10	2–7 × 10^9/L	Bilirubin	75	3–17 micromoles/L
Platelet	450	150–400 × 10^9/L	ALP	350	75–250 IU/L
			Alanine aminotransferase (ALT)	372	10–45 IU/L

He was admitted to a side room on the respiratory ward, and all TB chemotherapy was stopped. He was tested for hepatitis B and C viruses, in addition to HIV, which showed the presence of hepatitis B surface antigen. Fasting glucose was normal. His gastrointestinal symptoms settled quickly, and, when his liver function normalized, his TB treatment was reintroduced, according to the unit protocol, with daily blood monitoring. After 2 weeks, he was established on four anti-tuberculous medications and was discharged home. He was referred to the hepatologists for further tests and investigations.

Meanwhile, the TB keyworker had identified all possible TB contacts, and his wife, son, uncle, and aunt were all invited for screening. The patient's uncle had been treated for TB just 1 year before and had a chest radiograph that showed right upper lobe fibrotic change, consistent with his history of TB. The aunt had no radiological or clinical evidence of active disease, so they were encouraged to report any symptoms in the future should they occur.

The patient's son was 5 years old and had not had BCG vaccination. He had no evidence of active TB disease on clinical assessment, so he had a Mantoux test which was positive. He was given chemoprophylaxis with 6 months of isoniazid. The patient's wife was 35 weeks' pregnant with their second child. She had been vaccinated with BCG in childhood and had no symptoms of active TB on clinical assessment. Her Mantoux test was 20 mm, i.e. strongly positive, and so she was given chemoprophylaxis with isoniazid. Both she and her son were given pyridoxine to take with the isoniazid, to reduce the risk of peripheral neuritis and counteract any isoniazid in breast milk.

The keyworker assessed the patient's work colleagues also, because the kitchen in which they worked together was small and poorly ventilated, and the patient commented that the shifts were often longer than 8 hours in duration. None were found to require chemoprophylaxis.

Learning point Risk factors for multidrug-resistant TB

Staff should wear respiratory protection during routine interaction.

- Residence in London.
- Male.
- HIV-positive.
- Prior history of TB.
- Birth in a foreign country (sub-Saharan Africa/Indian subcontinent).
- Age 25–44.
- Contact with a resistant case.

Clinical tip

Rifampicin induces cytochrome P450 systems and increases the metabolism of a number of medications, including prednisolone. Thus, the active dose of prednisolone is approximately half that taken by the patient. Oestrogen contraceptive medication will not be effective at the usual lower doses used in the oral contraceptive pill.

Learning point

Each case of TB infects an average of two individuals. Infection risk increases with close proximity and longer duration of exposure.

NICE guidance [6] recommends that all household contacts are screened for active and latent TB infection. In addition, those who may be close contacts, e.g. spend >8 hours in the same domestic size

(Continued)

room, should be screened. If non-close contacts are at risk (e.g. HIV-positive, children), then screening should also be considered. If screening of close contacts picks up significant disease, this suggests the index case is particularly infectious, and a wider circle of contacts should be screened. If an index case is smear-positive, screening automatically includes a wider circle of contacts. In smear-negative or non-pulmonary cases, it is usually sufficient to screen only those within the household.

Screening involves an interview to identify symptoms of active TB. Adults over 35 years will be offered a chest radiograph to look for signs of TB, and those younger will have a TST (a Mantoux test). Those who have a positive test should be considered for treatment of latent TB with chemoprophylaxis. People over the age of 35 whose risk of developing active disease is higher than the risk of hepatotoxicity from the antituberculous drugs should also be offered chemoprophylaxis. This would include those who are HIV-positive, health-care workers, and those on immunosuppressive medication. Patients who are Mantoux-negative should be offered an IGRA after 6 weeks. If this is positive, then they should be offered chemoprophylaxis. If this remains negative and the contact has not had a BCG, this should be offered.

Newborn babies are at increased risk of developing TB if exposed to a smear-positive contact. It is particularly important therefore that the patient's wife is screened for active TB. If she had required treatment, the same four medications are safely used both in pregnancy and during breastfeeding. Ideally, initiate medications at least 2 weeks before the baby arrives, to reduce the possibility of infection in the infant.

The patient was seen in the clinic 2 months later, and his sweats and cough had dissipated. He had regained 6 kg in weight and was back at work. The initial sputum had grown a fully sensitive MTB, so treatment was changed to 'continuation phase' with rifampicin and isoniazid—given in combination as Rifinah 300®.

Discussion

This case highlights some of the commoner challenges involved in the diagnosis, management, and control of TB both on an individual and public health level.

The WHO estimates that one-third of the world's population has been infected with TB and the majority have latent disease. In the UK, 7892 people were identified as having TB in 2013 [7]. TB incidence in the UK as a whole is 12.3/100,000; However, London achieves a rate of 35.5/100,000 (with some of its areas exceeding 100 per 100,000). TB rates are higher in people born outside of the UK, and migrants are at most risk of presenting with TB in the first 5 years after arriving.

The presentation of TB is usually an indolent one, with non-specific pulmonary symptoms, often in a patient who remains well enough to work. However, in an individual at risk, the following should trigger a search for TB: night sweats (drenching the bed), weight loss, lymphadenopathy, prolonged course, e.g. longer than 2 weeks, and a productive cough with small-volume haemoptysis. TB is a great mimicker and should be considered in the differential of any number of presentations. Approximately 50% of TB in HIV-negative individuals is extrapulmonary and easily overlooked [8].

Microbiological confirmation of TB is the gold standard for diagnosis; however, other investigations can be supportive. Whilst TB can be seen on smear microscopy from 15% of people with a normal chest radiograph [9], it may demonstrate signs suggestive of TB. Parenchymal disease tends to present with apical patchy consolidation. Upper lobe cavities are seen in 40–80% of post-primary TB and are highly suggestive of TB. Lymphadenopathy is commoner in primary TB. Miliary changes

Expert comment

The presence of a normal chest radiograph should not be used to rule out active TB when the patient is symptomatic and especially in immunocompromised patients. It is therefore important to proceed to other tests (such as a CT thorax) if the symptoms are suggestive of TB.

Expert comment

At present, routine use of the IGRA as a 'rule-out' test in active TB cannot be advocated, but ongoing studies of additional antigens may, in the future, allow these tests to have a sufficiently high sensitivity to perform in this manner.

can be overlooked; the presence of an area of calcification representing a Ghon's focus (calcified TB in a lymph node) suggests previous exposure and therefore an increased risk of reactivation.

Classically, the appearances of TB on a CT scan are described as 'tree in bud'—the congestion of smaller bronchi with inflammatory tissue resembling a branch with furled leaf buds. It is also important to look for cavitation and miliary changes (bronchovascular concentric, seed-like nodules) and to review the lymph nodes—in TB, one would expect these to be enlarged and necrotic centrally.

There are two current tests for previous immune sensitization to TB. The Mantoux test is a skin test where the response to the intradermal purified protein tuberculin is measured. Tuberculin sensitivity can occur in response to environmental mycobacteria and to BCG. BCG is no longer performed routinely in the UK, except in infants born in high-risk areas or in high-risk populations. However, it forms part of the standard vaccination programme in most countries with a high incidence of TB. The vaccine is usually given at birth or in infancy, either in the left deltoid region or, if the country was involved in smallpox vaccination, it may be on the left forearm; it would usually leave a scar which is still visible in adulthood.

IGRAs measure the output of the patient's T cells in response to two TB-derived proteins that are not contained within BCG. The patient's blood is mixed with ESAT-6 and CFP-10 proteins, and the production of IFN-γ is measured. There are two commercially available tests whose sensitivity in active disease in a meta-analysis ranges between (compared with culture-positive TB) 70% and 90% [10]. A positive result from either test would suggest that the patient has been exposed to TB, but it cannot distinguish between active and latent infection. Importantly, given their high risk of TB reactivation or infection, studies have shown that these tests, in particular the ELISpot, perform better than the skin test in immunosuppressed groups (in particular, children, HIV-positive individuals, and those with autoimmune disease or chronic renal impairment). Work is ongoing to identify the role of the IGRA tests in diagnosing active TB, but currently their sensitivity is insufficient to use them as a single 'rule-out' test. Notably, one group has showed that, by adding a third TB-specific antigen to the test and combining the result with TST results in a HIV-negative population, the ELISpot plus has a sensitivity of 99% for active TB. In the case of a negative TST and negative ELISpot plus, then the negative likelihood of active TB is 0.02 (95% CI 0–0.06), meaning that this combined approach may, in the future, be a useful test of exclusion [11].

It is also important to note that, whilst the IGRA discriminates between exposure to TB and BCG, the proteins are shared with environmental NTM (*Mycobacterium kansasii*, *marinum*, and *szulgai*).

In the case described, a microbiological diagnosis was made from expectorated sputum; however, this is not always possible, and it may be necessary to obtain tissue where histology would be supportive and tissue can be sent for TB culture. Bronchoscopy, in addition to obtaining pulmonary secretions, provides an opportunity to sample lymph nodes, if a CT scan suggests that there is nodal involvement. EBUS has the ability to biopsy multiple mediastinal lymph node stations and achieves acceptable culture rates [12].

The gold standard for TB diagnosis is when *Mycobacterium* has been cultured. Sputum culture is more sensitive than smear (in the range of 80–93%) because only 10–100 organisms/mL are required for a positive culture. The culture also allows crucial drug sensitivity testing, so all samples should be sent for culture. This can take up to 6 weeks on solid culture media, such as Lowenstein Jensen media, but many laboratories now use a liquid broth system which uses automatic radiometric methods to detect mycobacterial growth, or the Mycobacterial Growth Indicator Tube (MGIT) which uses colorimetric methods. The use of liquid culture in the microscopic observation drug susceptibility (MODS) assay allows for simultaneous culture and drug sensitivity testing. In a head-to-head study with Lowenstein Jensen culture, the MODS assay reduced time to culture positivity to 6 days in HIV-negative patients and improved sensitivity to 97.8% [13].

Alternatives to smear microscopy and culture that have gained some recognition in recent years include the NAATs. The commercially available tests are sensitive and specific in the diagnosis of smear-positive pulmonary TB but perform less well in smear-negative or extrapulmonary TB. The novel molecular platform used in the Xpert MTB/RIF technology has shown great promise and is simple to use. It is highly specific and diagnosed 98.2% of smear-positive patients and 72.5% of smear-negative patients (90.2% if three tests were used) [14]. Within a 2-hour period, the test also identifies 97.6% of rifampicin resistance, which is usually strongly associated with multidrug-resistant (MDR) TB. On the basis of these results, the WHO has recommended that this technology be first-line tests in individuals suspected of MDR TB or who are HIV-positive, and as a second-line test if a patient is smear-negative.

Management challenges

Untreated TB has a mortality rate of approximately 50% as a result of both unchecked bacillus replication and a destructive immune response. The treatment consists of combination therapy to avoid the development of drug resistance. In TB, the drugs are split into those with early bactericidal activity, those that decrease the bacterial load rapidly in the first 2 weeks of treatment, and those with sterilizing activity that kill off any persistent organisms. The standard regime consists of four drugs for 2 months (isoniazid/rifampicin/pyrazinamide/ethambutol), then two drugs (isoniazid and rifampicin) for 4 months. Isoniazid and rifampicin have high early bactericidal activity; pyrazinamide is an effective sterilizing agent, and ethambutol is bacteriostatic. In patients at risk of peripheral neuritis (pregnant women, alcoholics, malnourished patients, cancer patients), pyridoxine should also be given with isoniazid.

The majority of patients tolerate TB chemotherapy well. However, there are side effects associated with each of the medication (Table 22.2).

Hepatotoxicity is the commonest reason to stop medication. NICE guidance suggests a rise in ALT to >5 times the normal (or three times the normal with clinical symptoms) should prompt the termination of treatment. To avoid the development

Table 22.2 Side effects seen with antituberculous therapy

Drug	Common side effects	Rarer side effects
Isoniazid	Rash, tingling in hands and feet, drowsiness	Hepatotoxicity
Rifampicin	Rash, anorexia, nausea, flu syndrome, orange urine (secretions)	Renal failure, shock, hepatotoxicity
Ethambutol		Optic neuritis
Pyrazinamide	Joint pains	Hepatic necrosis

of resistance, all drugs should be stopped. A rise in transaminases to less than twice the normal should simply prompt repeating blood tests in 2 weeks in the absence of symptoms. If ALT and AST are repeatedly raised to greater than twice the normal, then they should be monitored at 2-weekly intervals. Patients with underlying liver disease, alcohol dependency, cirrhosis, hepatitis B or C infection, or HIV infection, malnourished patients, or those at the extremes of age are more at risk of liver derangement during treatment and should have regular liver function monitoring.

When blood levels normalize, the medication can be reintroduced. If a patient has been on treatment for >2 weeks and has conversion to smear-negative sputum, then the medication can be reintroduced without covering with alternative therapy. However, if the patients are smear-positive, unwell, or within 2 weeks of starting treatment, then whilst medication is being reintroduced, antituberculous therapy should be maintained with at least three other medications that are unlikely to cause hepatic embarrassment (e.g. ethambutol and streptomycin/amikacin or moxifloxacin). Reintroduction of the first-line drugs in a stepwise fashion with increasing doses over time is then undertaken with careful monitoring of the liver function.

Isoniazid is reintroduced first, since hepatic toxicity is thought to be an idiosyncratic response. Rifampicin rarely causes severe hepatic failure but, via the enzyme induction pathway, can potentiate the toxicity caused by isoniazid. Pyrazinamide has been reported to cause fatal hepatic necrosis; therefore, if the transaminases rise following reintroduction, then it should be stopped and not reconsidered, and the patient receives either an alternative agent (e.g. moxifloxacin) for the induction phase, i.e. the first 2 months, or a prolonged continuation phase of rifampicin and isoniazid for a total of 9 months.

Ten to 25% of HIV-negative patients undergo a paradoxical reaction, usually associated with ART. Whilst the underlying pathological process is poorly understood, the phenomenon is widely recognized in association with cervical lymph node or CNS disease. It commonly occurs after 1 month on treatment; there is an apparent worsening of disease, with lymph node swelling; radiographic features can worsen, and patients can experience more cough, fevers, and sweats. This can be a challenge for the clinician. There is only one retrospective analysis of the use of steroids in these circumstances, and it found no association between the use of steroids and the length of the reaction, although many clinicians would favour their use.

There is ongoing interest in adjunctive medication to antituberculous chemotherapy. Work has shown that treating vitamin D-deficient TB patients with vitamin D shortens the time to sputum conversion in individuals with the *tt* genotype of the *TaqI* vitamin D receptor polymorphism, i.e. reducing their potential infectivity [15].

TB control challenges

NICE guidelines for management of TB in the UK recommend that, unless unwell, a patient with TB can be treated as an outpatient. They should, however, be encouraged to stay at home (away from new contacts) in the first 2 weeks of treatment. If a patient is homeless, lives with immunosuppressed or HIV-positive individuals, they can be admitted to protect their contacts. All patients suspected of active TB should be isolated and nursed in a side room. If the ward is also shared by patients who are HIV-positive or immunosuppressed, then the patient should be cared for in a negative-pressure side room. If the patient travels to X-ray, they are required to wear a respiratory mask. Staff should wear FFP3 respiratory masks during procedures where particles can be aerosolized, e.g. bronchoscopy or sputum induction.

For routine nursing care, a mask is not mandatory, UNLESS the patient is suspected of having MDR TB.

Patients should be isolated until either their sputum converts to negative on auramine staining or they have taken 2 weeks of antituberculous chemotherapy and have shown clinical improvement, e.g. remission of cough, dissipation of fever, or evidence of weight gain.

As in this case, the contacts of the individual must be screened for TB. The household will have been exposed to similar TB risks as the patient, as well as to the index case, hence the reason that, even in non-pulmonary TB cases, the household are invited for screening.

NICE has created a variety of algorithms for screening different populations particularly at risk. Where the Mantoux test is less sensitive, an IGRA should be the primary screening investigation, e.g. in HIV-positive patients. In the UK, NICE recommends either 3 months of isoniazid and rifampicin or 6 months of isoniazid as preventative therapy. In an unvaccinated child <2 years old with close contact to a smear-positive index case, the risk of TB meningitis is significant, and therefore isoniazid would be started whilst screening is being organized. Contacts of patients with MDR TB should be followed up but are not routinely given chemoprophylaxis.

In the UK, MDR TB is responsible for just 1% of cases. MDR means resistance to isoniazid and rifampicin. Rates of treatment success are much lower in MDR TB, and the financial burden is significant. Every identified case of TB should be tested microbiologically for drug resistance. In most cases, it is sufficient to send sputum on for drug sensitivity testing once MTB has been cultured. These results should be reviewed before the continuation phase of treatment. In the UK, isoniazid resistance occurs in approximately 6% of cases and would require a change in therapy. In cases where MDR TB is suspected, it is appropriate to request a line probe assay on a microbiologically identified sample to assess for the presence of a resistant mutation in the *rpoB* gene. Mutations in this gene are associated with isoniazid resistance (i.e. MDR) in 95% of cases. The management of MDR TB should only be undertaken by those with experience, and patients should therefore be referred to a local specialist. In the first instance, there is a national advisory service which can be contacted via mdrtb@brit-thoracic.org.uk.

In summary, this case illustrates the importance of confirming a diagnosis of TB and the implications for the patient, the clinical team, and society in adequately managing the disease.

A final word from the expert

The awareness of the symptoms and risk factors for TB are key to initiating the investigations. Delays in diagnosis are generally related to the lack of awareness of TB being a potential differential.

IGRAs have a higher specificity in latent TB infection and are not affected by prior BCG vaccination. These blood tests are easier to perform and record than the conventional tuberculin test but are costlier. There are ongoing studies to evaluate their prognostic value versus the TST in latent infection and also if it is more cost-effective to use these as the only screening modality for latent TB infection. Currently, IGRAs are insufficiently sensitive to use alone as a 'rule-out' test for TB in the active disease setting.

A normal plain CXR is insufficient to rule out a case of pulmonary TB, and, if symptoms are suggestive, more detailed investigation is warranted, in addition to sending sputum samples. In addition to the gold standard of bronchoscopy, induced sputum may be used if the patient is non-productive or smear-negative, but only if appropriate isolation facilities are available. Induced sputum should only be relied on in the context of TB being the only significant diagnosis, and bronchoscopy should still be used if there is more than one significant diagnosis or if induced sputum samples are negative.

The use of CT/MRI, and even PET, scans complements the use of plain radiology and allows the clinician to target sampling approaches. The finding of cavitation, in combination with tree-in-bud change or miliary shadowing, on a CT scan has a high predictive value for diagnosing TB. However, TB associated with HIV or immunosuppression can present with atypical radiological appearances.

The place of EBUS to target intrathoracic tuberculous nodes is now emerging and allows the respiratory physician to obtain a definitive diagnosis, whilst ruling out the other significant cause of mediastinal adenopathy, without resorting to a mediastinoscopy.

Microbiological proof of TB is critical not only to confirm the diagnosis, but also to elucidate the drug sensitivity of the organism. Although the level of MDR and extensively drug-resistant disease in the UK is currently low, poor management of single drug resistance may ultimately lead to this becoming an increasing issue. The newer PCR platforms allow for more rapid identification of such cases, as compared to culture-based techniques, and will increasingly be used in higher-risk settings to allow immediate initiation of appropriate second-line treatment and infection control measures.

References

1. Al Zahrani K, Al Jahdali H, Poirier L, René P, Menzies D. Yield of smear, culture and amplification tests from repeated sputum induction for the diagnosis of pulmonary tuberculosis. *Int J Tuberc Lung Dis* 2001;**5**:855–60.
2. McWilliams T, Wells AU, Harrison AC, Lindstrom S, Cameron RJ, Foskin E. Induced sputum and bronchoscopy in the diagnosis of pulmonary tuberculosis. *Thorax* 2002;**57**:1010–14.
3. Schoch OD, Rieder P, Tueller C *et al.* Diagnostic yield of sputum, induced sputum, and bronchoscopy after radiologic tuberculosis screening. *Am J Respir Crit Care Med* 2007;**175**:80–6.
4. Willcox PA, Potgieter PD, Bateman ED, Benatar SR. Rapid diagnosis of sputum negative miliary tuberculosis using the flexible fibreoptic bronchoscope. *Thorax* 1986;**41**:681–4.
5. Prasad K, Singh MB. Corticosteroids for managing tuberculous meningitis. *Cochrane Database Syst Rev* 2008;**1**:CD002244.
6. National Institute for Health and Care Excellence (2011). *Tuberculosis: clinical diagnosis and management of tuberculosis, and measures for its prevention and control.* NICE guidelines CG117. Available at: <https://www.nice.org.uk/Guidance/CG117>.
7. Public Health England (2014). *Tuberculosis in the UK 2014 report.* Available at: <https://www.gov.uk/government/uploads/system/uploads/attachment_data/file/360335/TB_Annual_report_4_0_300914.pdf>.
8. Okur E, Yilmaz A, Saygi A *et al.* Patterns of delays in diagnosis amongst patients with smear-positive pulmonary tuberculosis at a teaching hospital in Turkey. *Clin Microbiol Infect* 2006;**12**:90–2.

9. Geng E, Kreiswirth B, Burzynski J, Schluger NW. Clinical and radiographic correlates of primary and reactivation tuberculosis: a molecular epidemiology study. *JAMA* 2005;**293**:2740–5.
10. Lange C, Pai M, Drobniewski F, Migliori GB. Interferon-gamma release assays for the diagnosis of active tuberculosis: sensible or silly? *Eur Respir J* 2009;**33**:1250–3.
11. Dosanjh DPS, Hinks TSC, Innes JA *et al*. Improved diagnostic evaluation of suspected tuberculosis. *Ann Intern Med* 2008;**148**:325–36.
12. Navani N, Molyneaux PL, Breen RA *et al*. Utility of endobronchial ultrasound-guided transbronchial needle aspiration in patients with tuberculous intrathoracic lymphadenopathy: a multicentre study. *Thorax* 2011;**66**:889–93.
13. Moore DAJ, Mendoza D, Gilman RH *et al*. Microscopic observation drug susceptibility assay, a rapid, reliable diagnostic test for multidrug-resistant tuberculosis suitable for use in resource-poor settings. *J Clin Microbiol* 2004;**42**:4432–7.
14. Boehme CC, Nicol MP, Nabeta P *et al*. Feasibility, diagnostic accuracy, and effectiveness of decentralised use of the Xpert MTB/RIF test for diagnosis of tuberculosis and multidrug resistance: a multicentre implementation study. *Lancet* 2011;**377**:1495–505.
15. Martineau AR, Timms PM, Bothamley GH *et al*. High-dose vitamin D(3) during intensive-phase antimicrobial treatment of pulmonary tuberculosis: a double-blind randomised controlled trial. *Lancet* 2011;**377**:242–50.

INDEX

A

B

D

H

I

J

K

L

M

N

R

S

T